THE TEMPOROMANDIBULAR JOINT AND RELATED OROFACIAL DISORDERS

THE TEMPOROMANDIBULAR JOINT AND RELATED OROFACIAL DISORDERS

Francis M. Bush, D.M.D., Ph.D.

Professor
Department of General Practice
Medical College of Virginia
Virginia Commonwealth University
Richmond, Virginia

M. Franklin Dolwick, D.M.D., Ph.D.

Professor
Department of Oral and Maxillofacial Surgery
University of Florida School of Dentistry
Gainesville, Florida

Illustrated by Sue Lee

96017

J.B. Lippincott Company
Philadelphia

Acquisitions Editor: James D. Ryan
Sponsoring Editor: Delois Patterson
Project Editor: Ellen M. Campbell
Indexer: Lynne E. Mahan
Senior Design Coordinator: Kathy Kelley-Luedtke
Cover Designer: Larry Pezzato
Production Manager: Caren P. Erlichman
Senior Production Coordinator: Kevin P. Johnson
Compositor: Compset Inc.
Printer/Binder: Arcata Graphics/Kingsport

6   5   4   3   2   1

Library of Congress Cataloging-in-Publication Data

Bush, Francis M.
    The temporomandibular joint and related orofacial disorders /
Francis M. Bush, M. Franklin Dolwick.
        p.   cm.
    Includes bibliographical references and index.
    ISBN 0-397-50982-0
    1. Temporomandibular joint—Diseases.   2. Orofacial pain.
I. Dolwick, M. Franklin.   II. Title.
    [DNLM: 1. Temporomandibular Joint Diseases.   2. Temporomandibular
Joint—anatomy & histology.   3. Temporomandibular Joint—
physiopathology.   4. Facial Plan—therapy.   5. Diagnosis,
Differential.   WU 140 B9775t 1994]
RK470.B87   1994
617.5′2—dc20
DNLM/DLC
for Library of Congress   94-33796
                                                                  CIP

☉This Paper Meets the Requirements of ANSI/NISO Z39.48-1992 (Permanence of Paper).

The authors and publishers have exerted every effort to ensure that
drug selection and dosage set forth in this text are in accord with
current recommendations and practice at the time of publication.
However, in view of ongoing research, changes in government
regulations, and the constant flow of information relating to drug
therapy and drug reactions, the reader is urged to check the package
insert for each drug for any change in indications and dosage and for
added warnings and precautions. This is particularly important when
the recommended agent is a new or infrequently employed drug.

To Madge, to Nancy and Emily, and to Brenda, with love

Preface

This book was written for current and future practitioners of dentistry and medicine, and for health professionals in allied fields. We intend it to serve as a succinct and readable text that will have practical value in the diagnosis and treatment of individuals suffering from temporomandibular disorders. It is predicated on the premise that the affected individuals in the general population are primarily the concern of the general practitioner. While much of the complex treatment of these individuals can be managed by various specialists in dentistry and medicine, and then delegated to auxiliary service groups of these specialities, the widespread prevalence of temporomandibular disorders in the population makes it necessary for the general dentist to be responsible for the primary care of affected individuals.

The text begins with information on the history of temporomandibular disorders and clarification of some of the terminology used in the field. In addition, detailed descriptions of pertinent anatomy and physiology of the masticatory system are presented to reinforce practitioners' comprehension. Major symptoms and signs of TMJ disorders are delineated from incidental complaints and associated clinical findings.

Several possible etiologies are discussed because of differing opinions about the causes of temporomandibular disorders. This discussion leads to a review of epidemiological studies conducted on populations around the world. This review seeks to clarify some of the information associated with gender– and age–related relationships.

To reinforce the discussion of these fundamental concepts, practical methods are described that enable the practitioner to screen, examine, and differentially diagnose temporomandibular disorders from similarly presenting complaints. The text also discusses the concept of algorithms for keying temporomandibular disorders; in essence, these are decision-trees for identifying and evaluating signs and symptoms that lead to successful diagnosis of these disorders.

Conservative treatments are addressed which should help both the practitioner and the patient to manage the pain and the impairment of TMJ disorder. Wherever possible, the literature on therapies is reviewed to prevent practitioners from recommending obsolete and useless procedures. Surgical therapies are considered on the face of available evidence regarding success and failure outcomes.

The text also presents details about record keeping, management of insurance claims, quality assurance, and potential litigation. Information about insurance claims is discussed so that practitioners can identify appropriate codes for services rendered. Instructions are given for writing a narrative report. The need for detailed and accurate treatment records, which may prevent legal action, is discussed.

The book is devoted to improving self-confidence in management of temporomandibular disorders. We believe that when practitioners finish it, they will be wiser than they were. While no practitioner will possess all of the answers about temporomandibular disorders, each should develop a more authoritative professional image concerning care of these disorders. Instructions are presented that allow practitioners to effectively communicate useful information to their patients. From this base of information, they will be able to raise the level of consciousness of their patients. Practitioners and patients both will then be better equipped to understand significant symptoms and signs, to understand a diagnosis, and to select an appropriate treatment to improve temporomandibular health.

Acknowledgments

We owe much gratitude to our families. They have been patient and have provided much encouragement during the many hours devoted to this book. The senior author is particularly indebted to his wife, Madge. She has provided financial and loving support throughout his career beginning with the PhD program in Anatomy and extending beyond the DMD degree. Her generosity has allowed him to pursue this endeavour and avoid unnecessary intrusions.

Some of the material for the book has been constructively criticized by both professional colleagues and students. Many gave insightful and helpful suggestions or supplied illustrations. We extend our appreciation to Drs. David Abbott, James Butler, Robert Campbell, William Donlon, H. David Hall, Stephen Harkins, Walter Harrington, Claire Kaugers, Riley Lunn, Parker Mahan, Singh Salmi, Bruce Sanders, and M.P. Trutta.

Lastly, we thank the editors of other journals and books who allowed us permission to use source materials or illustrations.

Contents

THE TEMPOROMANDIBULAR JOINT AND RELATED OROFACIAL DISORDERS

The Temporomandibular Joint and Related Orofacial Disorders,
by Francis M. Bush and M. Franklin Dolwick.
J.B. Lippincott Company, Philadelphia, © 1995.

1

Scope of the Problem

The temporomandibular joint (TMJ) is the anatomic region where the lower jaw attaches to the skull. The term "TMJ" has been popularized in the modern world primarily as a complaint involving pain and discomfort of the jaws. It is considered an orofacial or masticatory disturbance because the complaints involve the mouth. Many vague physical complaints, including those somewhat removed from the oral cavity, also have been imputed to this condition.

Temporomandibular (TM) complaints have been difficult to subject to an accepted system of classification. When patterns of signs (what the doctor sees) and symptoms (what the patient reports) occur simultaneously, the condition is referred to as a *syndrome*. Because certain TM complaints are often characterized by both pain and abnormal function, these complaints at one time were broadly classified as *TMJ syndrome* or *TMJ dysfunction syndrome*. This classification was further divided into true joint (ie, TMJ) complaints and muscle-related complaints surrounding the TM region. Because painful symptoms have been associated with the covering or fascia on the muscles associated with the joint, this kind of disturbance has been referred to as myofascial pain dysfunction syndrome (MPDS), myofascial pain syndrome (MPS), and sometimes "myofacial" pain syndrome (because the face is involved).

Still other confusing terminologies have persisted in the literature, including mandibular dysfunction (MD), craniomandibular disorder (CMD), and craniofacial disorder (CFD), because the complaints involved the head, jaw, and face. Other terms, based on structural changes within the joint, have included internal derangement (ID) and degenerative joint disease (DJD). Pain dysfunction syndrome (PDS) has been linked to TMJ as a disease entity and thus has contributed to the present controversy about these complaints.

The considerable overlap among these signs and symptoms has prevented the establishment of a generally accepted classification. In 1982, a group of prominent health care practitioners met at the headquarters of the American Dental Association in Chicago and agreed that these complaints should be broadly classified as temporomandibular disorders (TMDs). Collectively, TM complaints seem to represent an

1

assemblage of disorders that can be divided into subcategories or subsets. To put it another way, disorders of the TM region probably are not a single disease entity but represent a family of clinical conditions. In many ways, TM disorders form a branch of the tree of musculoskeletal dysfunctions that affect the average person during his or her lifetime. These orofacial complaints are referred to as TM disorders or TMDs throughout this text.

In a short period of time, TM disorders have gone from a relatively unknown problem to one that is diagnosed in a significant number of cases. Although these symptoms have been recognized for more than 40 years, only since the 1970s have these disorders been widely diagnosed. Since then, the diagnosis has become common. Because the symptoms seem to mimic those of many other conditions, some dentists, physicians, chiropractors, and physical therapists have attributed many of the puzzling symptoms of their patients to these disorders. Practitioners in search of a way to explain confusing symptoms have thus developed a wastebasket diagnosis that comes in handy when no other seems appropriate. Even for many expert practitioners, it is frustrating trying to discern whether it is "just TMJ" or some other clinical condition.

TM disorders have been the subject of much research over the past few years. No "one cause–one disease" relation has been established. Most cases of TM disorders begin with a few symptoms. These mild symptoms can represent a disorder of the joint or of the muscles that control the joint. Increased tension of the muscles is the most frequent problem. Because muscle tension is often the first stage of response to difficult life events, anxiety or any stressful situation may provoke an episode of muscular tension about the face, jaw, head, or neck. Pain and stiffness can develop in the jaw and restrict the movement of the mouth.

For individuals who can open their mouths only halfway, hear a clicking sound when they move their jaws, or cannot chew their food, life may be a "living hell." Many have to live with the pain and discomfort for several years. They do not always appear to be in extreme pain, yet they spend a great deal of time trying to convince relatives and employers that they really suffer. Some are labeled "kooks" because they manifest symptoms suggestive of more complex illness behavior.

Practitioners who try to diagnose these disorders say that because there are so many different kinds of symptoms, treatment from various kinds of doctors may be necessary to reduce the complaints. Specialists from many disciplines, including dentistry, neurology, psychology, physical medicine, otolaryngology, and chiropractic care, are often involved in the management of these cases. With so many different kinds of treatment available, it is difficult for the patient, practitioner, and insurance company to tell which, if any, works and why it works.

For the practitioner, risk management is significant. No practitioner wants treatment failures that result in dissatisfaction by the patient, and if a practitioner does not use standard-of-care procedures, there is an increased risk for negligence in care.

Because of the disagreement about the diagnosis among practitioners, the potential for abuse from overdiagnosis, and the uncertainty about the need for treatment, insurance companies have rejected many claims that involve TM disorders. Many companies are willing to pay to obtain surgical treatment for patients, and some provide optional coverage for conditions that do not require surgery. Rejection thus has been common when there has been a nonsurgical claim for certain dental procedures. Even when this kind of treatment is considered, most companies require a lengthy, written diagnosis to explain patient complaints and the reason for treatment. Yet these same companies pay willingly for nonsurgical treatment of the hip, knee, ankle, or shoulder joints. This kind of indifferent thinking infuriates patients and irritates honest practitioners.

In cases of long-standing pain, TM disorders often have been a source of litigation in the determination of disability. Most of these cases have been associated with trauma following accidents. A few cases have been concerned with pain and disability purported to be caused by orthodontic or surgical treatment.

As a dental practitioner, you will be confronted with patients who have symptoms characteristic of musculoskeletal disorders. Some of these symptoms may appear in the form of a TM disorder. Your patients will want to know many things about this disorder. If you master the material in this textbook, you will be able to communicate this information to your patients, diagnose their complaints correctly, and manage them appropriately.

The Temporomandibular Joint and Related Orofacial Disorders,
by Francis M. Bush and M. Franklin Dolwick.
J.B. Lippincott Company, Philadelphia, © 1995.

2

General Anatomy

To become or remain competent in the treatment of TMD complaints, the clinician needs a basic understanding of head and neck anatomy. Knowledge of the general morphology makes basic examination of the TMJ region easier. Physical evaluation provides an appraisal of patient-related information with an anticipated therapeutic outcome.

The review in this chapter is not meant to be an all-encompassing textbook of anatomy. Bits of morphology are described to help the clinician visualize clinical problems (Table 2-1). Key anatomic landmarks are presented as points of reference for enhancing interpretation of physical findings.

General Description of the TMJ

The temporomandibular joint is located just anterior to the tragus of the ear (Fig. 2-1). The joint is considered an articulation between the base of the skull and the condyle of the mandible. The articular surface of the skull is the squamous part of the temporal bone. This bone has a concavity, the *articular (glenoid) fossa* (Fig. 2-2) and a convexity, the *articular tubercle (eminence;* see Fig. 2-1).

The *condyle* of the healthy mandible is convex on surfaces that bear force. It is widest mediolaterally and roundish anteroposteriorly (Fig. 2-3). Deviation in form (DIF) is common in young adults.[1]

Unlike the articular surfaces of most other joints, the articular surfaces of the TMJ are covered with dense fibrous connective tissue instead of hyaline cartilage. Occasionally cartilage cells occur within this tissue; then, the surface is termed *fibrocartilage.*[2] The surfaces are nonvascularized and noninnervated. The cartilage accommodates compressive force.

An *articular capsule* lies beneath the skin and encloses the lateral surface of the joint (Fig. 2-4). The circular fibers are attached superiorly and medially to the articular

5

Table 2-1
Partial Anatomy of the Head and the Neck

Temporomandibular Joint

General description
Mechanics of the healthy joint
Disk/condyle derangement
Progressive joint derangement

Muscles

Masticatory
Suprahyoid
Infrahyoid
Muscles moving scalp, head, and shoulders

Arteries

TMJ
Masticatory region
Anterior neck
Posterior neck, scalp, and shoulders

Nerves

TMJ
Masticatory region
Anterior neck
Posterior neck and shoulders

Larynx and thyroid gland

Paranasal sinuses

Salivary glands

Lymph nodes

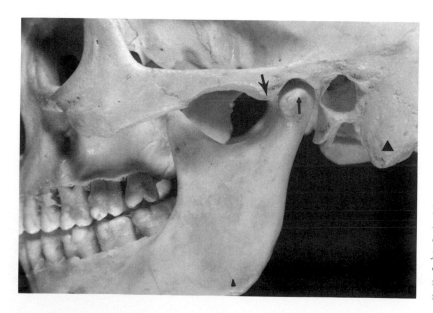

Figure 2-1.
Lateral view of skull showing the condyle articulating with articular fossa (small arrow); *the articular eminence* (large arrow); *the angle of mandible* (small triangle); *and the mastoid process* (large triangle).

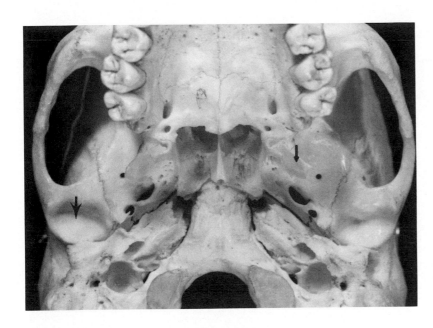

Figure 2-2.
Inferior view of skull showing the lateral pterygoid plate (small arrow) *and the articular fossa* (large arrow).

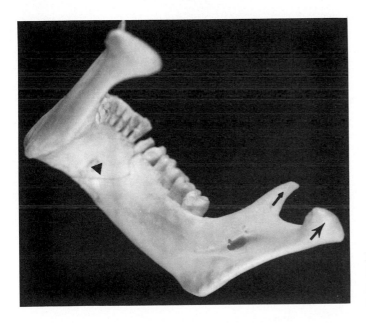

Figure 2-3.
Medial view of mandible showing the coronoid process (small arrow), *condyle* (large arrow), *and symphysis region* (triangle).

fossa and extend to the eminence and the neck of the condyle. The *lateral (temporomandibular) ligament* is anterior to the capsule and reinforces the joint laterally. Collagenous fibers are arranged obliquely in the lateral part of the ligament and horizontally in the medial part. No comparable reinforcement occurs along the medial surface of the joint. Capsular tissue is highly vascular and innervated.

The TMJ is a *synovial* joint. The soft tissue between the articular surfaces contains two synovial compartments (Fig. 2-5). The superior compartment is largest and contiguous with the fossa. The inferior compartment is smallest and reinforced by diskal

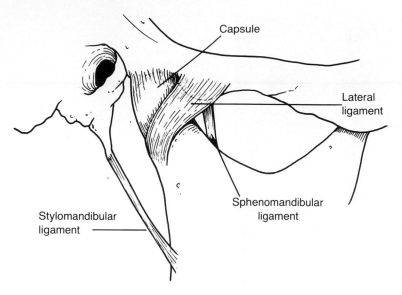

Figure 2-4.
Sagittal view of TMJ showing the articular capsule and the lateral, stylomandibular, and sphenomandibular ligaments.

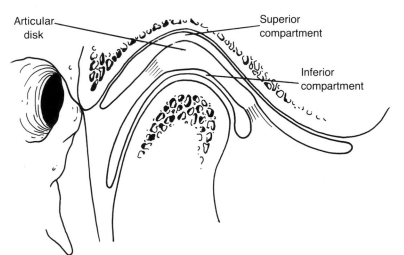

Figure 2-5.
Sagittal view of TMJ. Articular disk separates superior and inferior synovial compartments. Superior and inferior heads of lateral pterygoid muscle are anterior to joint.

attachments. The superior compartment extends more anteriorly than the lower compartment. These compartments contain fluid that has both lubricating and nutritional functions.

These compartments are divided by an *articular disk*, composed of dense fibroelastic connective tissue (Fig. 2-6). The disk encloses the superior surface of the condyle when the jaws are closed (Fig. 2-7). It fuses to the capsule and the lateral pterygoid muscle anteriorly (Fig. 2-8), joins the capsule mediolaterally, and attaches to loose, vascular connective tissue posteriorly.

The disk is divided into an *anterior band*, an *intermediate zone*, and a *posterior band*.[3] The anterior band has fibers interspersed with fibers of the lateral pterygoid

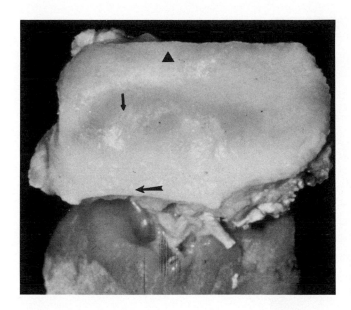

Figure 2-6.
Superior view of disk showing a thin intermediate zone (small arrow), *a dissected anterior extension* (large arrow), *and a posterior band* (triangle). *(Courtesy of Dr. James Butler, Richmond, VA.)*

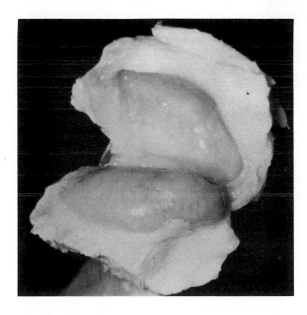

Figure 2-7.
Superior view of left condyle following dissection of the disk. The medial attachment is on the left and the lateral attachment on the right. (Courtesy of Dr. James Butler, Richmond, VA.)

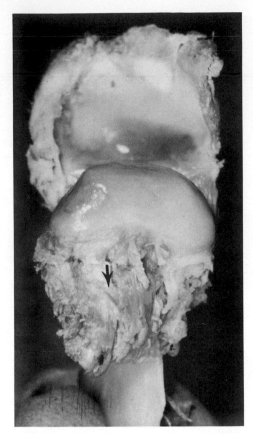

Figure 2-8.
Superior view of the condyle following dissection of the disk. Arrow indicates the anterior attachment of the lateral pterygoid muscle. (Courtesy of Dr. James Butler, Richmond, VA.)

muscle (Fig. 2-9). The intermediate zone is the thinnest part of the disk. During jaw opening, it forms the articulating surface between the condyle and fossa. The posterior band is the thickest and joins the posterior attachment, often termed the *bilaminar zone (retrodiskal pad*; Fig. 2-10).

Although the disk lacks neural tissue, finely branched fibers innervate the collateral diskal ligaments that attach the disk to the medial and lateral poles of the condyle, the retrodiskal tissue, and the posterior wall of the capsule. The condyle articulates with the disk to form a separate joint, often termed the *disk–condyle complex*. This complex articulates with the temporal bone to form a sliding joint.

The disk often is inappropriately termed a *meniscus,* a term that better applies to the crescent-shaped disk of fibrocartilage attached to the superior articular surface of the tibia.[4] One side of the meniscus of the knee joint attaches to the articular

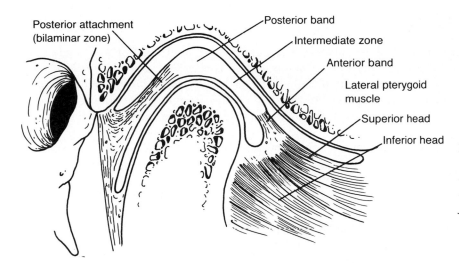

Figure 2-9.
Sagittal view of zones of the disk: anterior band, intermediate zone, and posterior band. (Adapted from Dolwick MF, Sanders B. TMJ internal derangement and arthrosis. St. Louis: CV Mosby, 1985:20.)

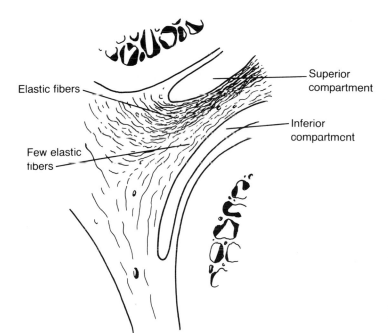

Figure 2-10.
Sagittal view of the superior and the inferior laminae of the bilaminar zone. Note the presence of elastic fibers in the superior lamina and scarcity of them in the inferior lamina.

capsule, and the other two sides extend into the joint, ending in a free edge. The disk of the TMJ does not fit this description.

Significance: The disk is an active structure that maintains contact of the joint surfaces with the mandible at rest, at intercuspation, and during function. Although innervated with somatic and visceral afferent (including nociceptive) fibers, retrodiskal tissue has no proprioceptive capability.[5] Inflammation may develop within the tissue if it is injured by excessive condylar force.

Mechanics of the Healthy Joint

The joint is a bilateral articulation. The right and left joint function as a single unit. Because of the capability of free movement, it is classified as a *diarthroidal* joint. Both hinge (ginglymus, rotation) and *gliding* (arthroidal, translatory) motions are possible. The hinge action relates to the disk–condyle complex; the gliding action, to the disk–temporal bone. Also, the joint is capable of *bodily* (side) movement.

There are close relations among the appearance of the disk, the shape of the synovial compartments, and the location of the condyle. Often, the thick posterior band may locate superior to the condyle when the jaws are closed. Yet the disk conforms to the shape of the fossa and is not restricted to this superior position.[3]

Movement involving the joints has been divided into different phases, namely the *occlusal, retruded opening, early protrusive, late protrusive, early closing,* and *retruded closing* phases.[3] Recently, more detail has been illustrated.[6]

The *occlusal* phase involves a static jaw position with the teeth in maximum intercuspation. The posterior band occupies the deepest part of the mandibular fossa. The intermediate zone and anterior band lie between the condyle and posterior slope of the eminence (Fig. 2-11*A*).

In the *retruded opening* phase, the condyle rotates and moves 5 to 6 mm inferior to the intermediate zone, which now becomes the articulating surface. The medial pole of the condyle moves anterosuperiorly, and the lateral pole moves posteroinferiorly. The shape of the inferior compartment changes the most. The movement continues with opening to about 18 mm.

In the *early protrusive opening* phase, the condyle moves inferiorly and anteriorly approximately 6 to 9 mm beneath the intermediate zone (Fig. 2-11*B*). The movement stretches the bilaminar zone. More space develops posteriorly as the condyle translates anteriorly. This change shifts the posterior band posteriorly.

In the *late protrusive opening* phase, the condyle moves inferiorly and anteriorly beneath the anterior band (Fig. 2-11*C*). More space develops in the superior compartment posteriorly than in the inferior compartment during rotation. Blood enters spaces of the posterior attachment.

The superior retrodiskal lamina contains elastic connective tissue (see Fig. 2-10). Apparently, during forward translation the lamina exerts posterior traction on the disk. This action limits anterior dislocation of the disk.

In the *early closing* phase, the condyle translates posteriorly, about 6 to 9 mm, to the intermediate zone. There is simultaneous reduction of space posteriorly in the superior compartment (see Fig. 2-11*B*).

In the *retrusive closing* phase, the condyle rotates superiorly but remains inferior to the posterior band. This movement reduces the space in the inferior compartment, tightens the mandibular attachment, and forces blood from the posterior attachment. The condyle returns near the occlusal phase (see Fig. 2-11*A*).

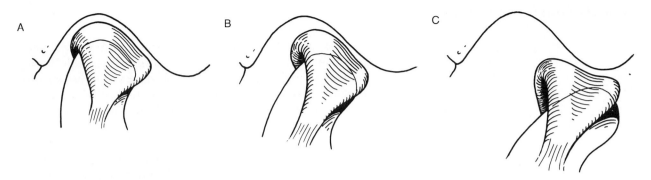

Figure 2-11.
*Disk–condyle assembly during opening (**A** to **C**) and closing (**C** to **A**) movements. (**A**) Condyle at occlusal phase beneath the posterior band. (**B**) Early protrusive phase with condyle beneath the intermediate zone. (**C**) Late protrusive phase with the condyle near the anterior band. Movement from **C** to **B** represents the closing phase and return to the occlusal phase at **A**. (Adapted from Dolwick MF, Sanders B. TMJ internal derangement and arthrosis. St. Louis: CV Mosby, 1985:23.)*

The width of the disk space is inconstant and changes with interarticular pressure. Disk space widens if the pressure is low (ie, during empty mouth movements). It narrows when pressure is high (ie, during maximal intercuspation of the teeth).

The *limitations* of specific ligaments and the lateral pterygoid muscle restrict movements of the condyle. The attachment of the lateral ligament at the lateral pole prevents condylar displacement posteriorly away from the eminence. Side shifting of the mandible is passively restricted. This movement also is controlled by activity of the lateral pterygoid muscle on the contralateral side of the mandible. Other prominent ligaments, including the stylomandibular and sphenomandibular ligaments (see Fig. 2-4), play little role in the mechanics of movement.[7]

During opening phases, the superior head of the lateral pterygoid muscle is inactive.[8] In one study, the superior head was inserted at the pterygoid fovea of the medial condyle in 70% of 26 human cadaveric joints.[9] Accessory fibers terminate under the foot of the disk. They join the anterior ligament and insert at the condyle. The foot of the anterior part of the disk joins the capsule. This arrangement indicates that the superior head has little role in movement of the disk.[9] The superior head is active during closing, assisting the elevator muscles in seating the condyle and the disk anterosuperiorly against the eminence.

The inferior head of the lateral pterygoid contracts during the early phase of closure.[9] Electromyographic studies show that it is inactive near initial tooth contact.[10]

Significance: The TMJ is considered a compound joint; the disk acts as an intermediate nonossified structure between the temporal bone and the condyle. The attachment of the superior lateral pterygoid muscle to the anterior part of the disk prevents the disk from dislocating posteriorly. The specific events concerning anterior displacement are unclear.

Disk–Condyle Derangement

Alteration in the healthy disk–condyle relation leads to the appearance of joint sounds. Different configurations and positions of the disk account for sounds during movement.[11] In *disk displacement with reduction*, the condyle may be either slightly delayed or blocked by the disk during forward movement. Usually, the disk is displaced anteromedially. The accounts for the hesitation or "hang" on opening. Ultimately, the disk self-reduces (see Fig. 7-69 in Chapter 7).

With reduction, the displacement lasts through rotation. The disk reduces posteriorly as the condyle translates (see Fig. 2-11*B*). This shift in disk position and configuration results in noise.

Different kinds of sounds have been identified.[12] A click is a distinct sound of brief duration with a clear beginning and an end. Fine crepitus is a fine grating sound that is continuous over a longer period of opening or closing. Coarse crepitus is a continuous noise over a longer period of time consistent with bone grinding on bone.

Clicking that occurs on opening and on closing is termed *reciprocal clicking*. This may be divided into reproducible reciprocal clicking, reproducible opening clicking, and reproducible closing clicking, based on presentation of sounds following two or more opening and closing movements.[12]

In *disk displacement without reduction*, the blocked disk persists (see Fig. 7-71 in Chapter 7). Hence, no reduction occurs. The condition is termed a *closed lock*. Without reduction, the posterior band is more anteriorly positioned with respect to the condyle than normal.[6] Because no translation occurs, no noise results.

Several conclusions have been made about joint sounds from electromyography of the lateral pterygoid muscle.[13] Apparently, the superior head hyperfunctions during the final closing sound, and the inferior head hyperfunctions during the opening sound. Presumably, closing sounds result from the contact between an anteriorly moving disk and a posterosuperiorly moving condyle. The hyperfunctional inferior head pulls the condyle anteriorly to contact the anterior band of the disk or the posterior slope of the eminence.

Progressive Joint Derangement

The anatomic, clinical, and radiologic evidence is ambiguous about a sequence leading to progressive dysfunction of the joint.

Argument for Progression

Otherwise healthy disks become displaced leading to reduction followed by a period of nonreduction. This progression has been described from combined dissection of joints and arthrography.[6]

The sequence proceeds as follows. The posterior band thickens, compressing the inferior compartment, which increases the space anteriorly. The intermediate zone lies inferior to the eminence. After more derangement, the shape of the anterior band diminishes and the superior compartment narrows. The posterior attachment thins initially, becomes denser from adaptation, then may perforate laterally (see Fig. 7-73 in Chapter 7). Once perforation occurs, bony changes may follow. Progressive and regressive remodeling occurs in the condyle and the eminence. If severe, the articular surfaces become osteoarthrotic. Crepitus results from friction of articular surfaces against one another.

Other clinical and arthroscopic findings confirm some of these changes. Arthroscopy showed osteoarthrosis was more frequently present in the temporal connective tissue than in the disk.[14] Reciprocal clicking was common in joints with slight or no osteoarthrosis. Crepitation correlated with advanced and not an early phase of osteoarthrosis. Lateral joint soreness correlated with synovitis. Posterior joint soreness was uncommon. When present, it was associated with lateral joint soreness.

Argument Against Progression

Evidence is lacking to support certain assumptions involving progression. Studies of dissected human cadaveric joints showed that anterior displacement was rare and may be a normal variant. The condyle does not force the disk anteriorly, and perforations of the posterior attachment are rare.[15]

Significance: A criticism of the argument for progression is that small groups of patients with joint disease have been studied. In the absence of widespread muscular tenderness, persistent soreness along the lateral surface of the joint likely means synovitis. If the joint remains tender to palpation, chronic inflammation is probable.

Muscles

The anatomy of major head and neck muscles is reviewed because muscular complaints may be referred to the TMJs. Because of their involvement in mandibular movement, the muscles of mastication are emphasized (Table 2-2).

Masticatory

The *masseter* is divided into two heads (Figs. 2-12 and 2-13). The superficial head originates on the anterior zygomatic arch and inserts on the angle and the ramus. The deep head originates from the posterior part of the zygoma and inserts on the ramus and the coronoid process.

The *medial pterygoid* arises from the medial surface of the lateral pterygoid plate and from the lateral surface of the palatine bone. Fibers run posteroinferiorly, inserting on the medial surface of the ramus and the angle (see Fig. 2-13).

The *lateral pterygoid* has two heads. The superior head originates on the infratemporal surface of the greater wing of the sphenoid bone (see Figs. 2-2 and 2-13). Nearly horizontal fibers insert at the pterygoid fovea of the medial condyle.[9] The inferior head arises from the lateral surface of the lateral pterygoid plate and inclines superiorly as fibers run posterolaterally inserting into the pterygoid fovea.

Table 2-2
Jaw Movements and Masticatory Muscles Involved

Movement	Muscle	Function
Elevation	Masseter	Supplies power during jaw closure
	Medial pterygoid	First muscles to contract during jaw closure
	Temporalis (posterior fibers)	Main positioner of jaw closure
	Lateral pterygoid	Superior head is active during final stage of jaw closure, especially during clenching; inferior head is active during early stage of jaw closure
Depression	Lateral pterygoid	Bilateral contraction of inferior head
	Digastric (anterior fibers)	Bilateral contraction
	Mylohyoid	Bilateral contraction
	Geniohyoid	Bilateral contraction
Retrusion	Digastric (posterior fibers)	Bilateral contraction
	Temporalis (posterior fibers)	Bilateral contraction
	Lateral pterygoid	Superior head is active during clenching
Protrusion	Lateral pterygoid	Bilateral contraction of inferior heads
	Medial pterygoid	Bilateral contraction
	Temporalis (anterior fibers)	Bilateral contraction
Lateral	Lateral pterygoid	Superior head is active during movement from contralateral position toward midline
	Medial pterygoid	Contracts with lateral pterygoid during movement from contralateral position toward midline
	Temporalis (middle and posterior fibers)	Ipsilateral contraction to side of movement

The *temporalis* arises from the frontal and parietal bones inferior to the superior temporal line (Fig. 2-14). Fibers converge into a tendinous band, which then divides into two parts. A superficial group of fibers inserts on the superolateral surface of the coronoid process. Deeper, larger fibers form a band along the inner coronoid process extending inferiorly to the anterior border of the ramus.

Suprahyoid

The suprahyoids are accessory muscles located superior to the hyoid bone (Fig. 2-15) They act during depression of the mandible or assist with elevation of the hyoid bone.

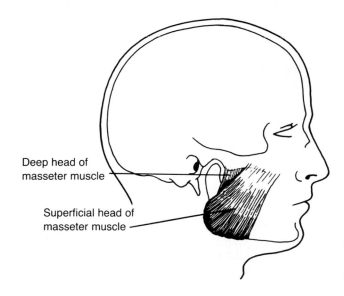

Deep head of
masseter muscle

Superficial head of
masseter muscle

Figure 2-12.
*The superficial head of the masseter muscle overlies
the deep head.*

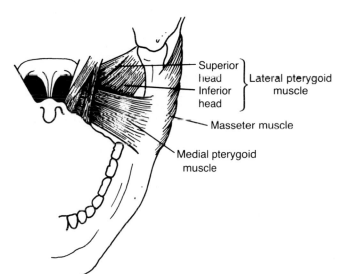

Superior
head
Inferior
head

Lateral pterygoid
muscle

Masseter muscle

Medial pterygoid
muscle

Figure 2-13.
*Inferior view of skull. Medial pterygoid muscle
attached to medial angle of the mandible. Superior
and inferior heads of the lateral pterygoid muscle
insert near the condyle. Masseter muscle is lateral
to angle to mandible.*

The *digastric* has two bellies. The anterior belly originates near the mandibular symphysis and inserts on the hyoid bone. The posterior belly originates on the mastoid notch and inserts on the hyoid bone. The anterior belly assists in depression of the mandible and the posterior belly in retrusion (or retraction).

The *geniohyoid* originates near the inner surface of the mandibular symphysis and inserts at the hyoid bone. The muscle assists in drawing the hyoid bone anteriorly.

The *mylohyoid* is inferior to the tongue and inserts at the body of the hyoid bone. This muscle assists in elevating the floor of the mouth.

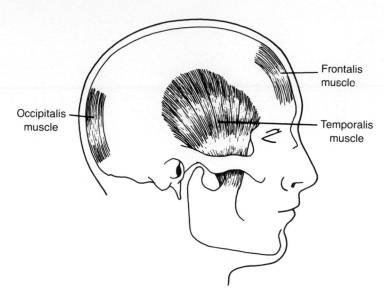

Figure 2-14.
Sagittal view of frontalis, temporalis, and occipitalis muscles.

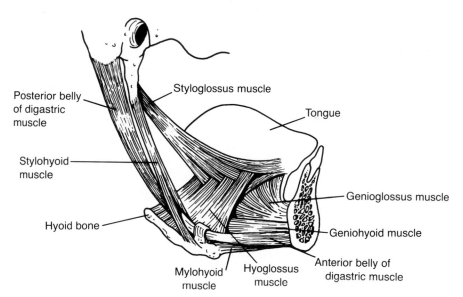

Figure 2-15.
Sagittal view of suprahyoid muscles, tongue, and hyoid bone.

The *stylohyoid* is located at the styloid process and inserts at the body of the hyoid bone. This muscle pulls the hyoid posterosuperiorly.

Infrahyoid

The infrahyoids are accessory muscles located inferior to the hyoid bone (Fig. 2-16). They act during depression of the hyoid bone or elevation of the larynx.

The *sternothyroid* originates on the manubrium of the sternum and inserts at the thyroid cartilage.

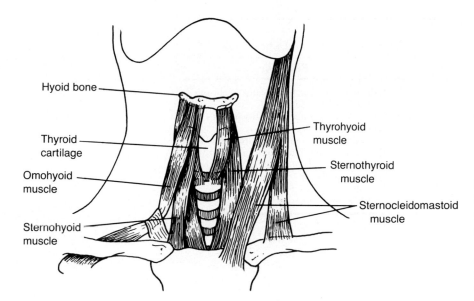

Hyoid bone

Thyroid
cartilage

Omohyoid
muscle

Sternohyoid
muscle

Thyrohyoid
muscle

Sternothyroid
muscle

Sternocleidomastoid
muscle

Figure 2-16.
Frontal view of mandible and neck. Left side shows intact sternocleidomastoid muscle. Right side shows sternocleiodmastoid muscle dissected away revealing deeper infrahyoid muscles.

The *thyrohyoid* originates on the thyroid cartilage and inserts on the hyoid bone.

The *omohyoid* originates on the superior part of the scapula and inserts at the lateral border of the hyoid bone.

The *sternohyoid* originates on the manubrium of the sternum and inserts on the body of the hyoid bone.

Muscles Moving the Scalp, Head, and Shoulders

Several muscles are responsible for movements of the scalp, head, and shoulders (Table 2-3).

The *frontalis* is the anterior half of the epicranius muscle. It originates on the galea aponeurotica, a tendinous sheath, and inserts into the skin along the orbit and the nose (see Fig. 2-14).

The *occipitalis* is the posterior half of the epicranius muscle. It originates at the occipital bone and the mastoid part of the temporal bone and inserts at the galea aponeurotica.

The *sternocleidomastoid* has two origins, the sternum and the clavicle. Both heads insert at the mastoid process and occipital bone (see Fig. 2-16).

The *splenius* muscle is divided into two parts. The capitis originates near the seventh cervical vertebra and inserts at the mastoid process and occipital bone. The cervicis joins at the first three cervical vertebrae (Fig. 2-17). Inferior to the splenius is the semispinalis capitis.

The *trapezius* is a triangular muscle that originates at the occipital bone and inserts at the acromian and spine of scapula.

Table 2-3
Muscles Moving the Scalp, Head, and Shoulders

Muscle	Function
Frontalis	Pulls scalp anteriorly, elevates eyebrows
Occipitalis	Pulls scalp posteriorly
Sternocleidomastoid	Flexes head and neck, rotates head to contralateral side
Splenius capitis	Extends head, turns head to the same side
Trapezius	Elevates and retracts shoulders, rotates scapula, extends head or pulls it to the contralateral side
Levator scapulae	Elevates scapula
Rhomboids	Moves scapula posteriorly

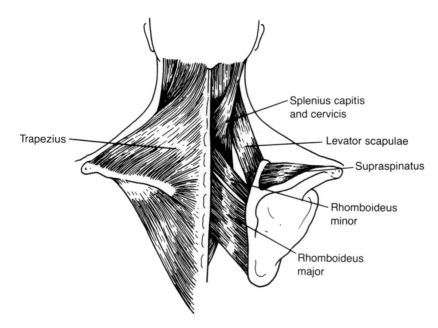

Figure 2-17.
Posterior view of neck and upper back. Left side shows intact trapezius muscle and right side with trapezius dissected away showing underlying musculature.

The *levator scapulae* originates at the fourth and fifth cervical vertebrae and inserts at the scapula.

The major and minor heads of the *rhomboids* originate along the first cervical vertebra and extend to the fifth thoracic vertebra.

   Significance: Specific head and neck muscles need to be identified appropriately by location. This facilitates correct palpation and, ultimately, treatment as required.

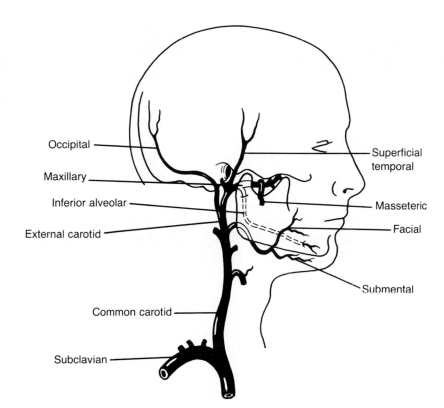

Occipital

Maxillary

Inferior alveolar

External carotid

Superficial temporal

Masseteric

Facial

Submental

Common carotid

Subclavian

Figure 2-18.
Arterial supply to TMJ and head and neck muscles.

Arteries

The main blood supply to the *TMJs* is derived from the external carotid artery (Fig. 2-18). The maxillary artery branches from it by way of the infratemporal fossa at the neck of the mandible. A lesser branch, the masseteric artery supplies the posterior attachment. The superficial temporal artery, which ascends through the parotid gland, also serves the joint.

The *masticatory muscles* are supplied by the maxillary artery. After branching from the external carotid, the maxillary artery divides into six branches. Each branch supplies the muscle of the same name: masseteric, lateral pterygoid, medial pterygoid, anterior and posterior deep temporal, and buccal (see Fig. 2-18).

In the region of the *anterior neck*, the facial artery supplies the posterior belly of the digastric muscle. A branch of this artery, the submental artery, supplies the anterior belly (see Fig. 2-18). The inferior alveolar artery divides into smaller vessels that supply the mylohyoid, geniohyoid, genioglossus, hyoglossus, and styloglossus muscles.

In the region of the *posterior neck and scalp*, the occipital artery supplies the sternocleidomastoid muscle and the deep muscles of the posterior neck and scalp (see Fig. 2-18). A dorsal branch of the subclavian artery supplies the trapezius, but neighboring sources also participate.

Significance: No definitive relation has been established between TM complaints and vascular disorders, including vascular kinds of headache. Nonetheless, there is still a need to assess the possibility of a relation.

Nerves

The *TMJ* region is innervated by the mandibular branch (V_3) of the trigeminal nerve (V). The main branch is the auriculotemporal nerve from the posterior division of V_3 (Fig. 2-19). The masseteric nerve also branches from the anterior division of V_3 to the joint.

The *masticatory muscles* are innervated by the anterior division (V_3) nerve. Numerous branches of the same name innervate the masseter, lateral pterygoid, and anterior and deep temporal muscles (Fig. 2-20). A lesser branch arising directly from the mandibular division innervates the medial pterygoid muscle.

In the region of the *anterior neck*, the anterior belly of the digastric and the mylohyoid are supplied by the V_3 division. The posterior belly and the stylohyoid are innervated by the facial nerve (Fig. 2-21). The geniohyoid is innervated by the branch of the first cranial nerve by way of the hypoglossal nerve (Fig. 2-22).

Along with the omohyoid and sternohyoid, the sternothyroid is innervated by the ansa cervicalis, a loop of nerves at the C1 to C2 vertebrae. The thyrohyoid is innervated by the C_1 spinal nerve by way of the hypoglossal nerve.

In the region of the *posterior neck and shoulders*, the frontalis and occipitalis muscles are innervated by the facial nerve. Cutaneous branches of C_2 to C_3 divide into

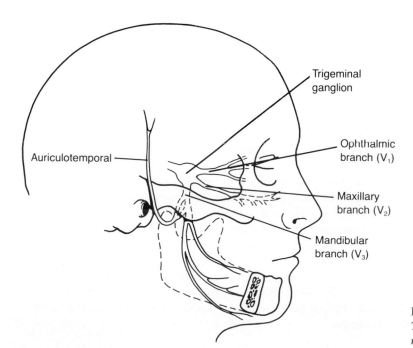

Trigeminal
ganglion

Ophthalmic
branch (V_1)

Auriculotemporal

Maxillary
branch (V_2)

Mandibular
branch (V_3)

Figure 2-19.
The trigeminal nerve with ophthalmic, maxillary, and mandibular branches.

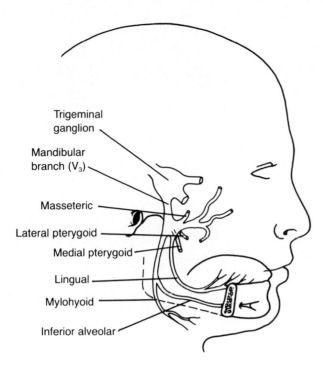

Trigeminal
ganglion

Mandibular
branch (V₃)

Masseteric

Lateral pterygoid

Medial pterygoid

Lingual

Mylohyoid

Inferior alveolar

Figure 2-20.
The mandibular division with branches to the TMJ, masticatory muscles, tongue, and mandible.

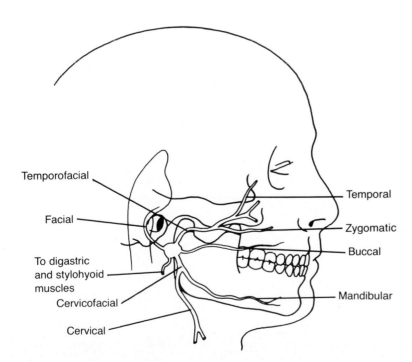

Temporofacial

Facial

To digastric
and stylohyoid
muscles

Cervicofacial

Cervical

Temporal

Zygomatic

Buccal

Mandibular

Figure 2-21.
The facial nerve with temporofacial and cervicofacial divisions.

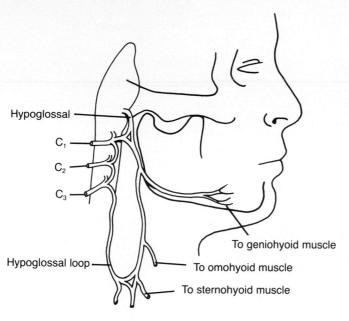

Hypoglossal

C₁

C₂

C₃

Hypoglossal loop

To geniohyoid muscle

To omohyoid muscle

To sternohyoid muscle

Figure 2-22.
The hypoglossal nerve with branches to tongue and infrahyoid muscles.

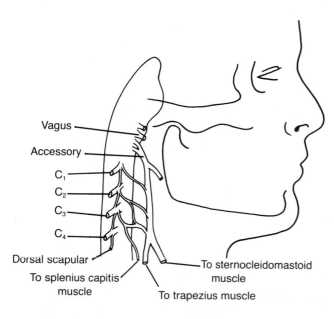

Vagus

Accessory

C₁

C₂

C₃

C₄

Dorsal scapular

To splenius capitis muscle

To sternocleidomastoid muscle

To trapezius muscle

Figure 2-23.
The spinal accessory nerve and branches to the sterno-cleidomastoid and trapezius muscles.

the lesser occipital, great auricular, and transverse cervical branches. The greater occipital nerve extends to the scalp branches from C_2.

The spinal accessory nerve supplies the sternocleidomastoid and trapezius muscles (Fig. 2-23). The splenius capitis is innervated by the lateral branches of the middle cervical spinal nerves, the levator scapulae by C_3 to C_4 (see Fig. 2-23), and the dorsal scapular nerves and rhomboid major and minor by the dorsal scapular nerve.

Significance: Certain nondental and dental disorders with neural origins mimic TMD. Visualization of alternate neural pathways enhances success of physical evaluation of the TMJs.

Larynx and Thyroid Gland

The larynx joins the pharynx superiorly and the trachea inferiorly (Fig. 2-24). It lies ventral to the C4 to C6 vertebrae. There are three paired and three unpaired cartilages. The thyroid and the cricoid cartilages are the easiest to palpate.

Bilateral thyroid cartilages unite to form a laryngeal prominence termed the *Adam's apple* (see Fig. 2-24). Superior to the thyroid cartilage is the epiglottis, a lid preventing aspiration of substances into the trachea. Inferior to the epiglottis is the hyoid bone. Between the body of the hyoid bone and the thyroid cartilage is a thyrohyoid

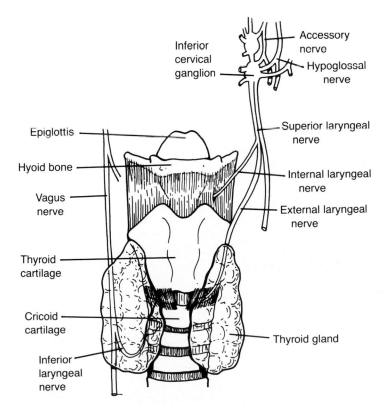

Figure 2-24.
The vagus nerve and branches supplying the larynx and thyroid gland.

membrane. Inferior to the thyroid cartilage is the cricoid cartilage that joins the trachea. Lateral to the cricoid cartilage and extending inferiorly along the trachea are the paired lobes of the thyroid gland.

Most muscles of the larynx are innervated by the inferior laryngeal nerve branching from the vagus (see Fig. 2-24). An exception is the cricothyroid muscle, which is supplied by the external branch of the superior laryngeal nerve dividing from the vagus.

Significance: This region should be palpated for tenderness or swelling, which may be confused with tenderness of the masticatory muscles. Chronic hoarseness suggests inflammation of the vocal folds.

Paranasal Sinuses

The paranasal sinuses are paired air-spaces that communicate with the nasal cavity. Antrums are present in the maxillary, frontal, ethmoid, and sphenoid regions of the skull (Fig. 2-25).

The *maxillary sinus* is the largest of the sinuses. This space occupies nearly two thirds of the maxilla. The superior wall forms most of the orbital floor and the anterolateral wall is bounded by the zygoma especially near the canine fossa. The infratemporal fossa abuts the posterior wall, and the lateral nasal septum abuts the medial wall. Usually the roots of the teeth do not contact the thick wall of the normal cavity. Some roots may be separated by a mucous membrane or thin lamina of bone if the antrum

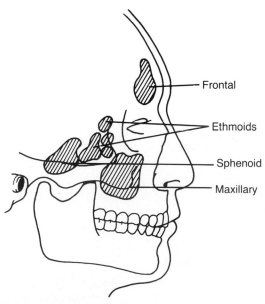

Frontal

Ethmoids

Sphenoid

Maxillary

Figure 2-25.
The paranasal sinuses.

is large. Drainage is variable, occurring mostly through the frontonasal duct in the anterior part of the middle meatus.

Posterior and anterior superior nerves, and sometimes the infraorbital nerve, innervate the antrum (see Fig. 2-19).

In the *frontal sinus*, the antrum is located mediosuperior to the orbit. Much variation and septation exists. The frontal bone separates the antrum from the anterior cranial fossa. The roof of the orbit forms the inferior wall. Drainage is mostly into the frontal recess of the nasal cavity, but ostia may open directly into the nose.

Branches from the V_1 division of the trigeminal nerve supply this region.

In the *ethmoid sinus*, the antrum fills the ethmoid bone. Numerous air cells are located posterior to the maxillary sinus and orbit. They drain into the nares anteriorly and posteriorly.

The antrum is innervated by the anterior ethmoidal nerve branching from the nasociliary nerve and, posteriorly, by the maxillary nerve.

The cavity of the *sphenoid sinus* is extremely variable in shape. In some instances, paired cavities may occur in the body of the sphenoid bone. Important boundaries include the middle cranial fossa, the posterior cranial fossa, the nasopharynx inferiorly, the optic nerve, and the cavernous sinus laterally. Drainage is by means of the sphenoethmoidal groove into the lateral nasal wall.

The antrum is innervated by the lateral posterosuperior nasal nerve.

Significance: The frontal sinus is the only paranasal sinus innervated by the trigeminal nerve. Dysfunction of neural origin associated with this sinus may relate to neural dysfunction of the TMJ and vice versa.

The bony floor of the maxillary sinus is thinnest above the roots of the molar teeth. The superior alveolar nerves approximate the lower margin of the maxillary sinus in some cases, making it difficult to determine whether pain emanates from the maxillary teeth or from infection of adjacent sinuses.

Salivary Glands

The proximity of the major salivary glands to the TMJ makes a review of their anatomy worthwhile. Pathology of the glands may mimic symptoms of TMD.

The *parotid glands* are paired glands of irregular triangular shape (Fig. 2-26). Each is divided into three surfaces. The lateral surface is bounded by parotid fascia, tela subcutanea, and skin. The gland passes anteriorly across the lateral surface of the masseter muscle and curves around the posterior border of the ramus just superior to the posterior belly of the digastric muscle. Posteromedially, the surface is adjacent to the sternocleidomastoid and digastric muscles and the mastoid process. Stensen's duct exits into the oral cavity near the maxillary second molar region.

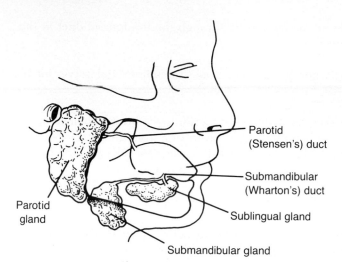

Parotid
(Stensen's) duct

Submandibular
(Wharton's) duct

Sublingual gland

Parotid
gland

Submandibular gland

Figure 2-26.
The major salivary glands.

The afferent nerve supply is from the auriculotemporal nerve. The efferent supply is from the glossopharyngeal nerve (Fig. 2-27). Parasympathetic fibers reach the gland by way of the auriculotemporal nerve. The sympathetic fibers probably travel by various arteries from the external carotid plexus.

The *submandibular glands* are paired glands that occupy most of the submandibular triangle. They are bordered by the bellies of the digastric muscle and the inferior border of the mandible (see Fig. 2-26). The fascial covering joins the parotid sheath. The thickened fascia between the paired glands forms the stylomandibular ligament. Laterally, the gland abuts with the mandibular branch of the facial nerve and vein. Along the anteromedial surface, it rests on the mylohyoid muscle and nerve and then extends posteriorly to the posterior belly of the digastric muscle, hypoglossal nerve, and sometimes the lingual nerve. The facial artery covers the superior part of the gland. Wharton's duct terminates at each salivary caruncula lateral to the lingual frenum.

The gland is innervated by the facial nerve. Parasympathetic fibers enter the chorda tympani branch and course with the lingual nerve of the V_3 to the submandibular ganglion. Presynaptic fibers synapse with postganglionic fibers to supply both the submandibular and sublingual glands.

The paired *sublingual glands* lie inferior to the mucosa of the floor of the mouth, superior to the mylohyoid muscle, and between the mandible and the hyoglossus and genioglossus muscles (see Fig. 2-26). The lingual nerve lies lateral, inferior, and medial to each gland. Many small ducts open into the oral cavity by way of the sublingual folds. Some anterior ostia join to form Bartholin's duct, which communicates with Wharton's duct and empties into the floor of the mouth.

Significance: The salivary glands may become obstructed or infected. Salivary calculi occur mainly in the submandibular gland (85%) and less often in the parotid gland.[16] Their presence may lead to swelling and pain. There may be insufficient or excess saliva because secretion is exclusively under nervous control.

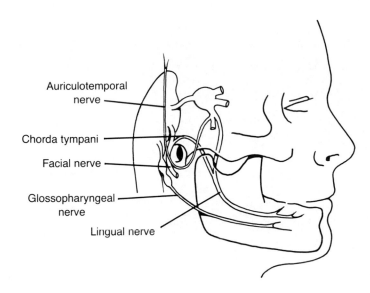

Auriculotemporal
nerve

Chorda tympani

Facial nerve

Glossopharyngeal
nerve

Lingual nerve

Figure 2-27.
The glossopharyngeal nerve.

Most tumors of salivary glands occur in the parotid.[17] Fortunately, few are malignant.

Frey's syndrome, identified by redness and gustatory sweating over the distribution of the auriculotemporal nerve, may be related to parotid trauma or to a complication of parotidectomy. There may be alteration of the parasympathetic fibers that would normally evoke parotid secretion.

Lymph Nodes

Lymph of the head drains into superficial lymph nodes (Fig. 2-28), whereas lymph of the neck drains mainly into deep cervical nodes and less often into superficial nodes (Figs. 2-29 and 2-30).[18–20] The head and neck are served by groups of nodes named after anatomic regions of the body (Table 2-4).

Head

The *retroauricular, anterior auricular,* and *superficial parotid* lymph nodes surround the ear.

The *facial* lymph nodes are scattered along the distribution of the facial artery. Lesser designations are the infraorbital, buccal, and mandibular nodes.

The *occipital* lymph nodes are located at the base of the skull and are associated with the occipital artery.

Neck

Superficial Groups

The *submental* lymph nodes are located inferior to the chin, along the mylohyoid muscle at the junction of the symphysis and the hyoid bone.

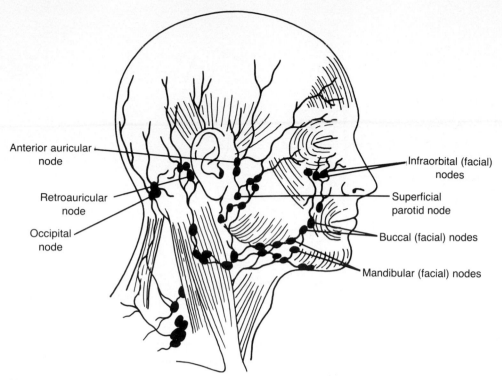

Anterior auricular
node

Retroauricular
node

Occipital
node

Infraorbital (facial)
nodes

Superficial
parotid node

Buccal (facial) nodes

Mandibular (facial) nodes

Figure 2-28.
The superficial lymph nodes of the head. (Adapted from Reed GM, Sheppard VF. Basic structures of the head and neck. Philadelphia: WB Saunders, 1976:497.)

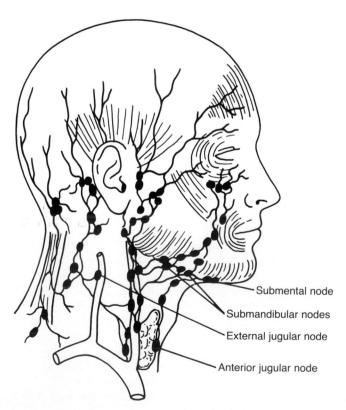

Submental node

Submandibular nodes

External jugular node

Anterior jugular node

Figure 2-29.
The superficial lymph nodes of the neck. (Adapted from Reed GM, Sheppard VF. Basic structures of the head and neck. Philadelphia: WB Saunders, 1976:501.)

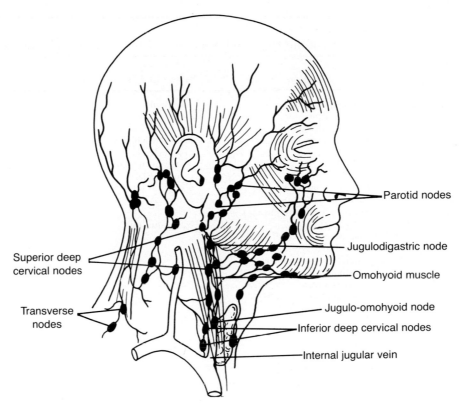

Figure 2-30.
The deep cervical lymph nodes. (Adapted from Reed GM, Sheppard VF Basic structures of the head and neck. Philadelphia: WB Saunders, 1976:504.)

The *submandibular* nodes lie near the inferior border of the ramus of the mandible along the submandibular gland.

The *jugular* nodes lie along the external jugular vein at the sternocleidomastoid muscle and abut with the anterior jugular vein.

Deep Groups

The *superior cervical* lymph nodes lie along the internal jugular vein and superior to the omohyoid muscle. Largest of this group is the jugulodigastric node. The jugulo-omohyoid node crosses at the junction of the vein and muscle.

The *inferior cervical* lymph nodes lie along the internal jugular vein and inferior to the omohyoid muscle. Lymph from the superior cervical nodes drains into the inferior cervical nodes or into the jugular trunk leading to the thoracic duct.

The *retropharyngeal* and *parotid* nodes most likely belong to the superior cervical group. The retropharyngeal nodes drain the nose, paranasal sinuses, pharynx, and palate. The parotid nodes drain the external auditory meatus, tympanic cavity, parotid gland, and TMJs.

Table 2-4

Regions of the Head and Neck, Associated Lymph Nodes and Patterns of Drainage

Region	Afferent Lymph to Nodes	Efferent Lymph to Nodes
Scalp—posterior Neck—upper	Occipital	Deep cervical
Scalp—anterior Ear—external	Anteroauricular, retroauricular, parotid (superficial)	Deep cervical, superior and accessory
TMJ	Anteroaurucular, parotid (superficial)	Deep cervical, superior
Maxillary anterior teeth and periodontium Skin—mucous membranes	Facial	Deep cervical, superior
Palate—hard Tongue—anterior Mandibular teeth—most molars and premolars Maxillary molars and periodontium—posterior Submandibular glands Sublingual glands Nose Cheeks Chin	Submandibular	Deep cervical, superior and other deep nodes
Gingiva—mandibular Premolars—mandibular Lips	Submental, submandibular	Deep cervical
Incisors—mandibular Canines—mandibular Cheeks Lip—mandibular Chin Tongue—tip	Submental	Submandibular and jugulodigastric
Nose Palate—soft Paranasal sinuses Pharynx Tongue—posterior	Retropharyngeal	Deep cervical, superior
External auditory meatus Auditory tube Tympanic cavity Parotid gland	Parotid (superficial)	Deep cervical, superior
Ear—lower parotid region	Jugular	Deep cervical, superior
Larynx Trachea Thyroid gland	Juxtavisceral	Deep cervical, superior and inferior

The *accessory* lymph nodes are members of the posteroinferior deep cervical chain. They lie posterior to the sternocleidomastoid muscle.

The *transverse cervical* nodes lie along the lateral surface of the neck and the trapezius muscle.

The *juxtavisceral* lymph nodes lie along the structures that they drain, including the larynx, trachea, esophagus, and thyroid gland.

Significance: Visualization of location and drainage patterns allows the clinician to discriminate dental-related or sinus infections from TMD complaints. The external surface of the TMJ region is drained by superficial anteroauricular nodes. Deeper structures are drained by the deep parotid nodes, which ultimately drain to the deep cervical nodes. Most maxillary anterior teeth drain into the facial nodes, whereas the molars drain into the submandibular nodes. Mandibular teeth drain into the submental or submandibular nodes. Paranasal sinus drainage is by way of the retropharyngeal nodes.

References

1. Hansson T, Solberg WK, Penn MK, Oberg, T. Anatomic study of the TMJs of young adults: A pilot investigation. J Prosthet Dent 1979;41:556.
2. Mohl N. Functional anatomy of the temporomandibular joint. In Laskin D, et al (eds). The President's conference on the examination, diagnosis and management of temporomandibular disorders. Chicago: American Dental Association, 1982:3.
3. Rees LA. The structure and function of the mandibular joint. Br Dent J 1954;56:125.
4. Bell WE. Understanding temporomandibular biomechanics. J Craniomandib Pract 1983;1:27.
5. Bell WE. Orofacial pains: classification, diagnosis, management, 3rd ed. Chicago: Year Book, 1985.
6. Dolwick MF, Sanders B. TMJ internal derangement and arthrosis. St Louis: CV Mosby, 1985.
7. Burch JG. Activity of the accessory ligaments of the temporomandibular joint. J Prosthet Dent 1970;24:621.
8. McNamara JA Jr. The independent functions of the two heads of the lateral pterygoid muscle. Am J Anat 1973;138:197.
9. Wilkinson TM. The relationship between the disk and the lateral pterygoid muscle in the human temporomandibular joint. J Prosthet Dent 1988;60:715.
10. Mahan PE, Wilkinson TM, Gibbs CH, Mauderli A, Brannon LS. Superior and interior bellies of the lateral pterygoid EMG activity at basic jaw positions. J Prosthet Dent 1983;50:710.
11. Westesson PL, Rohlin M. Internal derangement related to osteoarthrosis in temporomandibular joint autopsy specimens. Oral Surg Oral Med Oral Pathol 1984;57:17.
12. Widmer CG, Huggins KH, Fricton J. Examination and history data collection, part III, J Craniomandib Disord Fac Oral Pain 1992;4:335.
13. Zijun L, Huiyun W, Weiya P. A comparative electromyographic study of the lateral pterygoid muscle and arthrography in patients with temporomandibular joint disturbance syndrome sounds. J Prosthet Dent 1989;62:229.
14. Holmlund A, Hellsing G, Axelsson S. The temporomandibular joint: a comparison of clinical and arthroscopic findings. J Prosthet Dent 1989;62:61.
15. Hellsing G, Holmlund H. Development of anterior disk displacement in the temporomandibular joint: an autopsy study. J Prosthet Dent 1985;53:397.

16. Bodner L. Surgical gland calculi: diagnostic imaging and surgical removal. Compend Contin Educ Dent 1993;14:572.

17. Shklar G. Oral cancer. Philadelphia: WB Saunders, 1984.

18. Reed GM, Sheppard VF. Basic structures of the head and neck. Philadelphia: WB Saunders, 1976.

19. Crafts RC. A textbook of human anatomy. New York: John Wiley, 1985.

20. Woodburne RT, Burkell WE. Essentials of human anatomy. New York: Oxford University Press, 1988.

The Temporomandibular Joint and Related Orofacial Disorders,
by Francis M. Bush and M. Franklin Dolwick.
J.B. Lippincott Company, Philadelphia, © 1995.

3

Signs and Symptoms

Textbooks and clinicians generally agree that there are four cardinal signs and symptoms of TM disorders:

- Pain in the TM joints, muscles of mastication, and adjacent soft tissues
- TM joint sounds that occur during mouth opening and closing and moving the lower jaw to either side or forward
- Tenderness of the TM joints, muscles of mastication, and adjacent soft tissues on digital palpation
- Limitation on opening the mouth and moving the lower jaw to either side or forward

Other signs and symptoms that have been associated with TM disorders include the following:

- Headache
- Neckache
- Ear problems (eg, tinnitus, earache, stuffiness, impaired hearing)
- Dizziness
- Visual disturbances
- Paresthesias (eg, burning mouth, tongue, throat)
- Gastrointestinal distress
- Sinus complaints

However, there is limited evidence to establish a positive relation between these symptoms and the major signs and symptoms.

Pain: The Chief Symptom

Pain is the most obvious symptom identified by the person with a TM disorder. Usually, it is pain that brings the individual to the doctor. From a scientific perspective, pain can be thought of as an experience evoked by stimuli causing or warning of impending tissue damage and "defined introspectively by every person as that which hurts."[1] According to the International Association for Study of Pain, pain is "an unpleasant sensory and emotional experience associated with either actual or potential tissue damage, or described in terms of such damage."

Dimensions of Pain

Pain is a subjective phenomenon, recognized either by verbal communication or by nonverbal behaviors of the person in pain. This subjective nature complicates diagnosis and treatment of the patient.

Different dimensions of the pain experience have been recognized, including the sensory, affective, and evaluative qualities.[2] The sensory component reflects variation in intensity, quality, or duration of pain. The affective dimension deals with the degree of pain unpleasantness. Words that trigger tension, fear, or autonomic response fit this part of the pain experience. The evaluative dimension describes the overall subjective intensity of the experience. These dimensions depend on numerous cognitive and motivational experiences and are influenced by psychological factors.[3] An astute clinician must recognize the differences among these dimensions, particularly when interviewing the patient with pain.

Attacks of Pain

Nearly everyone suffers pain from time to time. Fortunately, for most sufferers of TMD pain, each episode ends with resolution of the symptoms. If the pain resolves in a short period of time, the person is said to suffer from acute pain. If the pain persists for long periods of time, the person suffers from chronic pain. A small but significant number of individuals may have recurrent, frequent episodes of pain (Table 3-1).

Chronic pain afflicts many individuals of the general population. Its course and the resulting disability are interwoven with social, psychological, economic, and cultural factors.[4] Chronic pain also is related to changes in the body due to normal processes such as aging. These factors must be weighed in the diagnosis and treatment of the individual.

Chronic pain accompanies many musculoskeletal disorders. Musculoskeletal pain, primarily in the upper or lower back, accounted for the largest percentage of all disorders found at the initial visit by physicians. According to the 1980 National Ambulatory Medical Care Survey, approximately 70 million (41%) of 1.2 billion initial visits to nonfederal, office based physicians practicing in the United States were for these disorders.[5]

Many work days are lost from pain. According to the *Nuprin Pain Report*,[6] Americans lose 550 million work days each year because of pain. If routine activities besides full-time work are included, adults lose more than 4 billion days each year because of pain (Table 3-2). The clinician should be aware of the hierarchy of these numbers. Orofacial pain may arise from joint, muscle, headache, or dental complaints. Based

Table 3-1
Temporal Characteristics of Pain

Acute Pain	Chronic Pain
Recent onset	Present for 3 months or more
Limited duration	May occur regularly or frequently over long period
Temporary	Appears to be permanent
Usually patient can localize	Difficult for patient to localize
Typically responds well to treatment	Simple therapies mostly ineffective
No persistent psychological reactions in behavior	Often accompanied by psychological changes

on the number of days lost, the typical patient is more likely to suffer from somatic pain of the joints than from pain of the muscles. Headache proved the most frequent pain problem. Some 73% of adults suffered one or more headaches in the past 12 months. The average patient would be expected to suffer less from dental pain than from these other pains.

Significance: When the patient presents for examination or telephones with a complaint of pain, ask the patient to identify the tissue system responsible for the pain. The problem for the clinician is predicting the course that the pain will follow for each individual. No one can predict with any great degree of accuracy the likelihood of recovery, the response to different therapies, or the potential for rehabilitation. Any correlation between the severity of pain and the level of disability at any given time is difficult, if not impossible to predict. Each case must be assessed on an individual basis.

Table 3-2
Numbers in Millions of Lost Work Days from Pain

Pain	Days/Adults	Days/Adults Employed Full Time
Backache	1307.8	88.8
Joint	961.3	107.8
Headache	637.9	156.9
Muscle	617.3	58.2
Stomach	394.1	98.7
Premenstrual or menstrual	74.3	24.5
Dental	70.3	15.1
Total	4063.0	550.0

Modified from Taylor H, Curran NM. The Nuprin pain report. New York: Louis Harris and Associates, 1985.

Pain of TM Disorders: Self Report

Clinicians have great difficulty in identifying the kind of pain present with TM disorders. Like musculoskeletal pain of the back, most TM pain is musculoskeletal in origin. This disorder has been classified as a group III craniofacial pain of musculoskeletal origin.[7] A diagnosis of this syndrome may be made after dental disease has been excluded by history, physical examination, and appropriate diagnostic tests of the teeth.

The individual with a TM disorder may complain of various kinds of pain. They may speak of pain on chewing, pain when opening the mouth wide, pain of the ears, pain that incapacitates or prevents them from functioning with daily activities, sleeping pain, or headache pain.

Typically, TM disorders are characterized by pain just in front of the ear or preauricular area. The pain is usually aggravated by functional jaw movements. If the pain arises from the joint, it is termed *arthralgia*. The pain may originate from the muscles (*myalgia*) or from a nerve (*neuralgia*). Some orofacial pains arise from vascular sources. Although orofacial pain may result from neoplasia, few complaints arise from this morbid condition. If the condition does not fit these descriptions, it is defined as *atypical facial pain*.

Word Descriptors

Word descriptors are terms used by patients to express the kinds of pain they are experiencing (Table 3-3). The intensity of TM pain generally has been referred to by patient self-report as dull and aching. The quality has been characterized as cramping, locking, and penetrating.[8–11] Among 164 patients with myofascial pain of the head and neck, the most commonly expressed words were pressure (48%), dull (27%), throbbing (26%), sharp (18%), burning (16%), and heavy (14%).[12] This list of descriptors does not fully embrace the gamut of words used by sufferers to describe TM pain. Research has shown a relation between certain symptoms and the kind of words chosen by the TMD sufferer.[13]

Some word descriptors are clinically significant. Although there is some overlap in selection by patients, most words have diagnostic importance. An individual with joint noise or joint locking is annoyed by the persistence of these complaints. Pain on chewing is annoying, but movement of the joints causes pain. Pain from headache or face-ache throbs or feels sharp. Knowledge of these associations is vital in communicating with patients.

The difficulty in identifying the source of the pain is complicated by patterns of referred pain. The individual with *referred pain* feels the pain at one anatomic site, such as the neck, ear, or shoulder, rather than at the site of the pathology (eg, the joint). An often overlooked pattern is the referral of pain of the masticatory muscles surrounding the joints to the teeth.

Table 3-3

Words Chosen with Symptoms

Throbbing	Face-ache, headache
Pulsing	
Sharp	Headache
Intense	
Hurting	
Sharp	Earache
	Pain on chewing
	Pain on opening the mouth wide
Aching	Pain on chewing
Shooting	
Annoying	
Tightness	Pain on opening the mouth wide
Nauseating	
Shooting	Jaw stiffness, soreness, tiredness
Tender	Jaw soreness
Tiring	
Exhausting	
Nagging	Joint noise
Cramping	
Annoying	
Annoying	Joint locking
Radiating	
Tiring	

Data from Bush FM, Chinchilli VM, Martelli MF. Pain perception and assessment among patients with temporomandibular (TM) disorders. Pain 1087; 4(suppl): 124. Abstract 236.

Numeric Index of Pain

The present level of any pain can be ascertained from a numeric rating index as follows: 1, mild; 2, discomforting; 3, distressing; 4, horrible; and 5, excruciating.[14] In contrast to other known painful syndromes, such as back and cancer pain, the intensity of TM pain has proved low. Among 85 TM patients admitted to a TMJ–Orofacial Pain Center, the pain was rated as mild at low intensity, discomforting at usual intensity, and distressing at high intensity.[15]

Frequency of Pain

The frequency of TM pain as reported by many sufferers varies greatly. In 85 TMD patients examined at a TMJ–Facial Pain Center, 42.5% rated their pain as frequent, 42.5% as constant, and 15% as occasional.[15] These variable findings contribute to the problems that practitioners experience in diagnosing and treating these individuals.

Severity of Pain

In a study that attempted to estimate the severity of TM pain, severity was graded according to six categories (Table 3-4).[16] From this information, approximately two thirds of patients with TMD complaints could be expected to suffer from recurrent

Table 3-4
Pain Grading

Grade	Patients (%)
0—no pain	2.1
1—nonrecurrent pain	9.1
2—recurrent pain	45.0
3—severe, persistent pain, no limitation on activity	21.1
4—persistent pain, limitation on activity 1–6 days	7.0
5—severe, persistent pain, limitation greater than 6 days	15.7

Data from Von Korff M, Dworkin SF, Le Resche L. Graded chronic pain status: an epidemiologic evaluation. Pain 1990;40:279.

or severe, persistent pain which would not limit their activities. Nearly 16% would suffer a severe, persistent pain and would require considerable limitation of activities.

Significance: From a clinical standpoint, pain is difficult to assess in the suffering individual. There are few reliable ways to measure pain. What pain means to the patient may not mean the same to the doctor and vice versa. During an interview of the patient, the clinician must be aware that the patient may be talking about pain of the entire body and not specifically about the orofacial pain. This difference in interpretation can significantly influence diagnosis and treatment outcome.

Muscular Pain

The primary source of most TM complaints is masticatory muscle. The exact cause of pain is enigmatic. Patients may complain of fatigue, tension, aching (myalgia), discomfort, soreness, tenderness, or cramping in these jaw muscles. Like other skeletal muscle, masticatory muscle is subject to strains and sprains. *Strain* implies overstretching of tissue. *Sprain* involves rupture of fibers, but continuity of the muscle remains intact. Some strains and sprains are acute; others become chronic. Most acute complaints are caused by single injuries, whereas chronic problems develop after repetitive or overuse activities.

For purpose of comparison, information about patients with TMD is interspersed with reviews of the present research about another musculoskeletal syndrome, so-called fibromyalgia, to extend the reader's knowledge on the extant literature. Fibromyalgia is a common rheumatologic syndrome.[17] It manifests as chronic, diffuse musculoskeletal aching and soreness. The sufferer complains of fatigue and morning stiffness among other problems, many of which are identical to the complaints of patients with TMD. If these complaints reflect muscle pain and the pain reflects pathology, one would expect to find muscular abnormalities in both TMD and fibromyalgia patients.

Muscular Fatigue

Fatigue is defined as an inability to produce a preexisting level of tension, or velocity of contraction, after either static or dynamic activities. This subjective perception represents an increased exertion of physical effort.[18] The sensation is one of localized slight discomfort and weakness. Although patients with either overuse or pain of the jaws may complain of fatigue, on an average, masticatory muscle fibers exhibit low fatigability (they do not tire easily).

Overuse Complaints

The experience of muscle pain within 1 or 2 days of unaccustomed or excessive exertion is a classic phenomenon. Localized tenderness and increased fatigability follow. Initially, fatigue results from muscles that contract concentrically. Concentric contractions shorten muscle fibers. Repetitive clenching of the teeth causes facial discomfort from this kind of isometric contraction. Among healthy adults, an average pain threshold is reached within 51 seconds of voluntary clenching.[19] Swift recovery occurs after clenching: 80% of the pain decreases within 1 minute.[20] Thus, static activities such as clenching give rise initially to fatigue and then to pain.

Grinding of the teeth is a dynamic activity that causes eccentric changes involving the lengthening of muscle fibers. After 20 minutes of working the jaw muscles by bruxing, there is gradual onset of pain.[19] The pain evolves from negative work that has not been equalized by positive work. Usually, spontaneous pain develops within 8 hours; pain is detectable by digital palpation in approximately 20 hours. Weak to moderate deep pain may last for 2 or 3 days.

Loss of Muscle Strength

The effect of fatigue on the induction of pain has been demonstrated after eccentric contractions of the elbow flexor muscles.[21] Strength was reduced 30% by exercise of muscles at long length and by 10% at short length. Force fell 65% at long length and 30% at short length. The level of pain was worse at long length than short length, and the authors concluded that the development of pain depended on length.

Patients with fibromyalgia had a 60% reduction in isometric and isokinetic muscle strength compared with healthy control persons.[22] Fatigue was figured a significant factor in this loss.[23]

Muscular Tension

Tension is defined as a tightening from prolonged contraction of muscle fibers. There is no motor unit activity associated with tension. Historically, hyperactivity leading to increased tension (hypertonicity) has been hypothesized as one source of jaw pain, although data supporting this hypothesis are meager.[24] Extensive discussion on hyperactivity as the cause of muscle pain is included in Chapter 4.

Based on the hypothesis that hyperactivity leads to tension, electromyography (EMG) is a method to assess changes in muscular activity. Studies have revealed no differences that relate pain with hyperactivity. EMG patterns differed little between patients with fibromyalgia and those with no symptoms.[25] Tonic and phasic EMG muscle tension of patients with fibromyalgia did not prove different from muscular tension of matched asymptomatic control patients.[23] Finally, muscle tension was ruled out as a prominent factor in fibromyalgia.[26] Compared with the EMG patterns of 9 healthy control patients, the EMG patterns of painful muscles of 22 women diagnosed with fibromyalgia showed only minor changes.

Muscular Tenderness and Soreness

Tenderness of the masticatory muscles is a common finding among patients with TMD. Generally, tenderness on palpation signifies muscle soreness. Soreness is a localized pain that can be induced by repeated strain or excessive movements of the muscles. It implies damaged muscle fibers.[19] The damage is not related to metabolic energy demands but has been attributed to the mechanic forces of eccentric contractions.

Muscle Architecture

Microtrauma characterizes the muscle tissue of fibromyalgia patients. Microscopic examination of muscle reveals inflammatory changes, including increased tissue fluids, fat, and numbers of mast cells; swollen mitochondria; and degenerated or compressed muscle filaments.[27–31]

The same kind of muscle fiber dissolution and extensive inflammation has been found in rat masseter muscle following repetitive lengthening contractions.[32] The authors of this study speculated that the repetitive lengthening contractions may be the mechanism for pain in human masticatory muscle.

Tenderness on Palpation

Lateral joint soreness has been claimed to be of muscular origin.[33] Evidence confirmed that patients with TMD decrease their use of tender muscles because of the pain. EMG recordings of several types of jaw movements showed that 43 patients with temporalis pain used the anterior fibers with less frequency and less intensity than did 17 control subjects.[34] Furthermore, clenching of the teeth significantly related to the degree of muscular tenderness. During maximal clenching, EMG activity of masseter muscle decreased as the severity of tenderness increased.[35] This reduction in activity indicated that the patients avoided jaw closure as tenderness of the masseter increased.

Muscle soreness proved difficult to induce in healthy men after repeated sustained isometric protrusion.[36] Neither jaw pain nor tenderness was found in the masseter and temporalis muscles of eight normal men who performed a series of protrusive exercises. The authors argued that soreness would result if previous underlying pathophysiologic changes occurred in the muscle.

Myofascial Pain

Myofascial pain is the hallmark of many generalized muscle pain syndromes. Hyperactivity leading to muscle spasm has long been considered important in the genesis of TM myofascial pain,[37] but no true spasms have been found. Muscle spindle sensitivity has been demonstrated to increase,[38] which suggests failure in the large contractile properties of the muscle. No pain has been related to this enhanced sensitivity.

The pain has been characterized as continuous, and usually dull, in one or more muscles. The regional aching seems to be associated with localized tenderness of firm bands of muscle and tendon termed *trigger points*. They are nodes of degenerated tissue. Usually dormant, they may become tender.

The belief that trigger points cause significant pain is controversial. Some clinicians believe that trigger points develop when the fibers are not stretched through the normal range of motion.[39] This shortening can result from lack of use, mechanical overload, misuse, or repeated minor injury. Any excessive strain or overuse may contribute to already shortened fibers and lead to pain. The pain is faithful at a referred site on palpation of a point.[40]

Trigger points have been found both in masticatory muscles and muscles of the neck and shoulders. Clinical judgments made by various health practitioners indicate that people with TM pain also have a high prevalence of neck and shoulder pain. Likewise, many individuals with neck and shoulder pain have a high prevalence of TM pain. The commonality of trigger points in these different anatomic locations suggests that muscle is the primary source of pain.

Each set of masticatory muscle tissue has its own referral pattern of pain.[41] In the illustrations that follow, trigger points are marked by X, " essential" referred areas of pain are shown in black, and "spillover" areas are stippled (Figs. 3-1 through 3-10). Pain does not occur in all patients with spillover areas. The muscle groups are masseter, temporalis, lateral pterygoid, and medial pterygoid. Other muscle groups with pain referral to or near the orofacial region are illustrated. These include the sternocleidomastoid, trapezius, occipitofrontalis, suboccipitalis, splenius capitis, splenius cervicis, medial posterior cervical muscles (semispinalis cervicis and semispinalis capitis).

Myositis

Myositis (myofibrositis) is defined as an inflammation or general change in consistency of muscle and attached connective tissue.[38] No focal muscle spasms occur. Lesions are present along the borders of muscle fasciae and may result from rupture of collagen fibers. Damage occurs in the contractile fibers. Usually, acute pain is accompanied by some localized swelling. Tenderness may occur over the entire region of the muscle.

Myositis of the TMJ region must be differentiated from fibromyalgia or systemic myofibrositic pain. It is uncommon among TMD sufferers.

Myospasm and Trismus

Spasm implies cramping, a sudden involuntary contraction of the muscle. *Trismus* is a motor disturbance of the trigeminal nerve. Acute pain signifies spasm, a complication of trismus that is usually caused by overstretching or overuse. This painful

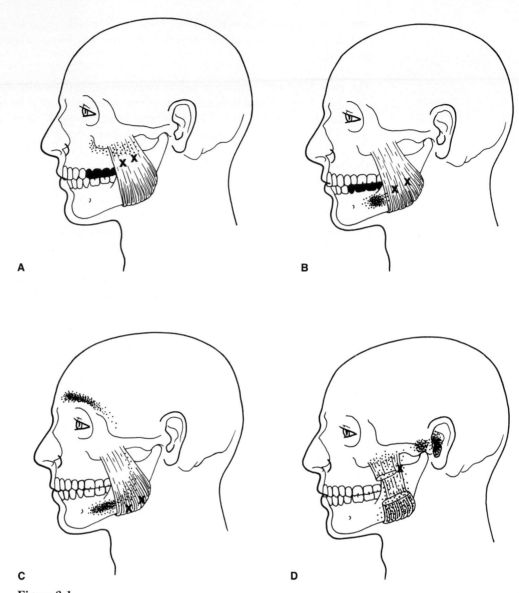

Figure 3-1.
*Pain reference patterns for masseter muscle: (**A**) superficial layer-upper, (**B**) mid-belly, (**C**) lower, and (**D**) deep. Trigger points are marked X.*

state may prevent the affected individual from opening the mouth, and there may be marked limited range of mandibular motion. Fasciculation is identified by continuous muscular contraction. Palpation reveals a firm, linear band within the affected muscle.

Speculation is that microspasms cause masticatory muscle pain. Groups of fibers can spasm without immobilizing the entire muscle.[42] Intermittent pain can be relieved by gentle stretching. Spasm is too painful to be considered a major cause of chronic jaw pain.

(text continues on p. 49)

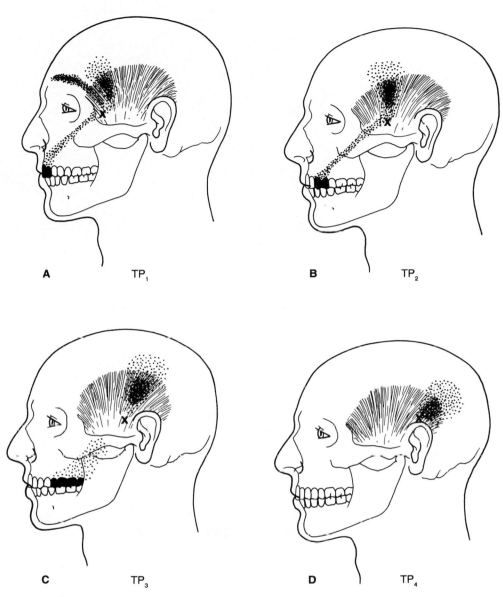

A TP₁ **B** TP₂

C TP₃ **D** TP₄

Figure 3-2.
*Pain reference patterns for temporalis muscle: (**A**) anterior fiber trigger point, TP₁;*
*(**B**, **C**) middle, TP₂ and TP₃; and (**D**) posterior, TP₄.*

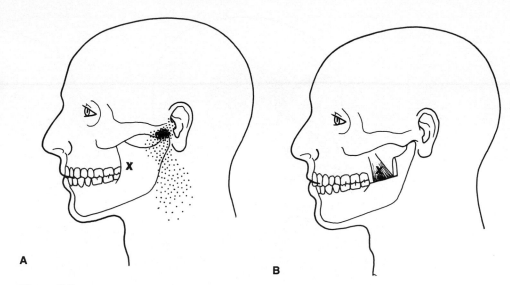

Figure 3-3.
*Pain reference pattern for medial pterygoid. Trigger points are shown before (**A**) and after (**B**) removal of coronoid process.*

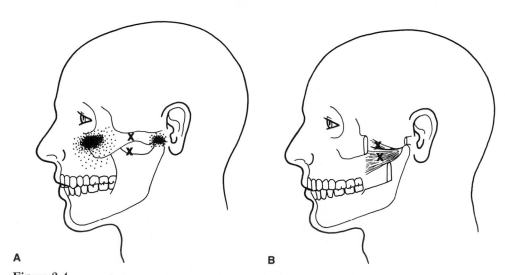

Figure 3-4.
*Pain reference pattern for lateral pterygoid. Trigger points are shown in (**A**) and after removal of superficial masseter (**B**).*

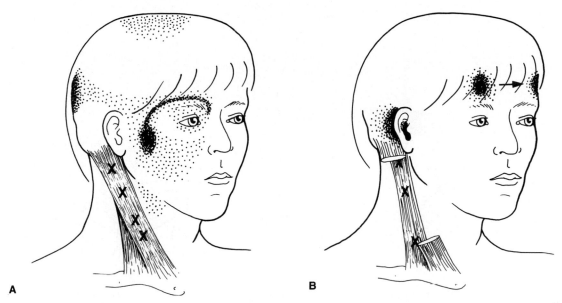

Figure 3-5.
*Pain reference pattern for right sternocleidomastoid, sternal division (**A**) and clavicular division (**B**).*

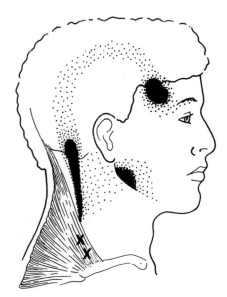

Figure 3-6.
Pain reference pattern in the upper right trapezius.

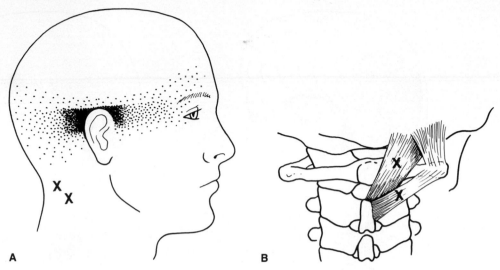

Figure 3-7.
*Pain reference pattern for the right suboccipitalis. (**A**) trigger points, (**B**) location of trigger points in obliquus capitis inferior and rectus capitis posterior major.*

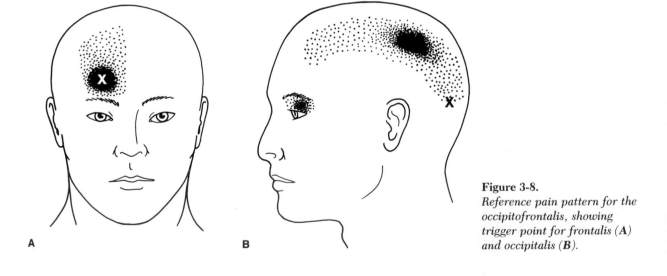

Figure 3-8.
*Reference pain pattern for the occipitofrontalis, showing trigger point for frontalis (**A**) and occipitalis (**B**).*

A

B

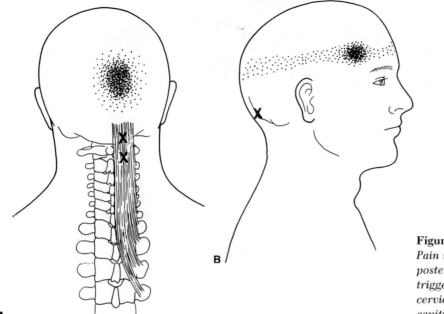

Figure 3-9.
Pain reference pattern for the medial posterior cervical muscles, showing trigger point for the semispinalis cervicis (A) and for the semispinalis capitis (B).

Contracture

Contracture is a chronic, usually painless, resistance to stretch that results from scarring or fibrosis. There is unyielding firmness on passive stretching. The limited range of motion is not associated with a joint disorder.

Up to 80% of patients with fibromyalgia have stiffness.[25] The content of energy-rich phosphates is reduced in painful muscles, suggesting that this form of contracture results from an energy crisis.[26]

Splinting

Splinting implies rigidity that is protective in nature. The patient guards against mandibular movement. Muscles may be tender on palpation. There is no evidence that prolonged splinting results in spasm.

Hypertrophy

Hypertrophy is a generalized abnormal enlargement of muscle tissue. Usually, no pain is involved. The condition is typically unilateral after persistent clenching. There may be a dull aching after extensive bruxing, and range of mandibular motion may be limited.

Significance: Muscle pain seems to account for most face and neck complaints of TMD sufferers. The presence of widespread tenderness on palpation suggests myofascial pain of the masticatory muscles. This pain results from specific tender areas

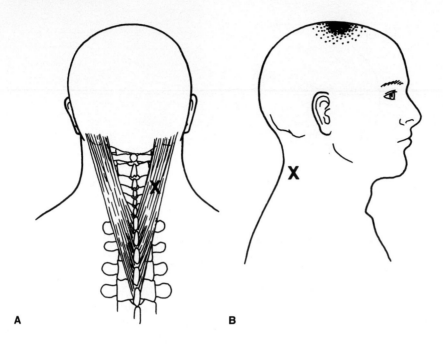

A   B

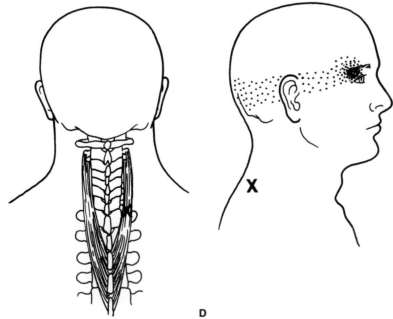

C   D

Figure 3-10.
*Pain reference pattern for the splenius muscles, showing trigger points in the splenius capitis (**A**, **B**) and in the splenius cervicis (**C**, **D**).*

termed *active* trigger points of pain referral. Often, those trigger points of the head and neck regions are a manifestation of myofascial syndrome of somatic origin. The astute clinician must master the technique of muscle palpation for proper diagnosis. Details of palpation are covered in Chapter 7. Appropriate identification of trigger points enhances treatment.

Joint Pain

The source of joint pain is difficult to establish. Conclusions drawn from the literature indicate that comments about the source of pain would be inferential. Most sensations from joint structures have been considered proprioceptive in nature. The fibrous tissue covering the mandibular condyle, the articular eminence, and the large central area of the disk lacks nerves and blood vessels. Few nerves have been found in the synovial tissues.

Branches of the trigeminal nerve supply the joint. The mandibular nerve branches into the auriculotemporal and masseteric nerves. Finer branches innervate the collateral diskal ligaments that attach the disk to the medial and lateral poles of the condyle, the retrodiskal tissue interposed between the disk and posterior wall of the capsule, and the capsule of the joint.

Most receptors are found in the lateral and posterior parts of the joint. Terminations have been found to be of three types:

1. Free nerve endings occur in ligaments, the joint capsule, and, to some extent, the synovial membrane.[43] Numerous sensory endings are pain-sensitive to tissue injury and are common near the junction of the capsule and periosteum;
2. Nonencapsulated endings are of the Rufini type and occur mainly in the capsule, primarily in regions that are compressed or otherwise deformed during movement.[44–46] These structures are designated *Golgi tendon organs* when located within ligaments and *Rufini-type endings* when present in the capsule. They are sensitive to stretch induced by movement or tension or by increase of intra-articular pressure.[47]
3. Encapsulated receptors are Pacinian-like corpuscles that are mostly involved in control of reflexes.

The actions of receptors are complex. Recordings of individual nerve fibers supplying the joint indicate two different kinds of receptors are involved with jaw movement. One type fires rapidly when the condylar head is rotated and provides information about mandibular movement. The other kind is slow adapting and fires when the condylar head is at a specific position.[48] The nociception probably derives primarily from contact or irritation of the free nerve endings.

Arthralgia may arise from several pain-sensitive structures. An early suggestion was that arthralgia resulted from stretching of the capsule during translation of the mandible.[49] Stretching of the capsule was not considered as important as condylar force directed against the synovial structures behind the disk.[50] Tearing of the fibers behind the disk from the condyle neck and poles has been hypothesized.[51] Maldirected condylar force could produce joint pain in cases of anterior disk displacement.[52] This primary source of pain could lead to protective muscle splinting.

Pain has been associated with inflammatory aspects of arthropathy. Synovitis and joint effusion frequently accompany derangement of the disk.[53] Pain referred to the face is a frequently observed symptom.

Significance: Although proof is lacking, irritation of free nerve endings is the likely cause of minor episodes of joint pain. Tenderness and soreness probably relate to stretching of tendinous attachments and localized muscle changes. Trauma to the joint may result in pain caused by swelling and effusion.

Arthritic Pain

Osteoarthrosis

Bony changes of the joint identify *osteoarthrosis,* a noninflammatory condition with neither pain nor associated tenderness. A hallmark is crepitus on mandibular movement.

Osteoarthritis

Osteoarthritis is often referred to as degenerative joint disease. It is a disease is of both articular cartilage and subchondral bone.[54] The joint lesion is primarily noninflammatory, characterized by deterioration of articular cartilage and remodeling of underlying bone.[55,56] Erosion results from pitting and fissuring of the cartilage. This destruction progresses to spiculation of subchondral bone. The bone collapses then undergoes sclerosis, with concomitant clinical disability of the joint. Advanced joint disease may lead to atrophy of associated muscles.

The pain of osteoarthritis has been hypothesized as arising from several sources. It has been attributed to synovitis, secondary to the original degeneration.[57,58] Joint soreness correlates with cases of synovitis.[59] Effusion results in swelling of surrounding tissues.[58] Irritation of the attachments, capsule, and possibly the superficial bone has been suggested as another cause.[56]

TMJ osteoarthritis may occur simultaneously with internal derangement of the disk[56] or may follow it.[60] Different stages of internal derangement with varying degrees of pain have been identified[61]: a few episodes of pain occur in the early stage; multiple episodes characterize an intermediate stage, followed by chronic, variable episodes in the late stage.

Most of the degeneration occurs in the lateral part of the joint. Morphologic study of human TMJs at autopsy showed that 56% of 102 individuals had some form of articular remodelling or arthritic lesions.[62] Twenty-two were judged with major arthritic changes, of which 4 involved all joint parts and 18 had local changes. Of the 18, 13 occurred laterally, 5 centrally, and none medially.

The clinical features of osteoarthritis are similar to those of other forms of joint dysfunction.[63,64] Typically, pain and crepitation occur during mandibular movement. The joint and surrounding masticatory muscles become tender to palpation.[65] Most people experience restriction of the mandible. Usually, crepitation remains after the

Table 3-5
Clinical Signs and Symptoms in 55 Patients With
Chronic Pain or Impairment of the TM Joints

Finding	Number Present
Limited opening	35
Crepitation	31
Joint soreness (lateral)	31
Limited protrusion	28
Muscle soreness	24
Reciprocal clicking	21
Reduced occlusal support	14
Joint soreness (lateral and posterior)	12

Modified from Holmlund A, Hellsing G, Axelsson S. The
temporomandibular joint: a comparison of clinical and arthroscopic findings.
J. Prosth Dent 1989; 62:61.

other symptoms disappear. It is one dominant clinical finding that can be expected
at follow-up examinations,[63,66] but it alone cannot be used as the determining clinical
feature of TMJ arthritis. Other bilateral symptoms are common with both[59,67] (Tables
3-5 and 3-6).

A long-term study of 119 patients observed for up to 10.5 years and examined for
pathology of the TMJs revealed well defined stages of degeneration in osteoarthritis[63]
(Table 3-7). The initial stage is characterized by mild symptoms. The intermediate
stage follows with mandibular pain at rest and during lateral and opening movements, and restriction of movement of the mandible. Patients generally seek care at
this stage. Individuals in the terminal stage may present with crepitation, slightly
reduced mandibular movement, and joint tenderness on palpation. As the symptoms
of arthropathy diminish, joint clicking may occur on the contralateral side.

Table 3-6
TM Findings in Patients With Rheumatoid Arthritis, Osteoarthritis, and Without
Joint Problems*

	Rheumatoid Arthritis (%)	Osteoarthritis (%)	Without Joint Problems (%)
Deviation of mandible	56	75	29
Decreased translation	52	50	2
Crepitus	76	76	19
Clicking	18	25	38
Locking	5	29	0
Painful movements	48	64	2
Lateral joint tenderness	40	40	4
Posterior joint tenderness	11	18	4
Masticatory muscle tenderness	81	93	21

Modified from Tegelberg A. Temporomandibular joint involvement in rheumatoid arthritis. A clinical study. Swed
Dent J Suppl 1987; 49:1.
*128 patients had rheumatoid arthritis, 28 patients had osteoarthritis, and 52 had no joint problems.

Table 3-7
Progressive Changes in Signs and Symptoms of the
TM Joints

Phase	Stage
1. Clicking	Initial
2. Periodic locking	Initial
3. Joint pain at rest	Intermediate
4. Joint pain on function	Intermediate
5. Residual symptoms other than pain	Final
6. Absence of symptoms	Final

Modified from Rasmussen OC. Clinical findings during the course of
temporomandibular arthropathy. Scand J Dent Res 1981; 89:283.

Arthritic lesions develop slowly over many years without any symptoms. Sometimes, they cause acute painful inflammation. Acute symptoms last about 9 months then gradually subside[66]; patients usually require treatment during these periods. Some severe symptoms may continue for 1 to 3 years. Study of 11 patients examined at a follow-up of 7 years showed 6 had no symptoms, 3 had slight symptoms, and 2 had moderate symptoms.[64]

In another study, TM symptoms appeared less than 1 year after general joint complaints in 55% of a group of patients with osteoarthritis.[67] They lasted for more than 2 years in 96% of these patients, compared with 12% for control patients. Other clinical findings are summarized in Table 3-6.

Some of these findings have been challenged by different groups of investigators.[68,69] These clinicians concluded that the evidence for clicking leading to osteoarthritis is too meager to make definitive statements. This conclusion is supported by the findings in two other studies. Clicking was more common in individuals lacking complex joint problems than in patients with osteoarthritis or rheumatoid arthritis[67] (see Table 3-6). Reciprocal clicking was found in joints with slight or no evidence of osteoarthritis.[59]

Rheumatoid Arthritis

After long-term study of patients with rheumatoid arthritis, the results showed 1 in 3 experienced TM symptoms and 1 in 10 developed TM symptoms.[67] TM symptoms appeared less than 1 year after general joint complaints in 38% of this group. The symptoms lasted for more than 2 years in 55%, compared with 12% for the control patients.

Skin surface temperature over the affected joint and the adjacent masseter muscle was low in patients with rheumatoid arthritis.[67] It was lower in the joint areas of these patients than in the joints of healthy patients, but higher than in patients with internal derangement. The low temperature in the masseter has been attributed to disuse atrophy and decreased muscular blood flow.

Comparison of 40 juveniles with rheumatoid arthritis matched by age and sex with 40 asymptomatic individuals showed few differences in symptoms reported by questionnaire.[70] Compared with control patients, arthritic patients more often experienced symptoms and crepitation in the cheek. Clinical examination revealed that the arthritic patients had more signs considered to be dysfunctional, including reduced maximum mouth opening. Crepitation occurred only in the arthritic patients (total of 6). Tenderness on palpation was more common in the arthritic patients for the posterior aspect of the TMJs, temporalis tendon, and lateral pterygoid areas. No differences were found for eight other areas palpated.

Various textbooks mention anterior open bite as a classic sign of rheumatoid arthritis. A recent review of the literature on occlusion and TMD problems concluded that skeletal anterior open bite was strongly associated with osteoarthritic patients and was rare in other populations.[71] Approximately 25% of 49 patients with TMJ arthrosis had anterior open bite.[72] Analysis conducted on juveniles with rheumatoid arthritis matched against nonarthritic control patients showed a significant difference only for those with class II (postnormal) occlusion.[70] Thirty-three percent of the arthritic group had occlusal problems compared with 8% of the control group. One cannot be too excited about this difference since the sample size was small. Also, for neutral occlusion, 93% of the control group had similar problems compared with 68% of the group with arthritis. Furthermore, just 7% to 11% of the 123 affected patients had open bites.[67] Thus, although open bite may occur frequently in arthritic populations, it should not be considered a main diagnostic feature. Adaptive changes may occur in some individuals and prevent the open bite.

Significance: Pain may arise from more than one area of the joint. Inflammation must be present, most likely synovitis. Joint soreness may represent synovitis or capsulitis, which are difficult to differentiate. The presence of crepitation signifies potential joint pathosis and correlates with advanced osteoarthrosis. The lateral surface of the joint degenerates most frequently. Radiographic, arthroscopic, or magnetic resonance analysis is required to establish the extent of degeneration.

Neurogenous Pain

The sensation of pain is perceived in the brain. Receptors in the body transmit impulses along nerve fibers to the spinal cord and then to the brain. Neurogenous pain usually occurs along the course of the involved cranial nerve.

Nociceptive Afferent Pathway

The nociceptive afferent pathway forms a third type of conduction system in the body. Sympathetic and parasympathetic systems form the basis for the fight-or-flight mechanisms. When appropriately stimulated, nociceptive fibers can transmit pain or cause a mitigation of pain.

Three different types of nerve fibers detect pain and other sensations; they are designated C, α-β, and α-δ. The thin C fibers form a network under the skin and transmit impulses slowly. The thick α-β fibers are few in number but transmit impulses quickly. α-δ Fibers are relatively thin and transmit impulses more quickly than C fibers but more slowly than α-β fibers.

C fibers carry pain to the spinal cord. Some α-δ fibers can carry pain and act in much the same way as C fibers. C fibers are capable of regeneration; α fibers are not. In a damaged area, impulses are transmitted through C and α-β fibers. α-β Fibers carry nonpainful sensations and block the painful signals of C fibers.

Spinal Gating System

This fibrous network participates in the operation of the "gate control system."[73,74] A specific area of the spinal column, the substantia gelatinosa of the dorsal horns, functions as the gate control system. This area modulates pain by influencing the afferent patterns. The effect of α-β fibers is to close the gate, and the effect of C fibers is to open the gate.

A simplified version demonstrates this system. When the mandible is abruptly displaced, the patient may feel a sharp sensation in the joint. This sensation travels quickly through the α-β fibers to the brain. A negative feedback mechanism is activated in the brain that reduces the original sensation. Shortly afterward, a second slow pain travels through the C fibers to the brain. Transmission by C fibers activates a positive feedback mechanism that exaggerates this slow pain effect. Now, the patient recognizes the pain as a dull ache.

The gate control system may be preset or reset any number of times. Specific neurons of the dorsal horn, so-called transmission cells, form the action system. Once triggered, this system elicits both conscious perception and physical reaction to the pain. Both pain perception and reaction act together to create suffering in the individual. Continued suffering becomes experience and subject to marked changes in reaction.

Significance: The gate control system may be modified by therapeutic modalities. Nerve blocking by local anesthesia is one method of influencing transmission of pain. Another method is transelectrical nerve stimulation (TENS). With TENS, an electric current of low intensity stimulates both large and small fibers. Activation of large - fibers closes the gate to pain transmission by small C fibers. Also, small fiber input, stimulated by the electrical current, activates the inhibitory areas of the brain and minimizes pain transmission.

Characteristics of Neurogenous Pain

Neurogenous pain is caused by structural abnormalities of nerves that innervate affected areas. Pain can arise without nociception.[75–77] The quality of pain is typically described as stimulating, bright, and burning. An abnormal sensation may occur along the nerve pathway. The patient usually can locate the pain, but the perceived area may not be the source. A pattern of referred pain may be absent. The severity of pain is almost always more intense than the degree of stimulation.

Peripheral and central mechanisms may be involved.[78,79] Peripherally, nociceptive neurons from primary afferent fibers may become hyperactive and elicit pain. Centrally, there may be less central inhibition or increased activity of the sympathetic efferent fibers.[75,77] Neurogenous pain can be classified into neuropathic and deafferentation categories.[76]

Neuropathy

Neuropathic pain is caused by a functional abnormality within a peripheral nerve. It can be divided into paroxysmal neuralgia, neuritic neuralgia, and traumatic neuroma pain. The last can also be classified as deafferentation pain.

Paroxysmal Neuralgia

Paroxysmal neuralgia represents a distinctive, severe, paroxysmal head pain that seems to arise from sudden episodic, intrinsic, and excessive discharges from a specific nerve.[80] The quality of pain is described as electric-like, jabbing, burning, or stabbing. Unilateral pain travels along the distribution of the nerve. Two examples of the orofacial region are trigeminal neuralgia and glossopharyngeal neuralgia.

Trigeminal Neuralgia

Trigeminal neuralgia (tic douloureux) is unilateral pain that involves the trigeminal (V) nerve. The highest frequency occurs in the mandibular division. Ten of 18 patients had pain limited to the V_3 branch, 3 each to the V_2 and V_1-V_2 branches, and 1 each to the V_1 and V_2-V_3 branches[81] (Table 3-8). A combination of peripheral and central factors seems to be involved.[82] The International Association for the Study of

Table 3-8
Pretrigeminal Symptoms in 18 Patients With Trigeminal Neuralgia

Dermatome of Nerve V (No.)	Pain Complaint		Gender	Age (years)
	Description	*Duration*		
V_1 (1)	Burning	9 mo	F	43
V_2 (3)	Toothache	3 mo	F	25
	Toothache	12 y	F	34
	Toothache	3 mo	F	55
V_3 (10)	Toothache	6 mo	F	68
	Toothache	6 mo	M	72
	Toothache	7 mo	F	52
	Dull	14 mo	M	76
	Dull	10 y	M	58
	Dull ache	2 y	M	67
	Deep ache	4 y	M	53
	Ache	4 y	F	42
	Ache	5 y	M	57
	Gnawing	2 y	F	67
V_1–V_2 (3)	Ache	3 mo	M	82
	Dull ache	3 y	F	65
	Tingling	16 mo	F	30
V_2–V_3 (1)	Dull–sharp	2 y	F	67

Modified from Fromm GH, Graff-Radford SB, Terrence CF, Sweet WH. Pretrigeminal neuralgia. Neurol 1990; 40:1493.

Pain recognizes two secondary forms of trigeminal neuralgia.[83] One arises from a lesion in the central nervous system and the other appears after facial trauma. Together, they account for less than 12% of all cases of this neuralgia.

The main features of trigeminal neuralgia are sharp, agonizing electric shock–like stabs of pain felt superficially in the skin or buccal mucosa.[83] Touching a trigger zone around the lips or jaw precipitates the brief, electric-like bursts. The pain lasts from seconds to minutes[84] and can be precipitated again after a refractory period of several seconds. Tic douloureux is probably one of the most intense of all acute pains.

Trigeminal neuralgia can be classified into symptomatic and idiopathic forms. The symptomatic form is experienced by most individuals who present to clinicians. A pathologic factor may be found, such as a tumor of the cerebellopontine angle, multiple sclerosis, or brain stem infarct.[79] The pain is probably caused by compression of the trigeminal nerve by surrounding arteries of the posterior fossa.[85,86] The idiopathic form has no known cause, but vascular, viral, neural, and dental origins have been suggested.[82] There may be demyelination of the nerve.

An argument has been made for dental involvement. Tooth extraction is the chief cause according to one investigator.[87] Presumably, extraction triggers ephaptic transmission (impulse conduction across nonsynaptic membranes) between the broken fibers for phasic pain of the tooth pulp and neighboring fibers of the epicritic (purposeful) and proprioceptive sensitivity. Remissions are explained by the theory of biorhythm neogenesis with the involvement of the antinociceptive and nociceptive subsystems. This proposition merits consideration, but it fails to explain affected individuals with no history of tooth removal. Also, few patients with typical trigeminal neuralgia present with toothache.

An early phase of the mature condition has been reported. This prodromal pain has been termed *pretrigeminal neuralgia*[81] (see Table 3-8). Just 6 of 18 patients with pretrigeminal neuralgia had tooth symptoms. This pain appears to be different than the typical neuralgia. Some patients reported a toothache or sinus-like pain that was triggered by chewing, talking, yawning, or drinking hot or cold liquids. They had little to no dental disease. The typical condition appeared a few days to 12 years later.

Glossopharyngeal Neuralgia

Glossopharyngeal neuralgia follows the distribution of the glossopharyngeal (IX) and vagus (X) nerves. A diffuse pain emanates from the pharynx and postmandibular areas.[76] It involves men and women equally, although there is a tendency for men more than women.[88] Most cases start after patient age 40.[79,88]

Swallowing, talking, and chewing are difficult and may trigger the pain. The trigger zone in the posterior pharynx causes pain to radiate toward the ear or angle of the mandible. The patient may sleep or swallow on the side opposite the trigger zone to avoid the discomfort.[88] A painful episode is not as severe as that with trigeminal neuralgia.

A serious complication of glossopharyngeal neuralgia is syncope, which may occur during an attack.[84] Probably, a spillover of impulses from the nerve to the dorsal motor nucleus of the vagus results in reflex bradycardia or asystole.

Neuritic Neuralgia

Neuritic pains result from inflammation of pain-conducting fibers.[76] Symptoms follow dermatome patterns. All painful effects are anatomically related to the specific peripheral nerve, and no patterns of pain referral occur. The main clinical feature of neuritic neuralgia is constant, dull, burning, or stimulating pain. The inflammation causes abnormal sensations along the distribution of the nerve.

The inferior and superior branches of the trigeminal nerve may be affected within the oral cavity.[70] Extraction of a mandibular third molar may traumatize the V_3 branch of the trigeminal nerve. An altered sensation or numbness may remain in the lip with neuritic-like pain in the teeth.[76] Pain of this sort following extraction of the maxillary teeth may be confused with a pain caused by inflammation in the maxillary sinus.

Postherpetic Neuralgia

Postherpetic neuralgia is a neuritic pain that affects the face and mouth. A history of varicella-zoster virus is diagnostic. The acute herpes zoster persists as a chronic burning pain. The pain precedes a rash (shingles) by a few days.[80] Dysesthesia along the involved dermatome confirms the diagnosis.

The ophthalmic branch of the trigeminal nerve may become involved. Lesions may form on the cornea. Vesicles occur on the tip of the nose. Postherpetic neuralgia generally follows shingles unless appropriate treatment is begun.

Geniculate Neuralgia

Geniculate neuralgia is extremely rare.[83] Infection of the geniculate ganglia of the facial nerve (VII) follows an attack of acute herpes zoster. Painful skin eruptions may occur within the auditory meatus and tympanic membrane. An ipsilateral palsy may result. A severe lancinating pain is felt deep within the auditory canal within several days to a week after eruption of vesicles.

Deafferentation Pain

Deafferentation pain is a neuropathic pain due to damage of a peripheral or central somatosensory pathway.[89] The sensory nerve supply to facial region may be partially or totally lost. The pain may arise after trauma as impulses are interrupted within afferent fibers. Highly emotional states tend to exacerbate the pain, which is severe and resistant to treatment.[79]

Within the orofacial region, deafferentation symptoms may be common after trauma.[76] Few elicit pain. Clinical features include burning pain and dysesthesia in the affected area. Occasionally, paresthesia or anesthesia develops after extraction of a posterior mandibular tooth. This altered feeling around the extraction site may not appear for several months. It may then spread to other orofacial fields. Trauma to the mandibular branch of nerve V must be suspected.

Deafferentation pain can be divided into traumatic neuromas, atypical odontalgia, and reflex sympathetic dystrophy.

Traumatic Neuroma Pain

Neuroma pain is rare in the orofacial area. Microscopy reveals an area of poorly integrated nervous tissue in the traumatized area, where successful healing has not occurred. Painful neuromas have been suspected for the trigeminal and facial nerves after surgery, fracture of the facial bone, or development of an area of scar tissue.[79] The pain of traumatic neuromas has been described as deep, aching, and burning. It can be induced by compression or stretching the neuroma and is relieved by local anesthesia.

Neuromas may be present at the surgical site of the TMJ, but no one has proved that they contribute significantly to the painful complaints associated with the joint.

Atypical Odontalgia

Atypical odontalgia has been characterized as toothache or tooth-site pain, with chronic occurrences of 4 months or longer, normal radiographs, and no observable cause.[90] This persistent pain occurs in apparently normal teeth and surrounding alveolar bone. Atypical odontalgia was formerly grouped under atypical facial pain or atypical neuralgia and included a host of unexplained disorders of the trigeminal–cervical 1 and 2 sensory fibers.[91]

The tooth pain appears to be a localized form of this syndrome.[92] It is marked by a dull, burning pain felt deep in the tooth that seems to radiate into soft tissues and bone[93] (Table 3-9). The pain may be throbbing of varying intensity but continuous in nature. It may move from tooth to tooth.[83] Unpredictable responses to percussion and pulp testing occur. Usually the teeth are hypersensitive to heat and cold. Radiographs of affected teeth and surrounding gingiva are within normal limits.

Most patients relate the onset of pain with minor tooth trauma or pulpal extirpation.[93] Unfortunately, the pain persists even after extraction of the offending tooth in nearly all cases. Most complaints involve premolars and molars. Maxillary teeth are affected more often than mandibular teeth (see Table 3-9).

A hypothesis has been suggested for the constancy of pain.[94] Apparently, the pain is sympathetically maintained from tonic activity in myelinated mechanoreceptor afferents. In some way, trauma serves to establish a high rate of firing in specific neurons and triggers the response in susceptible individuals.

Reflex Sympathetic Dystrophy

Reflex sympathetic dystrophy is sometimes referred to as causalgia (hot pain), but the International Association for the Study of Pain distinguishes these dystrophies

Table 3-9

Distribution of Atypical Odontalgia Pain in 37 Patients

Distribution	Percentage
Dermatome of nerve V	
V_2	68
V_3	19
V_2–V_3	13
Symmetry	
Unilateral	81
Bilateral	19
Tooth region	
Molar	41
Premolar	29
Canine	20
Anterior	10
Number of teeth	
1	38
2	24
3–5	24
6 or more	14

Modified from Solberg WK, Graff-Radford SB. Orodental considerations in facial pain. Sem Neurol 1988; 8:318.

from each other.[83] According to this classification, reflex sympathetic dystrophy does not involve a major nerve, whereas causalgia involves a nerve or its major branches.

The pain of reflex sympathetic dystrophy is continuous and has a burning quality. It usually follows mild trauma.[83] Some authors have attributed the dystrophy to deafferentation or nerve injury.[95] It is associated with sympathetic hyperactivity.

Areas of the limbs are affected first. The patient may experience severe hyperpathia on moving or touching the skin. The pain may spread to an entire extremity. Vasomotor changes may develop—first, vasodilation with increasing temperature and then later, vasoconstriction in the skin appendages. Disuse atrophy may follow.

Reflex sympathetic dystrophy has not been routinely associated with TMD. Degenerative TMJ disease was found in a 33-year-old woman who suffered from reflex sympathetic dystrophy. She presented with restricted mouth opening of 33 mm. Tomographic radiographs showed flattening of the left condyle.[95] A second case involved a 34-year-old woman with a maximum jaw opening of 33 mm.[96] She was diagnosed with otalgia, hypertonicity of the masticatory muscles, capsulitis, synovitis, and radiographic evidence of remodelling of the TMJs. These changes were considered secondary to the dystrophy.

A minor form may involve the mouth or face,[76,96] but few patients suffer from this complaint. It may follow minor oral surgical procedures or postsurgical infection. Facial edema and elevated skin temperature followed by cool, cyanotic skin and edema may terminate in atrophy.[78] Temporary reduction in pain may be achieved by stellate ganglion block.

Significance: Fortunately, orofacial neuralgias contribute little to most pain complaints associated with the TMJ apparatus. They are far less common than cervical neuralgias leading to frontal (cervicogenic-related) headache and facial pain.[97] This discomfort originates from the occipital area and ascends facially. An unpleasant dullness or cranial pressure results.

Vascular Pain

Vascular disease, either local or remote, probably is an uncommon cause of TMD pain. The degree to which vascular pain contributes to the genesis of TMD symptoms is unknown. Most of the information about head pain and face-ache has dealt with the involvement of vascular changes in headache. A few isolated cases have been reported in the literature involving hypertension, carotodynia, and cranial arteritis. These conditions are reviewed in Chapter 4.

Vascular pain has variable qualities. It has been the subject of various unconfirmed explanations for suffering in headache patients.[98] Moreover, the presence of TMJ symptoms in patients with concomitant headache has caused diagnostic confusion in both directions. TMD pain and the pain of acute and chronic tension headaches have the same system of origin. Each has been classified differently as subcategories of craniofacial pain of musculoskeletal origin.[83,99] Because the symptoms of patients with these separate pains share similar features, this review critiques the possible association between TM pain and pain of vascular origin.

Status of Fluid Exchanges in the Joint

Various areas of ischemia have been found in condyles subjected to trauma.[100] These condyles had undergone avascular necrosis, a sequela of an inflamed, deranged joint. Generally, pain is a consequence.

The disk is capable of large volumetric fluctuations.[101] Its posterior attachment seems to function as a device for rearrangement of blood, tissue fluid, and synovial fluid.

The superficial temporal and maxillary arteries supply the posterior attachment of the joint.[102] A profuse vasculature forms as branches of these vessels enter the intermediate zone.[101] Veins of this area are large and thin walled, and anastomose freely, forming a plexus mediolaterally. They dilate as the mandible opens. Vessels within the temporal and condylar parts of the posterior attachment are small and course randomly.

Theoretically, localized joint pain could arise as follows. Chronic overloading or frequent abrupt movement of the joint may compress the small arteries. Venous drainage slows, leading to swelling and pain. Alternately, excessive dilation of the veins might occur after sudden opening of the jaws. Arterial vasoconstriction could follow with the same consequences.

Alterations in the vascular layer of the synovial tissues may lead to pain. The synovium becomes expanded as the jaws open.[101] Folds (villi) lining the superior synovial cavity permit the disk to translate anteriorly as much as 2 cm. Similar folds line the inferior synovial cavity; they intermesh with diskal fibers, permitting rotation posteriorly as the condyle translates anteriorly. Speculation is that reduction in viscosity of synovial fluid could lead to frictional resistance within the capsule followed by joint noise, inflammation, and dysfunction.[103] Pain could develop in the associated masticatory muscles as a result of the dysfunctional joint.

Status of Vascular Changes and Some Head Pains

Headaches are viewed as a symptom, not a disease. They may originate from either peripheral or central mechanisms. Vascular structures about the head are pain sensitive, primarily the proximal cerebral arteries and the large veins and venous sinuses.[104] Apparently, noxious stimulation of sensory receptors and afferent fibers in vascular and perivascular tissue produces the pain.

Stretching or pulsation of arterial walls and muscle contraction have been suggested as affecting peripheral nerve receptors in these vessels, leading to head pain. Since the trigeminal nerve is the major innervation for these vessels[105] and the TMJs, overlap between TMD complaints and headache would be expected.

Migraine

The mechanism of the vascular headache, the so-called migraine, is not well understood.[98,106] Migraine has been considered a familial disorder with vasomotor instability of the extracranial and intracranial arteries, leading to excessive vasoreactivity.[107] Recent evidence shows that the symptoms of the migraine aura are caused by deficient cerebral blood flow,[99] although some argue that migraine may represent a neurologic disorder rather than a vascular disorder.[108] Little agreement exists about whether migraine is a single disorder or a set of related disorders. Hence, migraine has been used generically to include many chronic recurring forms of headache.

The throbbing, boring qualities of migraine have not been fully explained by arterial vasoconstriction and vasodilation.[109,110] The pain of migraine seems to arise from irritation of one or more branches of the carotid artery, with stimulation of nerve endings supplying the artery.

Supposedly, neurotransmitters released from nerve endings in the vessel walls lower the pain threshold, and pulsatile pain results. The release of vasoactive neurohumoral substances, including substance P, has been implicated in triggering the pain.[111] Platelet dysfunction has been suggested as another theory.[112]

Argument has been made for common migraine as a muscular disorder rather than a vascular disorder.[98] Other evidence seems to support this belief. Comparison of three subgroups of headache patients reveal many similarities of the common signs and symptoms. Among 19 TMD parameters studied in patients with migraines, tension headaches, or combination headaches, jaw pain on movement and tenderness of the masseter and temporalis muscles differed significantly.[113]

Tension-type Headache

Tension headache (scalp muscle contraction headache) has been designated craniofacial pain of musculoskeletal origin, but some opinions favor origin from either vascular or central nervous systems.[83] Continuous head pain in the form of nonpulsatile ache characterizes this myofascial disorder. Typically, the aching is symmetric and localized either frontally, frontotemporally, or occipitally. Patients may progress to photophobic, periorbital, or otologic complaints. Often, they are diagnosed as occipital neuralgia.[114] Apparently, fibers of the occipital nerve entrapped among tense cerviconuchal muscles cause the pain.

Cluster Headache

Review of the literature about other forms of vascular headache contributes little to understanding a relationship with TMD pain. Several hypotheses have been suggested for the pathophysiology of cluster headache, including vasomotor disturbances and changes in cerebral blood flow,[115] as well as altered levels of serotonin[116] and histamine.[117]

The pain of cluster headache may be stabbing, burning, or pulsating. It occurs unilaterally and almost always remains on the same side of the head.[118] The eye and frontotemporal region are the usual sites. Attacks may be accompanied by tearing, nasal congestion, rhinorrhea, and a partial Horner's syndrome.[114] Few of these symptoms fit TM pain.

Significance: There is the potential for pain of vascular origin to arise in the joint, probably after an inflammatory process. Attempts to differentiate joint complaints from pain referred from headache is difficult. Similar symptoms can be produced by various conditions. Diagnosis of headache is complex even for headache specialists. There are few reliable tests for diagnosis. It is doubtful whether treatment performed by dentists, such as occlusal adjustment, insertion of an occlusal guard, or rebuilding the occlusion, can solve the problems of headache.

Dental Pain

Toothache may be due to dentino-enamel defects, pulpitis, or periapical periodontitis and abscess. Most have throbbing, sharp, boring, and sickening qualities.[119] The boring and sickening qualities set toothache apart from other pains.

Compared with other types of pain, patients rated toothache less painful than postherpetic neuralgia and back pain and more painful than arthritic and menstrual pains (Table 3-10). Two characteristics make toothache rather dreadful: the sharp quality suggests that the intensity will last forever, and this sharpness causes considerable anxiety, which evokes the terror.[119]

Toothache From Dentino-Enamel Defects

Pain from dentino-enamel defects is short-lasting, diffuse, and evoked by local stimuli such as heat, cold, or air.[83] These stimuli cause movement of extracellular fluid

Table 3-10
Comparison of Toothache With Other Types of Pain

Pain	McGill Pain Rating*
Menstrual	17.5
Arthritis	18.8
Toothache	19.5
Postherpetic neuralgia	22.6
Phantom limb	25.0
Cancer	26.0
Back	26.3

After Melzack R. The language of pain. Dent Dimensions 1979; 3:2.
*The higher the rating, the greater the intensity.

that fills the dentinal tubules.[120] Dentinal pain occurs intermittently and lasts from seconds to minutes. Usually it is easy to identify the source of this pain either by radiograph or clinical examination. An exception may involve the so-called split-tooth syndrome. This pain may be sharp, lancinating, and with abrupt onset. Because there may be pulpal involvement, it may be poorly localized by both the patient and the dentist.

Toothache From Pulpitis

Pain caused by pulpitis may vary from mild to spontaneous if no external stimulus triggers it. Throbbing or burning may occur with moderate to severe intensity,[121] and bouts may last for minutes to hours. The tooth usually is not tender to percussion. Spontaneous pain confirms the diagnosis. If pulpitis is untreated, the pulp may die, with infection spreading into periapical tissues. Severe pain may result from acute periapical periodontitis.

Abscess causes the tooth to be tender to palpation, and biting on the tooth makes the pain worse. The abscess may track to the mucosal surface and drain. The pain may be sharp or dull with some throbbing and may last for hours or days. Pulpitis is identified by examination—radiologic, clinical, or both.

Toothache From Periodontal Abscess

Unlike a gingival abscess, which is confined to the marginal gingiva, the periodontal abscess involves the supporting periodontal structures. Periodontal pain is well localized by the patient.[122] Periodontal abscess can be differentiated from periapical abscess by the presence of a draining abscess on the lateral aspect rather than the apical part of the root. A radiolucent area along the lateral part of the root may be found in the early stages. A single lesion that can be probed from the gingival margin confirms the diagnosis.

Atypical Odontalgia

Atypical odontalgia is a form of toothache or tooth-site pain with no observable cause. Because the ache may persist even after the pulp of healthy teeth has been removed, this toothache is discussed in the section on neurogenous pain of deafferentation origin.

Significance: Most dental pains have observable causes. Peripheral stimuli evoke pathologic processes. The pain can be mitigated or eliminated by local anesthesia. Elimination of the pain leads to successful outcome. Some dental pains are obscured by the presence of simultaneous periapical and periodontal disease.

Psychogenic Pain

Many clinicians suspect a psychogenic component in the history in certain cases of TM pain. These conclusions usually are based on an absence of organic pathology following interview, clinical examination, and even special tests of the patient. The unanswered question in the minds of clinicians is, "Are these patients psychiatrically different from other non-pain patients that I treat, or is this a disorder of lesser behavior due to mental conflict?"

It is widely accepted that emotional processes play a central role in pain and that exposure to and manner of coping with stressful events contribute to the onset and exacerbation of a wide range of painful physical conditions, including TMD.[123,124] If the pain is chronic, one must determine whether the pain is of somatic delusion or if there is an underlying psychophysiologic disorder.

The pain of somatic delusion occurs in patients with profound psychiatric disturbances, such as psychotic depression or schizophrenia. (These are terms used in psychiatry to describe a conversion of mental experiences into bodily symptoms.) There is no evidence of structural disorder. Few patients with TM pain fall into this category.

Individuals with psychophysiologic disorders have psychological factors that engender physiologic changes. Often they may deny that any psychic factors are involved in their pain. Emotional stress may be a dominant factor. Structural disorders may not be obvious. Typically, these patients present as polysymptomatic with a diffuse pattern of complaints. The concept of "self" refers to a mental representation of what an individual thinks of him- or herself as a total person–a psychophysiologic total. Such images derive from experiences of emotions, sensations, and indirect perceptions of the bodily and mental self.[125]

The term *personality* refers to the predictable ways—attitudes or habits—in which an individual responds to life situations.[126] These ways evolve consciously and unconsciously and represent a compromise between a person's wishes and the need to restrict their expression. The chief function of personality is to maintain a stable relationship between the person and the surrounding environment.

A superb review of the literature that signaled the importance of psychological factors in TMD was published as part of the 1983 American Dental Association President's Conference on Temporomandibular Joint Disorders.[123] Psychological factors were considered under a number of different headings (Table 3-11). Based on information

---

Table 3-11
Psychological Characteristics in TMD

Psychological etiologic factors
    Personality and emotional characteristics
    Relationship between psychological stress and muscle tension
     pain
    Clinical observations
    Experimental studies
    Treatment outcome studies
Psychological characteristics of those seeking treatment
Psychological characteristics of unsuccessfully treated patients

---

After Rugh JD. Psychological factors in the etiology of masticatory pain and dysfunction. In Laskin DM et al (eds). The President's Conference on the Examination, Diagnosis and Management of Temporomandibular Disorders. Chicago: American Dental Association, 1983:85.

from that publication and review of the current literature, the present state of knowledge has been updated as discussed in the following sections.

Personality Traits of Pain Subjects

Differences between *personality* and *self* are vital for understanding that no single trait predisposes to TMD. Clinicians recognize many stereotypes of personality, which have been divided into normals, hypernormals, and psychoneurotics.[127] Normal persons are free of emotional problems, have a sense of humor, and relax easily. Hypernormal individuals are divisible into subgroups:

    Overly responsible—a person who feels responsible even for situations and events that are patently not his or her responsibility
    Career individual—a person with a high activity level who finds projects and is action oriented
    Explorer—a person who is driven to enhance himself or herself at the expense of others
    High approval motive—a person who carries the need for approval to extremes and who has an exaggerated fear of rejection
    Harridan—a person who rules by nagging, bullying, or cruelty.

The psychoneurotic is an individual handicapped in life by certain personality traits and is truly emotionally troubled. Although none of the three stereotypes has proved clinically useful, they give meaning to the way patients behave and enhance the diagnostic and treatment skills of the clinician. Every clinician knows individuals who subject themselves to much more external stress than normal. Many individuals with TM pain seem to fall into this category.

Problems in Testing for Emotions

Numerous scales and inventories have been used to assess the psychological status of individuals with TMD. These include the Minnesota Multiphasic Personality Inventory, Cornell Medical Index, Interpersonal Adjective Checklist, Edwards Personality Profile, Thematic Apperception Test, Cattell Personality Factors Question-

Table 3-12
Psychological Tests of Subjects With TMD

Test	Subjects	Findings	Reference
STAI	TMD vs asymptomatic subjects	Higher anxiety for TMD subjects	138
STAT	Facial pain subgroups—muscle, TMJ arthritis, trigeminal neuralgia	No difference for subgroups	137
STAI	TMD vs asymptomatic subjects	Higher anxiety for TMD subjects	140
STAI	Three subgroups—muscle, joint, and combined muscle–joint	Higher anxiety for muscle subgroup	136
BDI		Higher depression for muscle and combined subgroups	
VAS	Muscle subgroup vs joint subgroup	Higher anxiety and less ability to endure pain for muscle subgroup	15
VAS	TMD extroverts and neurotics	Higher emotion for high neurotics vs low neurotics, no difference between high vs low extroverts	139
MMPI	TMD vs asymptomatic subjects	No difference between groups	130
MMPI	TMD vs asymptomatic and medical clinic group	Higher stress level for TMD and clinic group	131
MMPI	Three subgroups—muscle, internal derangement, atypical facial pain	Higher hypochondriasis, depression, and hysteria in muscle and atypical facial pain subgroups	134
MMPI	TMD vs asymptomatic subjects	Higher hypochondriasis, depression, hysteria, and social introversion for men, all scores except hypomania for women	140
MMPI	Three subgroups—muscle, joint, combined muscle–joint	Higher scores in each category for muscle group	136
DSI	Orofacial pain vs arthritis, neurology, asymptomatic subjects	No difference between orofacial pain and asymptomatic subjects	137
BPI	TMD vs other pain and asymptomatic subjects	Higher depression and hypochondriasis for TMD and other pain subjects	143
PSS		No difference between groups	
MHLC		" " " "	
WC		" " " "	
CCEI	TMD vs other chronic orofacial pain patients	No difference between groups	141
GHQ			
CCEI	TMD vs asymptomatic subjects	Higher depression and somatization for TMD	144
CESD	TMD clinic patients	31% were significantly depressed	145
SCL	TMD clinic patients	Subgroups classified as normal, moderately, and severely distressed	135
SCL	TMD clinic patients	Three subgroups; somatization contributes to chronicity, depression may be premorbid or reactive	152
MPI	TMD clinic patients	Three subgroups; levels of distress, pain, and life interference depend on coping ability	151
MBHI	MPD clinic patients vs non-medical normals	Tendency toward psychological isolation and distress for MPD	150
CIC	TMD patients	Low score associated with amplification of symptoms	146
Chapman	TMD vs asymptomatic subjects	Higher stress level for TMD	148

(continued)

Table 3-12
(*continued*)

Test	Subjects	Findings	Reference
Chapman	TMD vs asymptomatic subjects	Higher stress and pain levels for TMD with poor control over stress	149
SRRS	TMD vs dental patients	Higher stress scores for TMD	147
SOS	TMD vs asymptomatic subjects	Higher stress level for TMD	144
IBQ	TMD, atypical facial pain, and facial neuralgia groups vs odontogenic pain group	Higher somatic preoccupation for TMD	153
IBQ	TMD vs asymptomatic subjects	TMD less likely to acknowledge psychological aspects of illness, high disease conviction, anxiety and depression	154
IBQ	TMD clinic patients	High disease conviction and inability to endure pain	155
IBQ	TMD extroverts vs neurotics	Higher affective inhibition for neurotics, higher affective disturbance, hypochondriasis, irritability and low denial for high vs low neurotics	139
IBQ	TMD populations—Australians vs Finnish	Lower affective disturbance for Finns	156
IBQ	TMD vs other pain subjects	No difference between groups	143

Key to tests: *BDI*, Beck Depression Inventory; *BPI*, Behavioral Health Inventory; *CCEI*, Crown Crisp Experimental Inventory; *CESD*, Center for Epidemiology Studies; *CIC*, Capacity for Interpersonal Contact; *DSI*, Depression Scale of the Institute of Personality and Ability Testing; *GHQ*, General Health Questionnaire; *IBQ*, Pilowsky Illness Behavior Questionnaire; *MBHI*, Million Behavioral Health Inventory; *MHLC*, Multidmensional Health Locus of Control; *MMPI*, Minnesota Multiphasic Personality Inventory; *MPI*, West-Haven-Yale Multipersonality Inventory; *PSS*, Perceived Stress Scale; *SLC-90 R*, Symptom Checklist 90 Revised; *SOS*, Symptoms of Stress Inventory; *SSRS*, Holmes and Rahe Social Readjustment Rating Scale; *STAI*, State/Trait Anxiety Inventory; *VAS*, Visual Analogue Scale for Emotion; *WC*, Ways of Coping.

naire, and Eysenck Personality Inventory.[123] Since the 1983 review by the American Dental Association, these and other inventories have been used (Table 3-12).

There have been several criticisms of the clinical significance of these tests. The general feeling is that clinicians should not waste their efforts on analyzing specific psychological characteristics of individual patients.[127] A second criticism asks the question whether higher scores reflect pain suffering caused by the disorder or if emotional disturbance leads to the suffering.[128] In addition, tests that inventory psychological factors have not yet been diagnostically applied successfully to patients with TMD.[129]

The first criticism has merit. There are many methodologic flaws in the interpretation of paper and pencil tests. Only a trend can be inferred by comparing results from a single profile against standardized values obtained from many profiles, and findings may differ between subjects even though the same inventory has been used. For example, consider the case for assessment with the Minnesota Multiphasic Personality Inventory (MMPI). About half of the patients with TM pain had an elevated score for anxiety on the MMPI compared with matched controls without TM pain.[130] Although the level of anxiety was higher for pain patients, it fell within the normal range for this test. In another study, MMPI scores for TMD patients were similar to scores of patients visiting a medical clinic for other disabilities.[131]

There may never be an answer to the second criticism. The problem of establishing cause and effect is not restricted to studies about TMD. Cross-sectional studies of 3023 individuals from the United States, aged 25 to 74 years, showed 14.4% suffered from well-defined chronic pain related to the joints and musculoskeletal system.[132] Pain of uncertain duration was present in another 7.4%. About 83% of the total had received treatment. Of the total, 18% had some degree of depression, compared with only 8% of those who did not have chronic pain. Although these differences were statistically significant, the investigators concluded that they still did not know whether the chronic pain caused the depressive illness or the contrary, or if there was comorbidity of both.

Other attempts have been made to resolve this dilemma. A well-controlled study compared 163 chronic, nonmalignant pain sufferers with 81 control subjects to determine whether emotional disturbance was the cause or the consequence of chronic pain.[133] Numerous measures, including personal history and psychological variables, were studied for both groups. The results suggested that emotional disturbances in the pain patients were more likely the consequence rather than the cause of chronic pain. The pain was related to more current depression and less current life satisfaction.

Evidence suggests that there may be some solutions to the third criticism, that tests that inventory psychological factors have not yet been diagnostically applied successfully to patients with TMD. Different psychological characteristics have been found among diagnostic subgroups of patients with orofacial pain. MMPI scores for hypochondriasis, depression, and hysteria were higher for patients suffering from myogenic facial pain and atypical facial pain than in patients suffering from internal derangement of the TMJ.[134] Three subgroups of psychologically different TMD patients have been identified using the SCL-90-R inventory[135]: normal, moderately distressed, and severely distressed. Patients with distress had high ratings of pain severity and interference with daily functioning.

Visual analogue scores for emotion in clinic patients with TM myogenous disorders were higher for disease conviction and inability to endure pain than for patients with TM arthrogenous disorders.[15] Similar results have been found in another study.

Evaluation of three subgroups of TMD patients (primarily myogenic, primarily TMJ, and combination myogenic and TMJ) confirmed psychological differences among the subgroups.[136] After differences in pain levels were adjusted for the groups, myogenic patients displayed higher concern for bodily functions and illness preoccupation compared with subjects of the other groups. Greater pain was not associated with anxiety and depression levels. Analysis of psychometric variables correctly identified 74% of structural patients and 46% of myalgia patients.

Anxiety

Anxiety is a feeling of apprehension, uncertainty and fear. Assessment with the same anxiety test has produced conflicting results in different groups (see Table 3-12). No difference was found between different subgroups of patients of orofacial pain with the State/Trait Test.[137] Higher levels were reported for TMD patients than for asymptomatic subjects[138] and for muscle-related TMD subjects than for TMJ-related subjects.[136] This same result was previously found using a visual analogue scale (VAS) for emotions.[15] Greater VAS levels were found in highly emotional TMD neurotics than in low neurotics.[139]

Depression

Depression is defined as loss of hope or cheerfulness. It is emotional dejection accompanied by decreased functional activity. Scores derived from studies on depression among TMD patients have varied (see Table 3-12). Most assessments have been made with the Minnesota Multiphasic Personality Inventory. Using this instrument, no difference was found between TMD and asymptomatic subjects.[130] Higher levels of stress were reported for TMD and medical clinic patients compared with pain-free subjects,[131,140] for muscle-related TMD and atypical facial pain patients versus patients with internal derangement,[134] and for muscle-related TMD patients versus patients with TMJ or combined muscle–joint problems using another scale.[136]

No difference was found between orofacial pain patients and asymptomatic subjects with other depression scales.[137,141,142] However, greater levels for depression and hypochondriasis discriminated TMD and other pain patients from pain-free subjects tested with one inventory[143] and between TMD patients and asymptomatic subjects with another inventory.[144]

Among 75 adult patients visiting a multidisciplinary orofacial pain clinic, 31% scored 16 or above on the CES-D scale, a score considered as being at risk for significant depression.[145]

Stress and Coping

Previous studies have suggested that TMD patients handle stress poorly (see Table 3-9). Such results must be viewed with caution in light of differences in the kind of tests used. Amplification of symptoms and disturbed capacity for interpersonal contact were reported for orofacial myofascial pain dysfunction (MPD) patients.[146] Other measurements of stress levels and ways of coping response showed TMD patients differed from asymptomatic subjects.[147] Higher levels of stress or difficulties in coping were found with three separate instruments,[144,148–150] but not with three others.[143]

Clearly, the interference of pain and levels of distress associated with life situations depends on the coping ability of TMD patients. Patients have been classified as normal, moderately distressed, or severely distressed[135]; as dysfunctional, interpersonally distressed, or adaptive copers[151]; and as highly emotionally distressed, moderately emotionally distressed, or nondistressed.[152] Somatization was the chief factor found by analysis of psychological variables among TMD patients.[152] The authors of that study concluded that the extent of somatization was a potent contributor to pain chronicity. These findings are consistent with results of other studies. A greater tendency toward distress and psychological isolation has been found among patients with chronic MPD syndrome of the total body than in asymptomatic subjects.[150]

Illness Behavior

Illness behavior embodies a broad range of pain-related complaints and responses. Several factors are embraced by the Illness Behavior Questionnaire: hypochondriasis, disease conviction, somatic versus psychological perception of illness, affective inhibition, affective disturbance, denial, and irritability.

Results with this instrument have been consistent for most studies (see Table 3-12). One or more factors have been identified as significantly different between TMD patients and asymptomatic subjects. TMD subjects had higher scores for somatic preoccupation, greater anxiety or depression, and inability to accept reassurance from the doctor easily, and were less likely to acknowledge psychological aspects of illness,[153,154] as well as disease conviction.[154,155] TMD patients with varying degrees of neuroticism differed significantly from TMD patients rated as extroverts.[139]

No significant differences were found between TMD subjects and patients with other bodily pains.[143] Populational differences have been reported. TMD patients from a Finnish population scored lower on affective disturbance than Australian patients.[156]

Psychological Stress Relationship and Muscle Tension

Several clinicians have reported that TM pain results from intense muscular activity that derives from emotional states. If one type of stress predominates over another, the condition may become pathologic, as when increased tension in the jaw muscles occurs after an emotionally stressful event. This is referred to as response specificity.[127] One theory is that psychological stress elicits muscular hyperactivity terminating in TMD pain. This logic forms the basis for the psychophysiologic theory of myofascial pain dysfunction syndrome in TMD.[157] The literature relating to this theory is divided and varies greatly in quality, and there is a persisting problem of distinguishing muscle pain syndromes from psychological illness.[158]

Clinical Correlational Studies

Many clinical observations suggest a relationship between psychological stress, increased muscle tension, and parafunctional habits. The classic example is the presence of bruxism and symptoms of the masticatory muscles. Most of these studies have focused on the presence of greater muscular tenderness and greater tooth wear in bruxers than in nonbruxers. A clinically relevant study compared self-reported frequency of nine oral habits in individuals with (1) facial pain, (2) tension headaches, or (3) no facial pain.[159] Clenching occurred most frequently in the facial pain group. Headache subjects reported a higher frequency of resting the hand on the chin and face than the group reporting no pain. It was hypothesized that one or a combination of oral habits could elicit muscular changes leading to head pain. In this case the mechanism by which patients became symptomatic seemed clarified, but not all causal relationships can be inferred from this kind of correlational study.

Experimental Studies

Numerous experimental studies suggest a relationship between stress-related muscular activity and TMD symptoms, and empirical findings support this notion.[160,161]

These studies fall into three categories: EMG activity of individuals in the natural environment; EMG activity under laboratory conditions; and the effect of experimental pain on individuals with muscular symptoms.

EMG activities of the jaw muscles of symptomatic individuals in the natural environment show that stressful life events create muscular tension. Bruxism and levels of nocturnal muscle activity become elevated during episodes of daytime stress and anticipation of stress.[123] Long-term study of patients diagnosed with chronic myogenous TMD showed that exacerbations of pain were preceded by increased EMG muscular activity.

Under laboratory-induced stress, differentially higher EMG levels occurred in the masseter and frontalis muscles of TMD patients compared with asymptomatic individuals.[162] EMG temporalis activity of TMD patients was different from the activity of matched controls when both were presented with timed psychomotor tasks. Stress, identified by finger temperature and skin admittance monitoring, showed TMD patients responded differently from controls in terms of habituation to stressful stimuli.[163] That is, they seemed to relax or became accustomed to the stimuli.

Other experimental findings suggest that chronic TM pain sufferers differ from asymptomatic individuals. For example, some investigators found lower pain thresholds, but only trends toward lower pain tolerance among individuals with TM pain, compared with controls.[164] Studies of young women (19 to 28 years of age) exposed to a slow-building pain under laboratory conditions tended to confirm psychophysiologic differences in women with myofascial pain. They had lower pain thresholds, poor discriminability, and greater proclivity to report pain, compared with asymptomatic controls.[165] These laboratory studies have been faulted for various reasons, including exposure of patients to unrealistic life situations and the argument that the response to stress has nothing to do with symptoms or etiology of TMD.

Treatment Outcome Studies

Outcome studies indicate that many TMD patients respond successfully to various kinds of treatments. Between 70% and 80% of all patients will improve regardless of the kind of treatment rendered.[166,167] Because patients can be managed with so many different therapies, something other than structural changes seems responsible for this success.[123] The findings do not necessarily mean that patients are rid of the pain or other clinical signs—they simply may not complain as much. An absence of evidence is not evidence of absence.

TMD pain complaints have been reduced using stress management techniques designed to reduce muscular activity, including biofeedback training and relaxation therapy.[168] Assessment of TM patients randomly divided into a group receiving biofeedback and a group receiving relaxation therapy showed no significant differences in report of pain. Both therapies were moderately successful in reducing complaints of pain immediately posttreatment and at a follow-up 2 years later. Although outcomes were not different, some characteristics of the groups were not similar. Patients receiving relaxation therapy were young, had TM pain of short duration, and had other psychophysiologic complaints. Those individuals treated by biofeedback were older, were married, and had pain of long duration. They also reported less tension of the facial musculature. Two predictors of outcome were presence of the disorder and pretreatment by occlusal adjustment of the teeth. Occlusal adjustment was negatively related to outcome and was not significant in the biofeedback group. Outcome of patients with bruxing habits was considered more successful in the relaxation group. No personality factors were associated with outcome. The study could have been improved by documentation of masticatory muscle tenderness to palpation before therapy, immediately posttreatment, and at the follow-up.

Another outcome study evaluated the effectiveness of psychotherapy and antidepressant medication on chronic, intractable, "psychogenic" pain.[169] A total of 129 patients, most with head and neck pain, were divided into four groups. During 12 weekly sessions, the groups were treated as follows: (1) amitriptyline plus psychotherapy, (2) amitriptyline plus support (reassurance), (3) psychotherapy plus placebo tablet, and (4) support plus placebo tablet. Results showed little difference in the effect on pain. Psychotherapy alone was ineffective in reducing pain, psychotherapy plus placebo slightly increased pain, and psychotherapy plus amitriptyline reduced the duration but not the intensity of pain. Some results were difficult to interpret, possibly due to the undetermined differences in initial baseline levels of pain for the groups.

An impressive study compared psychosocial correlates of TM pain among three groups.[143] TM patients, patients with other painful conditions, and a pain-free healthy group were subjected to a battery of psychological tests (see Table 3-12). This study showed no direct relationship between measures of personality, chronicity of pain, intensity of pain, or perceived severity of dysfunction. There was a weak relationship between chronicity and pain intensity of non-TM pain and perceived stress, hypochondriasis, depression, anxiety, and disease conviction. TM patients and patients with other painful conditions had significantly higher scores for hypochondriasis and depression than asymptomatic controls.

Furthermore, these and other illness traits decreased in patients who responded successfully to treatment. No changes occurred on the coping scales. This indicated that part of the distress resulted from the physical disability. It was suggested that although distress and symptoms may be unrelated, individuals seeking treatment may be more distressed and that reduction of pain after treatment lessens their total worry. The investigators concluded that TMD should not be considered a psychosomatic disorder. The patients did not differ from other pain patients on many psychological measures, but they did differ from pain-free controls. Neither did they differ from either pain patients or asymptomatic controls in illness behavior or manner of coping with stress. Furthermore, generalizations of greater emotional disturbances among TM patients have resulted from clinicians interacting with less manageable patients.

Significance: The findings suggest that there are psychologically different subgroups of patients with TMD. Some have personality characteristics that are different from asymptomatic individuals. Patients from one population may be psychologically different from patients of other populations. Although the inventories use different terms, in most of them affected individuals are found to be distressed.

Although pencil and paper tests have not always aided in diagnosis, it may be that the questions making up the test were inappropriate for diagnosis or were incomprehensible to the patient in the clinical setting. Certain questions appear to be of predictive value and give evidence of suffering or disability. The heterogeneity of these inventory findings shows no single specific pain-patient personality for the TMD patient.

Psychosocial Characteristics of Those Seeking Treatment

Practically every clinician has seen the patient who overreacts to rather minor symptoms. One of the mysteries about TMD is why some individuals cope effectively with the pain and others do not. It is unclear whether (1) TMD patients who are particularly maladaptive pain copers are confronted by a different class of intrinsically more problematic stressors that stretch their coping ability; (2) the stressors are of a particular type; or (3) the stressors are similar and the main problem is that TMD patients are poorer copers who habitually use ineffective strategies.[123]

An early attempt to classify TMD patients by their capacity for interpersonal contact showed that patients scoring low on the scale were more apt to overreport symptoms.[146] With increased severity of pain and other symptoms, there was an increasing severity of disturbed capacity for interpersonal contact. Patients with this disturbed capacity expected surgical treatment for their dysfunction and were less likely to improve with therapy.[170] A very sophisticated attempt has been made to identify which individuals can and which cannot cope with TM pain. The West Haven–Yale Multidimensional Pain Inventory (MPI) was used because it is comprehensive, demonstratedly reliable, and valid with heterogenous populations of chronic pain patients.[151] From this MPI, a taxonomy has been devised that provides a psychometrically sound heuristic framework for elucidating the mechanisms by which stress and coping processes influence TMD symptomatology. This typology was based on empirical integration of physical, psychosocial, and behavioral data.[151,171] Three different groups of TMD patients were identified. The crucial difference between groups was largely behavioral and psychosocial, with physical factors playing a secondary role. Physical factors were identified as common symptoms, age, or radiographic findings.

Group one was classified "dysfunctional" individuals; they accounted for 46% of the population studied. Dysfunctional individuals reported the highest levels of pain and affective distress and the greatest amount of life interference. Group two was designated "interpersonally distressed" individuals, who made up 22% of the population. They had intermediate levels of pain and were lowest on perceived social support. Individuals of group three were designated "adaptive copers" and constituted 32% of the population. These individuals had the lowest levels of pain, affective distress, and life interference, and the greatest perceptions of life control. None of the groups differed significantly based on any measures of structural abnormalities or oral dysfunction. Although division of TMD patients into these subgroups is significant, this classification critically limits diagnosis based on clinical findings.

Gender has not proved to be a prepotent variable for symptom presentation at the initial examination of TMD patients seeking treatment.[172] No significant differences were found between men and women with respect to pain experience or emotional state judged from numerous measures of pain intensity, pain unpleasantness, and psychological variables.

Significance: TMD patients differ in their ability to cope with the pain. Complaints may not relate to the number and degree of dysfunctional signs. Pain interference in daily living may relate to interpersonal conflicts.

Psychological Characteristics of Unsuccessfully Treated Patients

Clinicians worry about the 20% to 30% of patients who find little relief from complaints despite treatment. Clearly, these symptomatic individuals are more emotionally distressed than untreated individuals of the general population. Analysis of profiles of both successfully treated and unsuccessfully treated TMD patients showed elevated MMPI scores for both groups compared with untreated individuals.[173] For treated groups, there was a tendency toward somatization and repression. Unsuccessfully treated patients had higher scores for depression, agitation, and anger than successfully treated patients. These findings underscore the psychophysiologic characteristics of TMD.

The presence of psychological problems among treated patients does not mean that the treatment was necessarily a failure. Not all unsuccessfully treated patients should be considered failures because of the presence of pain. Survey of the literature showed 80% of patients undergoing surgery for TMJ pain were satisfied and would have the surgery again.[174] Approximately 70% were essentially pain-free; 18% had pain on chewing tough foods. Another study showed 90% of 300 patients treated surgically for internal derangement were generally pain-free.[175] Judged by surgical criteria, including clinical measurements for mouth opening and lateral jaw motions, reasonably good functional success had been attained.

These findings contrast sharply with a news release describing a National Institute of Dental Research—funded study completed on 200 TMD patients at the University of Washington dental school.[176] According to that release, 70% of the patients still reported TM pain after surgical treatment.

A central issue that must be addressed is whether clinicians can effectively identify psychosocial problems of TMD patients presenting for initial examination. Evaluation of the dentist's ability to detect psychological disturbances in these patients is fraught with problems. One study compared the dentist's clinical impression of the existence of psychological problems with criteria determined from standardized psychological tests.[177] Analysis of the results showed that judgments made from screening at the initial examination fail to satisfactorily identify psychosocial problems in these patients.

Comparison of pretreatment and posttreatment scores from five different kinds of personality questionnaires obtained on the same TMD patients illustrates the complexity of judging effectiveness of treatment. Significant differences were found with the Basic Personality Inventory and Illness Behavior Questionnaire, but not with the Perceived Stress Scale, Multidimensional Health Locus of Control, or the Ways of

Coping scales.[143] Lower scores were found after treatment for depression and hypochondriasis with the Basic Personality Inventory and the irritability, disease conviction, denial, and affective disturbance scales of the Illness Behavior Questionnaire. The authors concluded that some of the psychological distress may be a function of the physical condition.

Treatment approaches can be improved if dentists and physicians use some of the skills of psychologists.[178] Helping patients with skills for solving problems, approaching life's stressful events in a more rational manner, and dealing with interpersonal relations are a few of the more important areas that can be addressed in this way.

Significance: There is no stereotypic personality that characterizes a typical TMJ profile. Stress and coping are inextricably tied to every aspect of these patients. When imposed demands are perceived to exceed the ability to cope, distress arises.[179] Increases in physical distress do not appear to be linearly related to changes in psychological disturbance.[143] Proof is lacking that negative events always trigger psychological distress.[180]

The psychological status of TMD patients differs little from that of patients presenting with most other painful conditions. No major gender differences have been found in the pain experience and emotional state of subjects seeking treatment.

Many standardized tests are available for evaluating psychological status. This information may be used to determine whether the patient needs referral for psychological counseling. The practitioner should select a test that patients can complete easily and that can be graded easily.

Attempts have been made to clarify the problem of selecting an appropriate test for assessment. Eleven different kinds of questionnaires (seven for depression; four for anxiety) were given to approximately 132 TMD patients.[181] Factor analysis revealed that the different questionnaires measured a single factor. The authors concluded that a simplified two-item assessment was as appropriate as more complex depression and anxiety scales. Half of this two-item test was the Single Question Depression Assessment (SQDA); the other half was the Single Question Anxiety Assessment (SQAA). For the SQDA, the patient responds to the question "How depressed are you?" by rating on a continuum from 0 (never) to 4 (often). For the SQAA, the patient rates himself on the question "Do you consider yourself more tense than calm or more calm than tense?" on a continuum from (0) calm to (4) tense. This short form may be useful for providing immediate information about the emotional status of TMD patients.

A larger and more systematic data base is needed for the assessment of this instrument.

Treatment of TM pain demands careful consideration. There must be clear understanding between clinician and patient before treatment begins. A clinical result acceptable to the clinician but unacceptable to the patient reflects differences in expectations of the two parties.

References

1. Mountcastle VB. Pain and temperature sensibilities. In Mountcastle VB (ed). Medical physiology, 13th ed. St. Louis: CV Mosby, 1974:391.
2. Melzack R. The language of pain. Dental Dimensions 1979;3:1.
3. Gracely RHN, McGrath P, Dubner RT. Ratio scales of sensory and affective verbal pain descriptors. Pain 1978;5:5.
4. Osterweis M, Kleinman A, Mechanic D (eds). Pain and disability: clinical, behavioral and public policy perspectives. Washington, DC: National Academy Press, 1987:306.
5. Knapp DA, Koch H. The management of new pain in office-based ambulatory care. In National Ambulatory Medical Care Survey 1980 and 1981. Advance Data from Vital and Health Statistics (No. 97 DHHS publication 84-1250). Hyattsville MD: Public Health Service, 1984.
6. Taylor H, Curran NM. The Nuprin pain report. New York: Louis Harris and Associates, 1985.
7. Merskey H. Classification of chronic pain, descriptions of chronic pain syndromes and definitions of pain terms. Pain 1986;27(suppl):59.
8. Schwartz LL. Pain associated with the temporomandibular joint. J Am Dent Assoc 1955;51:394.
9. Molin C. Studies in mandibular pain dysfunction syndrome. Swed Dent J 1973;66(suppl 4):66.
10. Harris M, Davies G. Psychiatric disorders. In Jones JG, Mason MK (eds). Oral manifestation of systemic disease. Philadelphia: WB Saunders, 1980:439.
11. Feinmann C, Harris M, Cawley RM. Psychogenic facial pain. Presentation and treatment. Brit Med J 1984;288:436.
12. Fricton JR, Kroening R, Haley D, Siegert R. Myofascial pain syndrome of the head and neck: a review of clinical characteristics of 164 patients. Oral Surg Oral Med Oral Pathol 1985;60:615.
13. Bush FM, Chinchilli VM, Martelli MF. Pain perception and assessment among patients with temporomandibular (TM) disorders. Pain 1987;4(suppl):124. Abstract 236.
14. Melzack R. The McGill pain questionnaire: major properties and scoring methods. Pain 1975;1:277.
15. Bush FM, Whitehill JM, Martelli MF. Pain assessment in temporomandibular disorders. J Craniomandib Pract 1989;7:137.
16. Von Korff M, Dworkin SF, Le Resche L. Graded chronic pain status: an epidemiologic evaluation. Pain 1990;40:279.
17. Smythe HA. "Fibrositis" as a disorder of pain modulation. Clin Rheum Dis 1979;5:823.
18. Christensen LV. Physiology and pathophysiology of skeletal muscle contractions. Part II. Static activity. J Oral Rehabil 1986;13:463.
19. Christensen LV. Pains from the jaw muscles in children and adults. In Graber LW (ed). Orthodontics: state of the art. St. Louis: CV Mosby, 1986a:22.
20. Clark GT, Jow RW, Lee JJ. Jaw pain and stiffness levels after repeated maximum voluntary clenching. J Dent Res 1989;68:69.
21. Newham DJ, Jones DA, Ghosh G, Aurora P. Muscle fatigue and pain after eccentric contraction at long and short length. Clin Sci 1988;74:553.
22. Jacobsen S, Danneskiold-Samsoe B. Isometric and isokinetic muscle strength in patients with fibrositis syndrome. Scand J Rheumatol 1987;16:61.

23. Boissevain MD, McCain GA. Toward and integrated understanding of fibromyalgia syndrome. I. Medical and pathophysiological aspects. Pain 1991; 45:227.

24. Moss RA, Garrett JC. Temporomandibular joint dysfunction syndrome and myofascial pain dysfunction syndrome: a critical review. J Oral Rehabil 1984; 11:3.

25. Bengtsson A, Henriksson GG, Jorfeldt L, Kadedal B, Lennmarken C, Lindstrom F. Primary fibromyalgia: a clinical and laboratory study of 55 patients. Scand J Rheumatol 1986;15:340.

26. Zidar J, Backman E, Bengtsson A, Henriksson KG. Quantitative EMG and muscle tension in painful muscles in fibromyalgia. Pain 1990;40:249.

27. Brendstrup P, Jesperson K, Asbol-Hansen G. Morphological and chemical connective tissue changes in fibrositic muscles. Ann Rheum Dis 1957;176:438.

28. Henriksson KG, Bengtsson A, et al. Muscle biopsy findings of possible diagnostic importance in primary fibromyalgia (fibrositis, myofascial syndrome). Lancet 1982;2:1395.

29. Yunus MB, Kalyan-Raman UP, Kalyan-Raman K, Masi AT. Pathological changes in muscle in primary fibromyalgia syndrome. Am J Med 1986;81(suppl 3A):38.

30. Yunus MB, Kalyan-Raman UP. Muscle biopsy findings in primary fibromyalgia and other forms of nonarticular rheumatism. Rheum Dis Clin North Am 1989;15:115.

31. Bartels EM, Danneskiold-Samsoe B. Histological abnormalities in muscle from patients with certain types of fibrositis. Lancet 1986;1:755.

32. Hutchins MO, Skjonsby HS. Microtrauma to rat superficial masseter muscles following lengthening contractions. J Dent Res 1990;69:1580.

33. Krough-Poulsen WG. Klinisk undersogelse. In: Krough-Poulsen, WG (ed). Patofunktion, Bidfunktion, Bettfkysiologi, 2nd ed. Copenhagen: Munksgard, 1979:107.

34. Nielsen IL, McNeill C, Danzig W, Goldman S, Levy J, Miller AJ. Adaptation of craniofacial muscles in subjects with craniomandibular disorders. Am J Orthod Dentofacial Orthop 1990;97:20.

35. Sorini M, Pasero F, Rapetti A, et al. Masticatory muscle tenderness and masseteric maximal clenching EMG activity. J Dent Res 1991;70:330.

36. Clark GT, Adler RC, Lee JJ. Jaw pain and tenderness levels during and after repeated sustained maximum voluntary protrusion. Pain 1991;45:17.

37. Laskin DM. Etiology of the pain-dysfunction syndrome. J Am Dent Assoc 1969;79:147.

38. Christensen LV. Physiology and pathophysiology of skeletal muscle contractions. Part I. Dynamic activity. J Oral Rehabil 1986b;13:451.

39. Simons DG. Myofascial pain syndromes due to trigger points. In Osterweis M, Kleinman A, Mechanic D (eds). Pain and disability. Washington DC: National Academy Press, 1987:285.

40. Travell J, Rinzler SH. The myofascial genesis of pain. Postgrad Med 1952; 11:425.

41. Travell J, Simons DG. Myofascial pain and dysfunction: the trigger point manual. Baltimore: Williams & Wilkins, 1983.

42. Thomson H. Occlusion. Bristol: John Wright and Sons, 1975:43.

43. Olsson A. Temporomandibular joint function and functional disturbances. Dent Clin North Am 1969;13:643.

44. Thilander B. Innervation of the temporomandibular joint capsule in man. Trans R Sch Dent Stockh Umea 1961;7:9.

45. Griffen CJ, Harris R. Innervation of the temporomandibular joint. Aust Dent J 1975;20:78.

46. De Laat A. Reflexes elicitable in jaw muscles and their role during function and dysfunction: a review of the literature. Part I. Receptors associated with the masticatory system. J Craniomand Pract 1987;5:140.

47. Yavelow I, Arnold GS. Temporomandibular joint clicking. Oral Surg Oral Med Oral Pathol 1971;32:708.

48. Kawamura T, Abe K. Role of sensory information from temporomandibular joint. Bull Tokyo Med Dent Univ 1974;21(suppl):78.

49. Toller PA. Temporomandibular capsular rearrangement. Br J Oral Surg 1974; 11:207.

50. Leopard PJ. Anterior dislocation of the temporomandibular disc. Br J Oral Maxillofac Surg 1984;22:9.

51. Juniper RP. Temporomandibular joint dysfunction: a theory based upon electromyographic studies of the lateral pterygoid muscle. Br J Oral Maxillofac Surg 1984;22:1.

52. Eversole LR, Machado L. Temporomandibular joint internal derangements and associated neuromuscular disorders. J Am Dent Assoc 1985;110:69.

53. Schellhas KP, Wilkes CH. Temporomandibular joint inflammation: comparison of MR fast scanning with T-1 and T-2 weighted imaging techniques. Am J Neuroradiol 1989;10:589.

54. Howell SA. Osteoarthritis (degenerative joint disease). In Wyngaarden JB, Smith LH Jr (eds). Cecil textbook of medicine, 18th ed. Philadelphia, WB Saunders, 1988:2039.

55. Sokoloff L. The biology of degenerative joint disease. Chicago, University of Chicago Press, 1969.

56. Stengenga B, Lambert GMB, Boering G. Osteoarthritis as the cause of craniomandibular pain and dysfunction: a unifying concept. J Oral Maxillofac Surg 1989;47:249.

57. Holmlund A, Helsing G. Arthroscopy of the temporomandibular joint: occurrence and location of osteoarthrosis and synovitis in a patient material. Int J Oral Surg 1988;17:36.

58. Schellhas KP, Wilkes CH. Temporomandibular joint inflammation: comparison of MR fast scanning with T1- and T2-weighted imaging techniques. Am J Neuroradiol 1989;10:589.

59. Holmlund A, Hellsing G, Axelsson S. The temporomandibular joint: a comparison of clinical and arthroscopic findings. J Prosth Dent 1989;62:61.

60. Schellhas KP, Piper MA, Omlie MR. Facial skeletal remodeling due to temporomandibular joint degeneration: an imaging study of 100 patients. Am J Neuroradiol 1990;11:541.

61. Wilkes CH. Internal derangement of the temporomandibular joint: pathological variations. Arch Otolaryngol Head Neck Surg 1989;115:469.

62. Oberg T, Carlsson GE, Fajers C-M. The temporomandibular joint: a morphologic study of human autopsy material. Acta Odontol Scand 1971;29:393.

63. Rasmussen OC. Clinical findings during the course of temporomandibular arthropathy. Scand J Dent Res 1981;89:283.

64. Mejersjo C. Therapeutic and prognostic considerations in TMJ osteoarthrosis:

a literature review and a long-term study in 11 subjects. J Craniomand Pract 1987;5:70.

65. Clark GT, Adachi NY, Dornan MR. Physical medicine procedures affect temporomandibular disorders: a review. J Am Dent Assoc 1990;121:151.

66. Stewart CL, Standish SM. Osteoarthritis of the TMJ in teenaged females: report of cases. J Am Dent Assoc 1983;106:638.

67. Tegelberg A. Temporomandibular joint involvement in rheumatoid arthritis: a clinical study. Swed Dent J Suppl 1987;49:1.

68. Greene CS, Marbach JJ. Epidemiologic studies of mandibular dysfunction: a critical review. J Prosthet Dent 1982;48:184.

69. Gale EN, Gross A. An evaluation of temporomandibular joint sounds. J Am Dent Assoc 1985;111:62.

70. Forsberg M, Agerberg G, Persson M. Mandibular dysfunction in patients with juvenile rheumatoid arthritis. J Craniomand Disorder Facial Oral Pain 1988; 2:201.

71. Seligman DA, Pullinger AG. The role of intercuspal occlusal relationships in temporomandibular disorders: a review. J Craniomand Disorder Facial Oral Pain 1991;5:96.

72. Larheim TA, Storhaug K, Tveito L. Temporomandibular joint involvement and dental occlusion in a group of adults with rheumatoid arthritis. Acta Odontol Scand 1983;41:301.

73. Melzack R, Wall PD. Pain mechanisms: a new theory. Science 1965;150:971.

74. Wall PD. The gate control theory of pain mechanisms: a reexamination and restatement. Brain 1978;101:1.

75. Fields HL. Pain. New York, McGraw-Hill, 1987.

76. Bell WE. Orofacial pains: classification, diagnosis, management, 4th ed. Chicago, Year Book medical Publishers, 1989.

77. Portenoy RK. Mechanisms of clinical pain. Neurol Clin 1989;7:205.

78. Pertes RA. A practical approach to the diagnosis of chronic orofacial pain. Part II. Neurogenous and psychogenic pain. Compend Contin Educ Dent 1988; 9:622.

79. Pertes RA, Heir GM. Chronic orofacial pain: a practical approach to differential diagnosis. Dent Clin North Am 1991;35:123.

80. Andreoli TE, Carpenter CC, Plum F, Smith LH Jr. Cecil essentials of medicine, 2nd ed. Philadelphia: WB Saunders, 1990.

81. Fromm GH. Pre-trigeminal neuralgia. Neurology 1990;40:1493.

82. Olin RJ. The etiologies of tic doulolureux: trigeminal neuralgia. J Craniomand Pract 1990;8:319.

83. International Association for the Study of Pain, Subcommittee on Taxonomy. Classification of chronic pain. Pain 1986;suppl 3.

84. Stevens JC. Cranial neuralgias. J Craniomand Disord Facial Oral Pain 1987; 1:51.

85. Jenetta PJ. Treatment of trigeminal neuralgia by suboccipital and transtentorial cranial operation. Clin Neurosurg 1977;24:538.

86. Janetta PJ. Microvascular decompression for trigeminal neuralgia. Surg Rounds 1983;6:24.

87. Zurak N. Primary trigeminal neuralgia. Neurologia 1990;39:75.

88. Esposito CJ, Crim GA, Binkley TK. Headaches: a differential diagnosis. J Craniomand Pract 1986;4:317.

89. Davar G, Maciewicz, RJ. Deafferentation pain syndromes. Neurol Clin 1989; 7:289.

90. Graff-Radford SB, Solberg WK. Atypical odontalgia. Cal Dent Assoc J 1986; 14:27.

91. Atypical facial pain. Curr Concepts Pain Analg 1979;6:1.

92. Reik L. Atypical odontalgia: a localized form of atypical facial pain. Headache 1984;24:222.

93. Solberg WK, Graff-Radford SB. Orodental considerations in facial pain. Semin Neurol 1988;8:318.

94. Roberts WJ. A hypothesis on the physiological basis of causalgia and related pains. Pain 1986;24:297.

95. Jaeger B, Singer E, Kroening R. Reflex sympathetic dystrophy of the face: report of two cases and a review of the literature. Arch Neurol 1986;43:693.

96. Cohan BL. Reflex sympathetic dystrophy syndrome. J Craniomand Pract 1991; 9:76.

97. Heyck H. Headache and facial pain. Chicago: Year Book Medical Publishers, 1981.

98. Ruff GA, Moss RA, Lombardo TW. Common migraine: a review and proposal for a non-vascular aetiology. J Oral Rehabil 1986;13:499.

99. Olesen J. The classification and diagnosis of headache disorders. In: Headache: assessment and management. 7th World Congress on Pain, International Association for the Study of Pain, Paris, 1993:107.

100. Schellhas KP, Piper MA, Omlie MR. Facial skeletal remodeling due to temporomandibular joint degeneration: an imaging study of 100 patients. AJR 1990;155:373.

101. Scapino RP. The posterior attachment: its structure, function, and appearance in TMJ imaging studies. Part 1. J Craniomand Disord Facial Oral Pain 1991; 5:83.

102. Stingl J. Blood supply of the temporomandibular joint in man. Folia Morphol 1965;13:20.

103. Toller PA. Synovial apparatus and temporomandibular function. Br Dent J 1961;3:356.

104. Ray BS, Wolff HG. Experimental studies on headache. Pain-sensitive structures of the head and their significance in headache. Arch Surg 1940;41:813.

105. Moskowitz MA, Beyerl BD, Henrikson GM. Approach to vascular head pain. In Asbury AK, McKhann W, McDonaldl (eds). Diseases of the nervous system. Philadelphia: WB Saunders, 1986:941.

106. Vieyra MAB, Hoag NL, Maskek BJ. Migraine in childhood: development aspects of biobehavioral treatment. In Bush JP, Harkins SW (eds). Children in pain: clinical and research issues from a development perspective. New York: Springer-Verlag, 1991:374.

107. Barlow CF. Headaches and migraine in childhood. London: Spastics International Medical Publications, 1984.

108. Edmeads J. Symposium on the prelude to the migraine attack. Natl Migraine Found Newslett 1986;55:3.

109. Edmeads J. Vascular headache and the cranial circulation: another look. Headache 1979;19:127.

110. Solomon GD. The actions and use of calcium channel blockers in migraine and cluster headache. Headache Q Curr Treat Res 1990;1:152.

111. Moskowitz MA. The neurobiology of vascular head pain. Ann Neurol 1984; 16:157.

112. Hannington E. Viewpoint: the platelet and migraine. Headache 1986;26:411.

113. Schokker RP, Hansson TL, Ansink BJJ. Craniomandibular disorders in patients with different types of headache. J Craniomand Disord Facial Oral Pain 1990;1:47.

114. McDonald JS, Pensak ML, Phero JC. Part 1. Differential diagnosis of chronic facial, head, and neck pain complaints. Am J Otol 1990;11:299.

115. Nelson RF, duBopulay GH, Marshal J, et al. Cerebral blood flow in patients with cluster headache. Headache 1980;20:184.

116. Medina JA, Diamond S, Fareed J. The nature of cluster headache. Headache 1979;19:309.

117. Sjaastad O. Histamine metabolism in cluster headache and migraine. J Neurol 1977;216:105.

118. Campbell JK. Cluster headache. J Craniomand Disord Facial Oral Pain 1987; 1:27.

119. Melzack R. The language of pain. Dent Dimens 1979;3:2.

120. Brannstrom M. Dentin sensitivity and aspiration of odontoblasts. J Am Dent Assoc 1963;66:366.

121. Brightman VJ. Oral symptoms without apparent physical abnormality. In Lynch MA, Brightman VJ, Greenberg (eds). Burket's oral medicine: diagnosis and treatment, 8th ed. Philadelphia: JB Lippincott, 1984:616.

122. Solberg WK, Graff-Radford SB. Orodental considerations in facial pain. Semin Neurol 1988;8:313.

123. Rugh JD. Psychological factors in the etiology of masticatory pain and dysfunction. In Laskin DM, Greenfield W, Gale E, et al (eds). The president's conference on the examination, diagnosis and management of temporomandibular disorders. Chicago: American Dental Association, 1983:85.

124. Parker MW. A dynamic model of etiology in temporomandibular disorders. J Am Dent Assoc 1990;120:283.

125. Jacobson E. The self and the object world. New York: International Universities Press, 1965.

126. Moore BE, Fine BD. A glossary of psychoanalytic terms and concepts, 2nd ed. New York: American Psychoanalytic Association, 1968.

127. Greene CS, Olson RE, Laskin DM. Psychological factors in the etiology, progression, and treatment of MPD syndrome. J Am Dent Assoc 1982;105:443.

128. Gale EN. Psychological characteristics of long-term female temporomandibular joint pain patients. J Dent Res 1978;57:481.

129. Dworkin SF, Truelove EL, Bonica JJ, Sola S. Facial and head pain caused by myofascial and temporomandibular disorders. In Bonica JJ (ed). The management of pain. Philadelphia: Lea & Febiger, 1990:733.

130. Solberg WK, Flint RT, Brantner J. Temporomandibular joint pain and dysfunction: a clinical study of emotional and occlusal components. J Prosthet Dent 1972;28:412.

131. Olson RE, Schwartz RA. Depression in patients with myofascial pain-dysfunction syndrome. J Dent Res 1977;56:160.

132. Magni G, Caldieron C, Rigatti-Luchini S, Merskey, H. Chronic musculoskeletal pain and depressive symptoms in the general population: an analysis of the 1st National Health and Nutrition Examination Survey data. Pain 1990;43:299.

133. Gamsa A. Is emotional disturbance a precipitator or a consequence of chronic pain? Pain 1990;42:183.

134. Eversole LR, Stone CE, Matheson D, Kaplan H. Psychometric profiles of facial pain. Oral Surg Oral Med Oral Pathol 1985;60:269.

135. Butterworth JC, Deardorf WW. Psychometric profiles of craniomandibular pain patients: identifying specific subgroups. J Craniomand Pract 1987;5:226.

136. McCreary CP, Clark GT, Merrill RL, Flack V, Oakley ME. Psychological distress and diagnostic subgroups of temporomandibular disorder patients. Pain 1991;44:29.

137. Marbach JJ, Lund P. Depression, anhedonia and anxiety in the temporomandibular joint and other facial pain syndromes. Pain 1981;11:73.

138. Molin C, Edman G, Schalling D. Psychological studies of patients with mandibular pain dysfunction syndrome. 1. Personality traits in patients and controls. Sven-Tandlak-Tidskr 1973;66:1.

139. Harkins SW, Price DD, Braith J. Effects of extraversion and neuroticism on experimental pain, clinical pain, and illness behavior. Pain 1989;36:209.

140. Conserva E, Bosio A, Mongini F. Relevance of psychologic factors in craniofacial pain and dysfunction. J Dent Res 1990;69.

141. Salter M, Brooke RI, Merskey H, Fichter GF, Kapusianyk DH. Is the temporomandibular pain and dysfunction syndrome a disorder of the mind? Pain 1983;17:151.

142. Andreasen KH, Zach GA. Evaluation of the psychological profile of temporomandibular joint dysfunction patients. J Dent Res 1990;69.

143. Schnurr RF, Brooke RI, Rollman GB. Psychosocial correlates of temporomandibular joint pain and dysfunction. Pain 1990;42:153.

144. Beaton RD, Egan KJ, Nakagawa-Kogan H, Morrison KN. Self-reported symptoms of stress with temporomandibular disorders: comparison to healthy men and women. J Prosthet Dent 1991;65:289.

145. Bush FM, Harkins SW, Welleford EA. Depression in orofacial pain: relation to activities of daily living (ADL) and neuroticism. International Association for the Study of Pain, 7th World Congress on Pain, 1993:51.

146. Heloe B, Heiberg AN. A multiprofessional study of patients with myofascial pain-dysfunction syndrome. II. Acta Odontol Scand 1980;38:119.

147. Feron CG, Serwatka W. Stress: a common denominator for nonorganic TMJ pain-dysfunction. J Prosthet Dent 1983;49:805.

148. Moody PM, Calhoun TC, Okeson JP, Kemper JT. Stress–pain relationship in MPD syndrome patients and non-MPD syndrome patients. J Prosthet Dent 1981;45:84.

149. Swart KM, Zeitler DL. The relationship of stress and pain in temporo-mandibular dysfunction patients. J Dent Res 1990;69:195.

150. Jorge M, Goldberg M, Fisbain D, et al. Millon Behavioral Health Inventory (MBHI) norms for male and female chronic myofascial pain patients. Pain 1990;suppl 5:S305.

151. Rudy TE, Turk DC, Zaki HS, Curtin HD. An empirical taxometric alternative to traditional classification of temporomandibular disorders. Pain 1989;36:311.

152. Grzesiak R, Attanasio V, Attanasio R, et al. Somatization and depression in TMJ/orofacial pain. J Dent Res 1990;69.

153. Speculand B, Goss AN, Spence ND, Pilowsky I. Intractable facial pain and illness behavior. Pain 1981;11:213.

154. Speculand B, Goss AN, Hughes A, Spence ND, Pilowsky I. Temporo-mandibular joint dysfunction: pain and illness behavior. Pain 1983;17:139.

155. Bush FM, Harkins SW, Price DD. Subjective signs of temporomandibular (TM) dysfunction: chronic pain, experimental pain and pain behavior. Pain 1990;suppl 5.

156. Suvinen T, Sunden B, Reade PC, Gerschman J. Coping strategies and illness behaviour in temporomandibular joint pain-dysfunction syndrome (TMJPDS). Pain 1990;suppl 5.

157. Laskin DM. Etiology of the pain-dysfunction syndrome. J Am Dent Assoc 1969;79:147.

158. Merskey, H. Psychosocial factors and muscular pain. 1st International Symposium on Myofascial Pain and Fibromyalgia. University of Minnesota, May 8-10, 1989.

159. Moss RA, Ruff MH, Sturgis, E.T. Oral behavioral patterns in facial pain, headache and non-headache populations. Behav Res Ther 1984;22:683.

160. Moss RA, Garrett J, Chiodo JF. Temporomandibular joint dysfunction and myofascial pain dysfunction syndromes: parameters, etiology, and treatment. Psychol Bull 1982;92:331.

161. Haber JD, Moss RA, Kuczmierczyk AR, Garrett JG. Assessment and treatment of stress in myofascial pain-dysfunction syndrome. J Oral Rehabil 1983;10:187.

162. Kapel L, Glaros AG, McGlynn F.D. Psychophysiological responses to stress in patients with myofascial pain-dysfunction. J Behav Med 1989;12:397.

163. Katz JO, Rugh JD, Hatch JP, et al. Effect of experimental stress on masseter and temporalis muscle activity in human subjects with temporomandibular disorders. Arch Oral Biol 1989;34:393.

164. Molin C, Edman G, Schalling D. Psychological studies of patients with mandibular pain dysfunction syndrome. 2. Tolerance for experimentally induced pain. Sven-Tandlak-Tidskr 1973;66:15.

165. Malow RM, Grimm L, Olson RE. Differences in pain perception between myofascial pain dysfunction patients and normal subjects: a signal detection analysis. J Psychosom Res 1980;24:303.

166. Greene CS, Markovic M. Response to nonsurgical treatment of patients with positive radiographic findings in the temporomandibular joint. J Oral Surg 1976;34:692.

167. Mejersjo C, Carlsson GE. Long term results of treatment for temporomandibular pain-dysfunction. J Prosthet Dent 1983;49:809.

168. Funch DP, Gale EN. Biofeedback and relaxation therapy for chronic temporomandibular joint pain: predicting successful outcome. J Consult Clin Psychol 1984;52:928.

169. Pilowsky I, Barrow CG. A controlled study of psychotherapy and amitriptyline used individually and in combination in the treatment of chronic, intractable "psychogenic" pain. Pain 1990;40:3.

170. Heloe B, Heiberg AN. A follow-up study of a group of female patients with myofascial pain-dysfunction syndrome. Acta Odontol Scand 1980a;38:129.

171. Turk DC, Rudy TE. Toward an empirically derived taxonomy of chronic pain patients: integration of psychological assessment data. J Consult Clin Psychol 1988;56:233.

172. Bush FM, Harkins SW, Harrington WG, Price DD. Analysis of gender effects

of pain perception and symptom presentation in temporomandibular pain. Pain 1994;53:73.

173. Schwartz RA, Greene CS, Laskin DM. Personality characteristics of patients with myofascial pain-dysfunction (MPD) syndrome unresponsive to conventional therapy. J Dent Res 1979;58:1435.

174. Bronstein SL, Tomasetti BJ. Temporomandibular joint surgery: patient-based assessment and evaluation. J Am Dent Assoc 1985;110:485.

175. Williamson EH, Sheffield JW. The treatment of internal derangement of the temporomandibular joint: a survey of 300 cases. J Craniomand Pract 1987; 5:120.

176. Dental researchers meet in San Francisco. ADA News 1989;20:35.

177. Oakley ME, McCreary CP, Flack VF, et al. Dentists' ability to detect psychological problems in patients with temporomandibular disorders and chronic pain. J Am Dent Assoc 1989;118:727.

178. Moss RA, Gramling SE. The role of clinical psychology in the treatment of craniomandibular disorders. J Craniomand Pract 1984;2:159.

179. Lazarus RS, Folkman S. Stress, appraisal, and coping. New York: Springer-Verlag, 1984.

180. Cohen S, Williamson GM. Stress and infectious disease in humans. Psychol Bull 1991;109:5.

181. Gale EN, Dixon DC. A simplified psychologic questionnaire as a treatment planning aid for patients with temporomandibular joint disorders. J Prosthet Dent 1989;61:235.

The Temporomandibular Joint and Related Orofacial Disorders,
by Francis M. Bush and M. Franklin Dolwick.
J.B. Lippincott Company, Philadelphia, © 1995.

4
Etiology

Etiology is the theory or study of the causation of a disease. Because there are many possible etiologies for TMD, a thorough history is crucial for making a decision. After a review of the patient's history, the clinician must decide if one factor or several factors seem plausible. Arriving at this decision is not easy.

Most TM disorders are idiopathic, that is, of unknown origin. Some TMD complaints have been associated with serious organic diseases. Yet the factors that make a person prone to developing TMD have not been carefully identified. Some factors that appear causal occur coincidentally in other individuals. Even in frank cases of pathology, little reliable information exists for differentiating joint changes from muscular changes during the natural course of development of TMD.

Single Versus Multifactorial Etiologies

Historically, the single etiology versus the multifactorial etiology abounds in controversy. This controversy continues even though few studies find a single etiologic factor. Extensive review of the literature suggests that a multifactorial etiology is the most reasonable solution.[1] Speculation is that distinct etiologies may be identified once an empiric classification for diagnosis is found.

Recently, an attempt has been made to clarify the single versus the multifactorial issue. The authors agreed on the multifactorial hypothesis, and factors including external trauma, intubation during general anesthesia, difficult dental extractions, and orthodontic procedures were evaluated in 195 TMD cases and 50 non-TMD controls.[2] Positive associations were found for TMD between the occurrence of factors versus no factors, between two or more factors versus one or no factor, and between multiple factors versus a history of general anesthesia. A trend was found between TMD and trauma with multiple factors versus single factors. No significant associations were found between TMD and the presence of one factor and between multiple factors and extractions.

Table 4-1
Factors That Contribute to TMD

Predisposing

Anatomic
Pathophysiologic

Precipitating

Microtrauma
Macrotrauma

Perpetuating

Behavioral
Emotional

Potential etiologic factors can be conceptualized as a continuum from the least severe to the most severe changes affecting the masticatory system. The least severe factors might include acute microtraumatic events, whereas the most severe factors would include degeneration of the TMJs.

The kinds of factors contributing to TMD can be divided into predisposing, precipitating, and perpetuating factors (Table 4-1). All must be regarded as potential factors. Predisposing factors are factors occurring naturally during the lifetime of an individual. Precipitating factors are initial events leading to onset of symptoms. Perpetuating factors are repetitive events that tend to create a continuing cycle of symptoms. Distinguishing one group of factors from another is not always easy. Considerable overlap may occur between factors.

Predisposing Factors

Several predisposing factors have been discussed in the literature. They primarily include anatomic and pathophysiologic conditions in the person's life.

Anatomic Conditions

Review of the etiology of anatomic conditions will find many possible etiologies. Some of the earlier literature viewed structural deformities as potential contributing factors. These factors mainly involved developmental abnormalities of the jaws. Most reports recognized abnormal maxillomandibular relations, dental or skeletal malocclusions, malalignment of the mandible, and improper position of the head and the spinal column.

Attempts to identify anatomic factors in the etiology of TMD are fraught with problems. Confusion arises because of difficulties in classifying different conditions.[3] For example, the same morphologic variants have been classified as tumors, congenital anomalies, and disturbances of postnatal growth. Most conditions are now classified on a morphologic basis because little to no information exists about anomalies.

Nonetheless, a thorough review has been conducted of the relation between facial anomalies and development of the TMJs.[4] Various prenatal and postnatal causes were discussed, but few etiologic factors were mentioned. None was related to TMD.

An impressive study has been conducted on the anatomy of the TMJs of young adults.[5] The study critically evaluated 95 autopsied joints of subjects in an age group (mean age 26.4 years) that comprises the largest segment of the population seeking TM treatment. These individuals might be considered the most susceptible to physical changes within the joint. Joints were examined for deviations in form (DIF), arthrosis, size, shape, and possible disk displacement. DIF was defined as a deviation from the normal rounded contours of the temporal and condylar surfaces and as deformation of the disk.

Most gross changes in DIF were attributable to adaptive phenomena occurring in response to articular fit and function. Most joints (83 of 95) had intracapsular changes, and 39% had mild-to-marked DIF of the three components, with condylar changes the most prevalent. Three percent showed arthritic lesions, and 12% showed disk displacement. Disk displacement was significantly higher in women than in men. It was greater overall when the disk was deformed or folded. The authors did not fully agree that such changes represented precursors to arthropathy.

Morphologic Malocclusions

Certain skeletal and dental malocclusions have been suggested as causing neuromuscular disturbances in the masticatory system, including TMJ disorders.[6,7] The aberrant functions may be either a direct result of the morphologic malocclusion or an indirect result of functional occlusal interferences. Potential causes have been categorized into vertical, horizontal, and lateral discrepancies.[8] Recognition of these categories is particularly useful if one accepts the theory that malocclusion plays a dominant role in TMD symptomatology (Table 4-2).

Table 4-2
Potential Extra-Articular Skeletal and Dental Causes
Leading to TMD

Vertical Discrepancy

Lack of posterior tooth support
Molar or bicuspid fulcruming

Horizontal Discrepancy

Anterior slide or anterior posturing
Distal displacement

Lateral Discrepancy

Functional side shift
True vertical asymmetry

After McLaughlin R.P. Malocclusion and the temporomandibular joint: an historical perspective. Angle Orthod 1988;58:185.

Classically, individuals with Angle class II, especially division 2, have been considered particularly vulnerable to TMD. Because of excessive overjet, it has been suggested that these individuals habitually posture the mandible during protrusive movements.[9] Presumably, this overuse causes chronic strain of the muscles and may be harmful to the TMJs. These individuals have been cited as commonly represented in many populational studies.[10,11] Other findings tend to support these conclusions. Morphologic malocclusion, class II and class III occlusions, frontal open bite, and cross bite, if correlated with functional malocclusion, may predispose to dysfunction.[12] A rather weak relation between dysfunctional symptoms and Angle malocclusions was demonstrated in children by regression analysis.[12]

Skeletal and dental variations and functional changes in the TMJs have been evaluated in patients examined from a private practice population. Clinical examination and cephalometric analysis of 33 variables were conducted on 62 patients with confirmed internal derangement of the TMJs.[13] Data were compared with identical parameters of 102 matched controls from the general population at large. Analysis showed no statistically significant differences in proportion of subjects in any Angle class, or in dental or occlusal parameters between the groups.

Several variables of morphologic malocclusion and anatomic characteristics have been studied in the TMJs of young adults.[14] Most associations proved age dependent. Autopsy of 96 cadavers showed that certain deviations in form (DIF) of the temporal bone, condyle, and position of the disk correlated significantly with some variables of malocclusion. Angle classes II and III dentitions correlated with DIF, and class II dentitions correlated with histologically evident morphologic changes in the TMJs. Cross bite was related to increasing presence of DIF in the three anatomic areas. Anterior cross bite correlated with DIF of the articular eminence.

Furthermore, abnormal overbite and overjet were associated with condylar DIF. Deep overbite was related to flat condyles and wide fossae. Excessive overjet was associated with DIF of the disk, particularly displacement. The authors argued that TMJ changes become more extensive the longer the exposure to malocclusion. They alluded to an association between malocclusion and TMD symptoms and noted that previous authors concluded these associations were weak.

Significance: The uncertainty of a precise definition for Angle classification, coupled with the findings of other investigations, weakens an argument that Angle malocclusion and a bevy of TMD symptoms are closely related.[15] No definitive correlations have been made between severity of morphologic malocclusion and TMD.

Functional Malocclusion and Occlusal Disharmonies

When clinicians define malocclusion as a change in bite position caused by occlusal disharmonies, the literature on TMD symptoms is replete with conjecture. Different kinds of occlusal interferences have been argued as being significant or insignificant in causing symptoms. The absence of any well-defined relation does not agree with the philosophy of some clinicians who consider that many TMD problems originate from occlusal interferences.

A consensus statement issued by a group of leading health care practitioners[16] confirms a previous statement[15] than an association between occlusal factors and certain symptoms of TMD is weak. Additional evidence refutes this single factor etiology. A study of many occlusal parameters and symptoms concluded that occlusion alone could not be responsible for etiology of TMD.[17] Stepwise logistic regression analysis of specific occlusal factors did not prove valuable in deciding whether specific symptoms would develop. These findings have been supported by other studies. A dysfunctional index system, devised from combinations of structural and neuromuscular factors, showed that structural factors are frequently related to some symptoms but that neuromuscular factors accounted for the head pain.[18]

A comparative study of 260 nursing students showed that differences in occlusion played no major role in TMD symptoms.[19] The students were diagnosed into the following subgroups: normal, joint disorder, muscle disorder, or joint and muscle disorder. Regression analysis revealed positive associations between the degree of dysfunction and parafunctional habits for the normal, muscle disorder, and joint and muscle disorder subgroups. Positive associations were found between dysfunction and emotional stress in the muscle subgroup. The authors concluded that any relation between potential etiologic factors and dysfunction depended on whether the subjects had muscle or joint disorders.

Significance: Although practitioners may conclude that occlusal disharmonies affect TM symptoms, the variation among studies suggests that no major change can be expected.

Malalignment of the Mandible

Some clinicians consider joint dysfunction as primarily a postural problem. They identify symptoms with malalignment of the condyle in the glenoid fossa. The position of the articular disk is considered deranged if the condyles are positioned improperly. Presumably, the dysfunction derives from a developmental problem concomitant with a dental malocclusion. According to this theoretical cause,[20] an unstable occlusion resulting from either premature tooth contacts or parafunctional oral habits causes malalignment of the mandible. Usually posterior displacement of the mandible results in compression of soft tissues. Undue stress is placed on muscles, ligaments, and bones. Pain, impairment of the blood supply, and degeneration of the joint follow. Based on this malalignment, TMD and malocclusion have been considered synonymous.[21]

This concept has remained popular. As late as 1990, a paper appeared in a leading journal supporting this concept. Condylar displacement originating from occlusal changes was endorsed as the probable cause of TMD, vertigo, tinnitus, and associated auditory symptoms.[22] Several recent papers were listed in the bibliography; none supported a relation between condylar displacement, occlusal prematurities, and TMD. Recognition of these symptoms resurrects Costen's syndrome,[23] a historical relation no longer considered meaningful or valid.[24]

The argument for condylar displacement as an etiology for TMD contrasts sharply with radiologic findings on condylar position in asymptomatic individuals. A critical analysis of 46 tomographs selected from a population of 441 individuals found that a diagnosis of dysfunction could not be based entirely on radiography of nonconcentric condyle–fossa relations.[25] Evaluation of eight additional studies confirmed an unidentifiable relation. Some patients in these studies were symptomatic, and judgments made from transcranial radiographs did not allow for variations in angulation of the condyle.

Another radiographic study of condyle position showed the subjective nature of interpretation. Interexaminer reliability and relation with clinical parameters were studied from transcranial radiographs and tomographs.[26] Observed eccentricity was not related to symptoms, clicking, or crepitation.

Significance: A conclusion that condylar displacement caused by altered occlusion leads to TMD symptomatology must be regarded cautiously. Statements that TMD and malocclusion are synonymous have little merit.

Improper Position of the Head and Spinal Column

The older literature on TMD is filled with descriptions of an orthopedic approach to management. Claims range from a need to clarify joint structure and neuromuscular function to correcting either occluso-muscle imbalance or jaw position. The modern literature has perpetuated many of these claims. The recognition that faulty curvature of the cervical spine may contribute to TMD has been especially noteworthy. Some clinicians may become confused by symptoms that arise from the neck and not the TMJs.

The position of the head is guided by information received from sensory innervations of the neck. Muscles of the dorsal neck region have rich sensory innervations, contain a high number of muscle spindles and Golgi tendon organs, and have many small afferents that conduct pain.[27] This sensory apparatus provides the central nervous system with vital information about the position of the head.

Because the TMJs are anatomically close to the spine, it is logical to argue that the complex of TMJ symptoms includes head, neck and shoulder problems. There is unsubstantiated opinion that subjects presenting with forward head posture and protracted shoulders are prone to TMD. Although poor mechanics between the head and neck may contribute to TMD-like symptoms, no well-controlled studies have been done.

Postural problems were assessed in 164 patients with myofascial pain of the head and neck.[28] The examinations were conducted under conditions considered standard in physical therapy. Most patients had postural problems (Table 4-3). This study would have been more meaningful if comparable data had been available on subjects without myofascial pain matched for age and gender.

Significance: The relation of these structural deviations to TMD remains controversial. Unfortunately, overlap in symptoms between the jaw and the neck has led to some exaggeration of treatment outcome. A letter to the editor of a leading TMJ journal typifies this kind of thinking. The letter states that "patients with scoliosis,

Table 4-3
Percentage of Postural Problems in 164 Patients With
Myofascial Pain

Postural Problem	Patients (%)
Poor sitting or standing posture	96.0
Forward head tilt	84.7
Rounded shoulders	82.3
Poor tongue position	67.7
Abnormal lordosis	46.3
Scoliosis	15.9
Leg length discrepancy	14.0

After Friction JR, Kroenig R, Haley D, Seigert R. Myofascial pain syndrome
of the head and neck: a review of clinical characteristics of 164 patients. Oral
Surg Oral Med Oral Pathol 1985;60:615.

especially those who are asymptomatic, have a highly complex compensatory
mechanism functioning in their bodies. Dental procedures tend to change the proprioceptive balance by either changing TMJ orientation or by totally stabilizing
TMJ migration and therefore eliminating further craniomandibular compensation to
further bodily change."[29] Although dental or TMJ treatment of some patients with
scoliosis may be compromised, such statements are questionable.

Pathophysiologic Conditions

Most etiologic theories concerned with the source of TM symptoms focus either on
pathology of the joints or on changes in the masticatory muscles.[20] A complete health
history followed by a screening radiographic examination may lead to the source of
potential TM pathology.

TMJ pathology may derive from various sources. Intra-articular disorders such as
internal derangement, osteoarthritis, and inflammatory arthritis have been widely
discussed in the literature. There is an ample literature on extra-articular pathology,
including muscular, vascular, and neurologic disorders. Neoplastic disease has been
addressed.

Joint Disorders

INTERNAL DERANGEMENT.   Internal derangement of the TM joint is defined as an
abnormal relation of the articular disk to the mandibular condyle, fossa, and articular
eminence.[30] It has been used to describe problems associated with the movement of
the disk between the head of the condyle and the eminence. Joint noise or a history
of joint sounds is the key symptom of this disorder. The kinds of joint noises are
described in another section of the text.

No aspect of TMD inquiry has become more controversial than the etiology of internal derangement. Little is known about predisposing factors, although numerous
precipitating factors have been postulated, including the following: macrotrauma to
the joint by impact or hyperextension injuries, microtrauma resulting from occlusal

changes, chronic muscular hyperactivity,[30] meniscal perforation secondary to muscle spasm, secondary ligamentous laxity with discontinuity, infection, and arthritis.[31]

The symptoms of internal derangement often mimic symptoms present in patients with myofascial pain. Myofascial pain dysfunction (MPD) syndrome is stress related,[32] and some clinicians have not recognized emotional stress as leading to TMD.[33] They argue that most TMD symptoms derive from internal derangements. The clinical features of internal derangement are essentially similar to features of MPD syndrome or TMJ arthropathy.[34] Malposition and altered position of the disk have been proposed as the basic lesions responsible for the clinical manifestations of these conditions. This argument has been based on an almost 100% correlation between disk displacement and the presence of signs and symptoms, on clinical expression in cases proportional to the degree of pathology found, and on findings of inflammation and mechanical signs and symptoms consistent with pathophysiologic mechanisms.

On the other hand, the view that internal derangement is the primary etiology has been criticized as too narrow. According to one noted clinician, "This is not to say that some percentage of patients with derangements will not develop more advanced problems or even have severe problems initially, but no one knows how large the subgroup is."[24] Most clinicians recognize muscular disorders as distinct from intrinsic joint derangement.[31]

Highly sophisticated studies suggest that TMD symptoms derive from internal derangements. Analyses of the TMJs of adult cadavers indicated that there is a progression of events during internal derangement.[35] Changes in both disk position and disk configuration have been found. The most common disk displacement was anteromedial, but posterior displacement also occurred. Oblique position with biconcave disks or disks of even thicknesses progressed to complete displacement with disks of biconvex configurations. Perforations were found in advanced stages. Advanced disk displacement characterized cases of osteoarthritis.

Three models have been proposed as causing disk displacement: hyperextension of the mandible, condylar displacement caused by trauma, and chronic muscular hypertonicity. In the first model, the mandible is hyperextended by a sudden event or a series of events with ultimate displacement (Fig. 4-1). Once the displacement occurs, arthralgia ensues and protective muscular splinting develops.[36] The second model presumes that the condyle is displaced superiorly and posteriorly in the fossa and that the disk prolapses anteromedially.[34] Usually a blow to the mandible precipitates the onset. The third model presumes that hypertonicity develops within the elevator and lateral pterygoid muscles (Fig. 4-2). Localized myalgia follows as the disk is pulled anteriorly by contracted lateral pterygoid muscles.[36] The disk is displaced anteriorly, and arthralgia develops.

The rationale for the first model appears more plausible than the rationales for the second and third models. Hyperextension of the mandible may result from minor or major events (Fig. 4-3). Sudden yawning or prolonged mouth opening are potential minor causes. Recurrent subluxation from hypermobility of the joint capsule could precede each. Effusion into the joint spaces may cause edema of soft tissues.

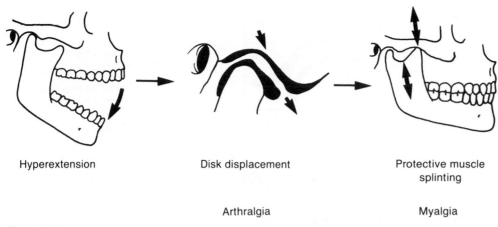

Figure 4-1.
Displacement of the temporomandibular joint disk caused by mandibular hyperextension.
(After Eversole LR, Machado L. Temporomandibular joint internal derangements and
associated neuromuscular disorders. J Am Dent Assoc 1985;110:69.)

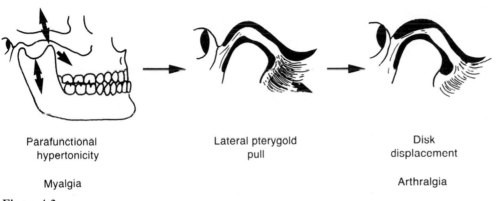

Figure 4-2.
Displacement of the temporomandibular joint disk caused by pull of the lateral pterygoid
muscle. (After Eversole LR, Machado L. Temporomandibular joint internal derangements
and associated neuromuscular disorders. J Am Dent Assoc 1985;110:69.)

An acceleration–deceleration force comparable to the force of whiplash could hyper-extend the mandible and induce displacement. A mechanism has been proposed for disk displacement resulting from whiplash (Fig. 4-3).[37] In a rear-end auto collision, the cranium and neck initially are hyperextended backward. The suprahyoid and infrahyoid muscles are too weak to prevent the backward motion. The mandible moves downward and forward. This hypertranslation occurs because the anterior cap-sule is weakly attached. The forward motion of the condyles stretches the posterior attachment of the disk. As the brakes are applied or the vehicle decelerates to a stop, the body and head move forward. The forward movement of the head causes hyper-flexion of the cervical spine. The condyle moves posteriorly and jams the stretched attachment against the posterior wall of the fossa. In effect, the soft tissues of the joint are subjected to a double whammy—hyperextension followed by hyperflexion.

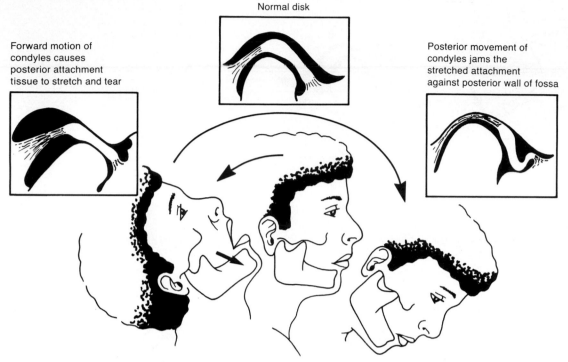

Normal disk

Forward motion of condyles causes posterior attachment tissue to stretch and tear

Posterior movement of condyles jams the stretched attachment against posterior wall of fossa

Figure 4-3.
Displacement of the temporomandibular joint disk by whiplash. Cervical hyperextension causes movement of the condyle, anteriorly stretching the posterior attachment of the disk (left). *Cervical hyperflexion forces the condyle posteriorly, crushing the posterior attachment* (right). *(After Weinberg S, Lapointe H. Cervical extension—flexion injury (whiplash) and internal derangement of the temporomandibular joint. J Oral Maxillofac Surg 1987;45:653.)*

Permanent disk displacement resulting from condylar luxation may be caused by a blow to the mandible. The force must be sufficient to drive the condyle superiorly and posteriorly. Because of the proximity of the condyle to the fossa, logic would have this be in a shearing direction to tear the disk. In light of the high frequency of disk dislocations reported in the literature, one hardly imagines that many displacements derive from injuries of this sort.

One study showed that incisal clenching stretches both the lateral diskal ligament and bilaminar zone.[38] Because of this relation, incisal clenching has been suggested as a major etiologic factor in anterior disk displacement. According to the author of this study, the bilaminar zone is not stretched excessively even on wide opening. The lateral diskal ligament would seem to have a greater role in diskal changes than that of the superior head of the lateral pterygoid muscle. Prolapse could occur only by detaching this muscle from the pterygoid fovea. This was not the case in any of the 26 cadaver TMJs dissected.

A view that the disk prolapses from pull of the lateral pterygoid holds little respect if one considers the anatomy of the lateral pterygoid muscle and its attachment to the disk. Dissection of 25 TM joints obtained from 22 cadavers showed that the upper head of the lateral pterygoid inserts at the medial half of the disk in 60% of the joints, whereas 40% had no muscular insertion to the disk.[39] Manual pull on irradiating fibers stretched the disk, but no forward movement occurred. The authors concluded that the function of the lateral pterygoid could be compared with that of an articular muscle. Thus, if pulling on the lateral pterygoid muscle with fingers fails to induce prolapse, any effect of incisal clenching on disk displacement should be considered minimal.

Significance: Although these studies are revealing, the etiology of internal derangement is unclear. Somehow, some way, the disk becomes displaced. There is no evidence to suggest spontaneous displacement or predisposition for displacement.

OSTEOARTHRITIS. Osteoarthritis is second to internal derangement as a common pathology of the TMJs. Although osteoarthritis can lead to major TMD complaints, most patients suffer mild symptoms. It has been predicted that, on average, 1 person in 10 with generalized osteoarthritis will experience TM joint symptoms.[40] Masticatory muscle tenderness has been the predominant symptom found in these patients (Table 3-6). The presence of other symptoms varies greatly from patient to patient.

The etiology of TMJ arthritis is unknown.[41] It can be differentiated into primary or secondary types. Reportedly, the etiologies differ between the two. Secondary osteoarthritis occurs in young individuals and derives from a prior incidence of trauma. Primary osteoarthritis may be found in the elderly. Usually this degeneration is an age-related deterioration of the articular surfaces and, sometimes, the disk.

A strong argument has been made that prior internal derangement leads to TMJ osteoarthritis.[42] The argument is that soft tissue derangement leads to features recognized as either osteoarthritis, avascular (aseptic) necrosis of the condyle, or regressive remodeling of the condyle (Fig. 4-4). Accordingly, osteoarthritis represents one of three possible degenerative and adaptive changes that occur after internal derangement.

Facial deformity may be an end product of these changes. Osteoarthritis may create insidious skeletal changes, simultaneous intrusion of the teeth, and realignment on the ipsilateral side. On the contralateral side, realignment or tooth eruption occurs as an adaptive response to the ipsilateral skeletal changes. Over the long term, little occlusal change is evident because of this adaptation. A posterior open bite may occur during an occasional episode of joint inflammation. Generally, most joints remain stable unless interrupted by trauma, systemic disease, or hyperextension of the mandible.

AVASCULAR NECROSIS. Avascular necrosis may occur in the mandibular condyle. According to the hypothesis, this may follow systemic disease, trauma, orthognathic surgery, or orthodontics, if the joint is previously deranged.[42] As the surface of the condyle degenerates, mechanical failure follows, leading to a reduction of vertical dimension. Occlusal changes, caused by the decreased vertical dimension, may in-

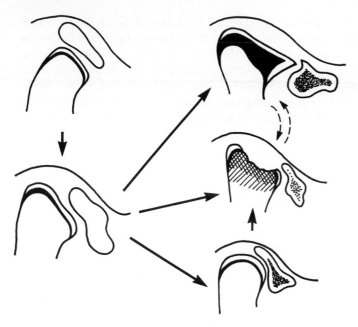

Figure 4-4.
Theoretical patterns of degeneration and remodeling associated with the temporomandibular joint: left, *anatomy of the normal joint;* middle, *disk derangement and early remodeling and deformity of the condyle and cartilage;* upper right, *osteoarthritis;* middle right, *avascular necrosis; and* lower right, *regressive remodeling. (After Schellhas KP, Piper MA, Omlie MR. Facial skeletal remodeling due to temporomandibular joint degeneration: an imaging study of 100 patients. AJR 1990;155:373.)*

clude contralateral anterior open bite with ipsilateral premature contact of the molars. Ultimately, these changes produce facial deformity and lateral shift of the mandible towards the affected joint on mouth opening.

This necrosis may develop in an otherwise metabolically inactive osteoarthritic joint. Potential triggers may include trauma, iatrogenic manipulation, systemic inflammatory illness, or administration of exogenous steroids. Secondary osteoarthritis may be a consequence of avascular necrosis.

REGRESSIVE REMODELING. This remodeling is the third presumed sequela of internal derangement. It is most frequently observed on the articular eminence and on the posterior part of the condyle.[43] There is loss of convexity or flattening of the contour of surfaces. It is both a degenerative and an adaptive process. In contrast to osteoarthritis and avascular necrosis, this remodeling is characterized by osseous remodeling and resorption with eventual decrease in condylar size. The process is slow developing, insidious, and without hypertrophic changes. Loss of vertical dimension is probably accomplished by osteoporosis.

Regressive changes start with early derangement of the disk. As the disk thickens, osteocartilaginous remodeling results. The articular surfaces of both the temporal bone and the condyle undergo this regressive-adaptive process. Occlusal changes may occur if condylar regression is rapid.

Tomographic films show stages of regressive remodeling that differ from stages of osteoarthritis. Unlike osteoarthritis, in which the joint space becomes narrow or obliterated, regressive remodeling shows either a widened or normal anterosuperior articular space.[42] Radiologic findings indicate that regressive remodeling may lead to avascular necrosis and structural deterioration.

On the other hand, there is conflicting evidence that internal derangement precedes the degenerative-adaptive processes. Symptomatic internal derangements have not been associated with high levels of prostaglandins and thromboxane, two inflammatory mediators present in rheumatoid synovial fluid.[44] Cases of osteoarthritis have been found without internal derangement.[45] Some authors argue that prior internal derangement may be regarded as an accompanying sign of osteoarthritis rather than as its cause.[46] For this reason, they consider osteoarthritis a primary rather than secondary pathology.

Some evidence supports this assertion. The microscopic anatomy of osteoarthritic joints resembles the histology of joints with internal derangement. The usual sequence of signs and symptoms of osteoarthritic TMJs is similar to the sequence found in other bodily joints undergoing osteoarthritis. In cases of internal derangement caused by laxity of soft tissues or direct trauma to the joint, osteoarthritis may develop secondarily.

Although the above conclusions merit consideration, other features rule against osteoarthritis as the primary factor in TMD. Osteoarthritis occurs in a much lower frequency than other diagnosed conditions among populations of clinic patients. One example illustrates this point. In 274 patients examined with TMD symptoms, diagnoses were as follows: MPD syndrome (71%), osteoarthritis (9%), symptomless clicking, recurrent subluxation, and rheumatoid arthritis (8%), and conditions unrelated to the TMJs (12%).[47] It is not likely that 7 of 10 patients with MPD syndrome convert to osteoarthritis.

Significance: No one has identified with any degree of certainty a predisposing factor for osteoarthritis. It is not clear if disk displacement precedes osteoarthritic changes, if they occur simultaneously, or if osteoarthritis initiates diskal derangement. The goal of every clinician will be to discover the sequence.

RHEUMATOID ARTHRITIS. Rheumatoid arthritis is an example of an inflammatory synovitis of unknown etiology. Inflammation develops mainly within the synovial membranes of the joints. Involvement of numerous extra-articular organs makes this condition a systemic disorder. Although diverse TMD symptoms have been found in patients with rheumatoid arthritis, some are less pronounced than those found in osteoarthritic patients (Table 3-6). As in osteoarthritis, the major TMD symptoms are masticatory muscle tenderness and joint crepitation. A chief difference is that rheumatoid arthritis is a symmetric synovitis affecting joints bilaterally. Usually joints of the hands and feet are affected first. The cervical spine may become involved late in the course of the disease. Patients may suffer from lateral neck pain as inflammation develops at the C1–C2 articulation.[48] Orofacial pain may be referred from the neck.

Rheumatoid arthritis affects few individuals of the general population (about 3%).[48] Usually, the more the severe the disease, the greater the risk of TMJ involvement. A study of 123 patients with rheumatoid arthritis predicted that 1 in 3 individuals with generalized rheumatoid arthritis will experience TM symptoms.[40]

Significance: Any patient with TMD symptoms and simultaneous symmetric joint symptoms lasting for 3 weeks or longer should be referred to a rheumatologist for evaluation of possible rheumatoid arthritis.

Muscle Disorders

Judged purely from clinical impressions, changes in the masticatory muscles have been considered secondary to mechanical jamming of the disk[49] or to trauma-induced internal derangements.[34] Because many patients with internal derangement suffer from complaints of the masticatory muscles, alternate opinions favor muscle changes over joint problems. The logic is that the masticatory muscles initiate symptoms and subsequent joint pathology. The literature is replete with information about muscular changes involved in TMD. Some terms include hyperactivity, hypertonicity (splinting), myospasm, myalgia, and trigger points.

HYPERACTIVITY. Hyperactivity of the jaw muscles has long been considered a primary etiologic factor in TMD.[32,50–52] Theoretically, excessive emotional stress promotes the hyperactivity. The stress-related hyperactivity forms the basis for the Psychophysiological Model of the Etiology of Myofascial Pain Dysfunction Syndrome (Fig. 4-5).[32] A pain–dysfunction cycle is set off in patients already predisposed psychologically and physiologically to inner stress. Hyperactivity also may develop secondarily if one is subjected to physical stresses.

Some of the problems in accepting hyperactivity as a prime etiologic factor derive from semantics. Traditionally, hyperactivity means abnormally sustained muscle tension, but it also may mean elevated muscle activity detected electromyographically. The reader is not always certain which definition is meant. The first definition is used here.

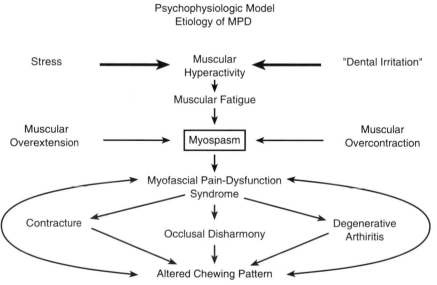

Figure 4-5.
The psychophysiologic model of etiology of myofascial pain dysfunction syndrome: larger arrows indicate greater importance than smaller arrows. (Adapted from Blasberg B, Chambers A, Temporomandibular pain and dysfunction syndrome associated with generalized musculoskeletal pain: a retrospective study, J Rheumatol 1989 (suppl 19); 16:87. After Laskin DM. Etiology of the pain-dysfunction syndrome. J Am Dent Assoc 1969;79:147.)

A thorough review of hyperactivity has been discussed from a theoretical basis.[20] The authors considered local causes and centrally mediated causes for this activity. They concluded that local factors exclusive of trauma appear unlikely to cause hyperactivity. Under centrally mediated causes, psychological and physical stresses were discussed. The authors summarized studies of subjects with MPD who were exposed to experimentally induced stress. They concluded that causal factors cannot be determined from these correlational studies and that methodologic problems make testing for differences between symptomatic and asymptomatic subjects appear futile.

Since publication of this review, a pathophysiologic model for masticatory muscle hyperactivity in TMD has been proposed. The model proposes a centrally mediated cause, yet it maintains support for present peripheral causes.[52] The authors hypothesize that the hyperactivity represents a mild extrapyramidal disorder distantly related to orofacial dyskinesias (eg, tardive dyskinesia). They consider this relation based on experimental evidence of an underlying neurotransmitter imbalance in the basal ganglia. This imbalance involves dopaminergic preponderance or cholinergic and gamma-aminobutyric acid-nergic hypofunction. Supposedly, during nonstressful periods, muscular activity remains in a subclinical state. During stressful periods, an imbalance results in hyperactivity. This hypothesis requires additional study.

Hyperactivity has been hypothesized as a contributing factor in disk displacement,[30,53] but recent investigations fail to support this assumption. Based on anatomic studies of the relation of the lateral pterygoid muscle and the disk, hyperactivity can be ruled out as a direct cause of disk displacement. Some disks lack direct connection with the lateral pterygoid muscle, and even pulling on this muscle did not cause significant prolapse.[39]

Although it is logical to expect a progressive increase in symptoms after prolonged hyperactivity, studies show that this does not occur. No progression of symptoms was found in a study of emotional stress among 39 subjects with combined muscle and TMJ pain compared with 24 subjects having only muscle pain or 28 with joint pain.[54] The lowest levels of stress occurred in the combined pain group. This group was rated lower than the muscle pain group by clinicians in terms of psychological factors, stress, and pain chronicity. Combined pain subjects and muscle pain subjects had comparable levels of visual analogue scores (VAS) for pain intensity and activity impairment. Comparable clinician ratings were found for the combined pain and joint pain groups. In summary, no well-defined relation has been established between hyperactivity and TM symptoms at this time.

MYOSPASM. The definition of muscle spasm does not seem to fit within the etiologic framework of the MPD theory. Muscular responses may include spasm, but to call an elevated tensional period a spasm is a misnomer.[46] Occasional trismus may occur. Under normal adaptive circumstances, however, there is no evidence that the masticatory muscle is predisposed to spasm. Many patients with TMD present with widespread tenderness of the muscles to palpation. Although some subjects may report that their face hurts, many are unaware that the muscles are sore. Few could tolerate the pain of sustained contraction diffusing throughout the orofacial musculature on a long-term basis.

FATIGUE.   Fatigue may be a significant factor in causing muscle pain. Levels of tension may build in the musculature, leading to chronic fatigue and, potentially, to dysfunction. Subjective reports of fatigue in the jaws have been evaluated in adolescents. A longitudinal study of 285 adolescents found that fatigue in the jaws was prevalent in 18% of 17 year olds.[55] Results obtained by questionnaire from 264 of these subjects at 19 years old showed higher percentages, with fatigue related to pain of the face or jaws, difficulties in chewing and opening wide, and recurrent headaches. Subjects who described themselves as being tense reported significantly more fatigue in the jaws. Awareness of clenching was related to fatigue, whereas teeth grinding and frequent chewing of gum were not. Clinical examination revealed that 56% of subjects reporting fatigue in the jaws had four or more sites tender to palpation. The authors concluded that subjective reports of fatigue in the jaw may be symptomatic of dysfunction in adolescents.

TRIGGER POINTS.   A trigger point is a tender area in a firm band of muscle tissue. These localized hyperirritable foci can be found in any skeletal muscle. They populate the muscles of the head, neck, shoulders, and lower back. Trigger points may refer pain. The referred area is the zone of reference. They can be active causing referred pain on palpation or can be latent (silent) with the potential for action.[56] There is a local twitch response to quick tapping. Generally speaking, the pattern of pain from a trigger point in any specific muscle is consistent from person to person. Details for specific trigger points and zones of referral are presented in the chapter under diagnosis.

Trigger points are thought to be activated by acute or chronic muscular overload, fatigue, or trauma. Speculation is that myofascial pain is the end product of this overload. Two different causes have been proposed for the origin of myofascial pain resulting from trigger points. Histologic examination has confirmed the presence of degenerated areas of muscle termed *fibrous nodules*. Most of the nodule consists of acid mucopolysaccharide.[57] In these areas, the muscle fascicle herniates, releasing histamine and 5-hydroxytryptamine from degrading mast cells. Presumably, hyperactive tonic contraction produces the structural modification. These areas may be active or silent. There is no agreement on how these tiny fibrous nodules elicit pain.

A modification of this hypothesis attributes the myofascial symptoms to release of noxious substances from chronically contracting muscles. Within the entire muscle or localized area, oxidative activities may increase. These activities release inflammatory substances (eg, bradykinin, prostaglandin) and potassium, which could cause excitation of type III and IV muscular nociceptors.[58] If this sustained contraction occurs locally, say at a trigger point, muscular fatigue may result. Steady contraction causes less blood flow, lowers ATP reserves, and slows the calcium pump. Free calcium interacts with ATP to trigger contractile activity, particularly if actin and myosin are overlapping in the shortened muscle.[28] A self-sustaining cycle develops so that noxious substances are released near the trigger point followed by a reduction in the activity of the calcium pump.

Feedback systems link trigger points and zones of referral to the central nervous system. This linkage establishes a reflex. When mechanical stresses, perhaps faulty body posture, are added to this reverberatory neural circuit, myofascial pain results.

Trigger point activity can be perpetuated by lesions in the joints or by remote visceral disease.

TENDER POINTS.   Like myofascial pain, fibromyalgia is a common cause of musculoskeletal pain and fatigue. This condition is a generalized disease with bilaterally symmetrical tender points. Tender points are the hallmark of fibromyalgia. Like active trigger points, they are tender when palpated. Unlike trigger points, the pain remains localized.[59] Usually trigger points of MPD are unilateral.

Tender points may occur within the same general area as trigger points. Because of this simultaneous presence, individuals with trigger points of the masticatory muscles may represent only a subgroup of patients with fibromyalgia. These subjects could be thought of as having masticatory fibromyalgia. A discussion of the overlapping characteristics of fibromyalgia and MPD has been published.[60]

An etiologic hypothesis has been suggested for fibromyalgia. Muscle microtrauma at the sarcomere has been proposed as the initiating factor.[61] This injury changes the permeability of the sarcolemmic membrane and permits an influx of calcium ions and an efflux of potassium. Contraction of contiguous sarcomeres results from this calcium influx. Normal mechanisms for decreasing calcium levels are overwhelmed, and the elevated levels of calcium maintain sarcomere contraction. The ATP becomes depleted leading to an uncoupling of actin-myosin cross-bridges. The involved sarcomeres remain contracted, causing a focal rigor mortis. Injured sarcomeres release potassium ions, activating type C unmyelinated nerve fibers causing pain. Eventually, localized response to injury results in the release of inflammatory substances that stimulate type C fibers. Pain continues. This mechanism may also explain the origin of pain at trigger points.

Significance: Muscle disorders account for most complaints reported by patients. Increased tension, rather than spasm or hyperactivity, would seemed to fit most muscular complaints of the jaw. Some tension may end in soreness, but not terminate in pain. Evidence suggests fatigue and trigger points relate to the genesis of pain. Some patients develop muscle complaints and joint complaints simultaneously. Few patients develop joint disorders independent of muscle disorders.

Cervical Spinal Disorders

Cervical spinal disorders may lead to complaints often associated with TMD (Table 4-4). Pain may be felt along the side of the head from disorders of the C2 to C3 vertebrae.[62] A possible mechanism whereby pathology of the cervical spine could lead to pain in the trigeminal system would include the input by way of the upper cervical nerve roots.[63] The descending tract of the trigeminal nerve passes ipsilaterally to the midcervical part of the spinal cord. A nociceptive impulse from degenerated cervical facets could refer pain to dermatomal distribution of the trigeminal nerve. Thus, this referred pain would not originate from the TMJs.

Cervical spine disorders may, in fact, result in bizarre symptoms.[62,64] These disorders may involve pain of the head, sinuses, face, ear, and throat. Sensory disturbances of the pharynx, vertigo, tinnitus, diminished hearing, sweating, flushing, lacrimation,

Table 4-4
Relation of Cervical Source of Pain and Referred
Location of Pain

Source	Referred Area
Occiput-atlas	Forehead, retro-orbital, may be bilateral
Cervical—2nd vertebra	Retro-orbital, temporal
Cervical—3rd vertebra	Occiput, lateral side of head
Cervical—4th–7th vertebra and thoracic—1st vertebra	Shoulder

After Bland JH. Disorders of the cervical spine: diagnosis and medical
management. Philadelphia: WB Saunders, 1987.

and salivation are possible symptoms. Because of the arrangement of the sympathetic
nervous system in the cervical spine, headache, nystagmus, nausea, vomiting, and
suboccipital tenderness may occur.[65] Some patients with TMD may experience these
symptoms. A thorough cervical neck examination may clarify the issue.

Headache

Because some patients with jaw symptoms have concomitant headache, the question
remains whether headache should be considered part of the overall TMD symptomatology. According to the *Guide to Dental Health* published by the American Dental
Association in 1985, TMD is often misdiagnosed because of an array of symptoms
common to several diseases.[66] Headaches, sometimes of migrainous proportions, are
listed as symptoms.

The etiology of most headaches remains complex and uncertain, and it is difficult to
clarify any probable relation. This uncertainty, coupled with the multifactorial etiologies of TMD, offers few opportunities for solving this puzzle.

Because the classification of headaches is subjective and many variants exist, this
discussion focuses on those painful cranial complaints neurologically diagnosed as
vascular (migraine, cluster), tension (muscle contraction), and cervicogenic headaches. Only those publications that suggest an association between headache and
TMD are discussed.[66]

Muscle contraction headache predominated in a study of patients who presented
with unsatisfactory dentures.[67] Forty percent of the 43 patients reported recurrent
headache. No patient was completely free of TMD symptoms. In two different
groups of 80 patients, the frequency of recurrent headache correlated with the frequency of masticatory muscle pain and TMJ pain on palpation, but not with several
other TMD symptoms.[68]

TMD symptoms were studied in three groups of 38 patients with different kinds of
headache and in 25 healthy subjects without headaches.[69] Subgroups of patients were
identified with either muscle contraction headache (13) common migraine (17), or a

combination of both (18). Tenderness on palpation of the pericranial muscles proved significantly greater in the headache patients than in the healthy subjects. The pain reported was least severe with migraine headaches, increased with muscle contraction headaches, and was most severe with combination headache. On an average, nine tender areas were found per headache patient. Twenty-nine of the 38 headache group had pain referred to other areas on palpation of the tender areas. Tenderness was blamed on abnormal tonic hyperactivity in the masticatory muscles and neck. Bruxism was greater in headache patients than in healthy subjects. No differences were found for malocclusion or loss of molars.

There is considerable support for a relation between common migraine and TMD symptoms. It has been argued that the common migraine is a muscular rather than vascular disorder.[70] Comparison of 100 patients referred to a hospital neurology clinic showed variability of TMD symptoms and the type of headache. Patients were diagnosed as having tension, migraine, or combination headaches.[71] Just three of 19 common signs and symptoms proved significantly different among the subgroups: tenderness on palpation of the masseter, tenderness of the temporalis muscles, and dynamic pain. This pain was identified as the patient performed mandibular movements with the examiner exerting slight manual resistance against the mandible. Several other differences were found between groups. Unfortunately, the data were marred by unacceptable statistics. The three significant symptoms should have been tested further. Only tenderness on palpation of the masseter proved greater for patients with combination headaches versus migraine patients. An acceptable level of significance should have been $P < 0.01$, not $P < 0.05$. Finally, the authors were unable to prove that the subgroups differed in myogenous or arthrogenous origins of pain. They concluded that patients with TMD pain suffered more from permanently present headache and subjective neck problems than patients without pain.

In contrast to the findings of the above-mentioned studies, no significant differences in TMD symptoms were found between groups with a different neurologic diagnosis of headache.[72]

There is considerable evidence that headache may arise from myofascial trigger points of masticatory, neck, and back muscles. Palpation studies illustrate the complexity of these relations. Both the location of the painful area and the respective trigger points were identified in 164 MPD patients who presented with headache.[28] About one third of these patients complained of postauricular pain traced to trigger points in the sternocleidomastoid, deep masseter, and digastric musculature. Just over one half complained of temporal pain that originated from four trigger point areas, namely, the temporalis, trapezius, and splenius capitis muscles (Table 4-5). Just less than one half had occipital pain emanating from the trapezius, semispinalis capitis, and levator scapulae.

A specific variant, cervicogenic headache, has been defined as a unilateral pain felt in the head but originating from the neck.[73] The anatomic proximity of certain cranial nerves and the trigeminal nerve may account for this pathophysiology. Because neurons of the trigeminal nerve and nerves VII, IX, and X share the same neuron pool with neurons of C_1 to C_3 of the cervical spine, pain emanating from the neck may be referred to the face and mandible.[74,75] Pain impulses may be felt at the trigeminal

Table 4-5

Relation of Painful Area with Trigger Point Location in Headache Patients

Pain Area	Trigger Point	Patients (%)
Supraorbital	Anterior temporalis Sternocleidomastoid Trapezius	9.8
Retro-orbital	Anterior temporalis Trapezius	29.9
Forehead	Sternocleidomastoid Splenius capitis	36.0
Temple	Anterior temporalis Middle temporalis Trapezius Splenius capitis	51.8
Postauricular	Sternocleidomastoid Deep masseter Digastric	36.6
Vertex	Splenius capitis Semispinalis capitis	34.7
Occipital	Trapezius Semispinalis capitis Levator scapulae	45.7

After Friction JR, Kroening R, Haley D, Siegert R. Myofascial pain syndrome of the head and neck: a review of clinical characteristics of 164 patients. Oral Surg Oral Med Oral Pathol 1985;60:615.

sclerotomes and dermatomes (V_1, V_2) from afferent pain fibers mediated by C2 rootlets,[74] (Fig. 4-6). Additional evidence to support this assertion is that surgical decompression or dissection of the C2 root eliminated or improved the cervicogenic headaches in 15 of 16 patients.[76]

Cervicogenic headache can be precipitated or intensified by head movement or by pressing on trigger points.[74] Palpation of several muscles of the neck, including the splenius capitis, splenius cervicis, and sternocleidomastoid, was conducted on 11 patients with cervicogenic headache.[77] Headache was reproduced in 8 patients by palpation. All had at least three trigger points on the symptomatic side. A comparison of symptomatic and asymptomatic sides found significant differences in the tender areas. Some 70 tender points (35 very tender and 35 tender) and 17 nonfascial tender points occurred on the symptomatic side, whereas there were 22 tender (one very tender and 21 tender) and 19 nonfascial tender points on the asymptomatic side. All patients had cervical dysfunction. Specific segmental dysfunction was found at the occiput on atlas or at the atlas on axis in 10 patients. The author concluded that trigger points may be a significant pain-producing mechanism in cervicogenic headache and segmental cervical dysfunction.

Some migraineurs present with TMD symptoms. Trigger factors, identified by patient self-report, have been studied in 217 migraineurs.[78] These trigger factors included the menstrual cycle (51.5% of the women), alcoholic beverages (51.6%), and psychic stress (48.8%). Alimentary triggers predominated in alcohol-susceptible patients compared with patients lacking these triggers. It was hypothesized that the

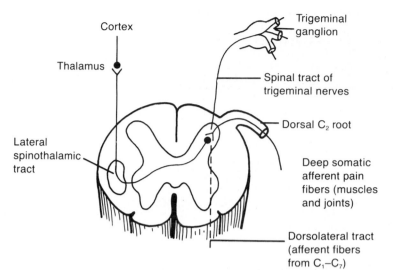

Figure 4-6.
Relation of cervical nerve 2 in the dorsal horn with the spinal tract of the trigeminal nerve. Cervical pain may be referred to the trigeminal tract at this junction. (After Pfaffenrath V, Dandekar R, Pollman W. Cervicogenic headache—the clinical picture, radiological findings and hypothesis on its pathophysiology. Headache 1987;27:495.)

gut of some migraineurs may be unduly permeable for certain substances. No significant difference was found between menstrual-related migraine and patients lacking triggers. Menstrual migraine attacks were often preceded by depressive symptoms. The authors speculated that migraineurs may share similar precipitating factors as individuals suffering from TMD.

Significance: The link between certain kinds of headaches and TMD symptoms seems plausible. Sufficient evidence exists to tie certain orofacial pains with dysfunctions originating from neck and masticatory musculature. Some trigger factors may be the same for both. Headaches are present in some patients with TMD symptoms and absent in others. Those of cervical origin should be considered distinct from the symptom complex of TMD.

Neoplastic Disease

The literature reveals few cases of malignant disease directly evolving from the TMJs. Therefore, most of these tumors should be classified as precipitating factors rather than as predisposing factors.

Malignant disease may disguise as TMD. A review of the literature found 42 cases of malignancy that mimicked TMD.[79,80] A summary of the symptoms showed that swelling was the chief problem, occurring in 54% of the cases (Table 4-6). An inability to open the mouth widely and deficits of the acoustic nerve were the next most prevalent symptoms. Pain did not prove to be a specific symptom, but altered motor sensory sensations (paresis or paresthesia) were common in just over one fourth of the cases.

These studies indicate that gender differences exist in the prevalence of these malignancies (Table 4-7). Women had more metastasis from the breast and pharynx than men. On the other hand, men were found with more squamous cell carcinomas of the maxillofacial area, sarcomas, and adenocarcinomas than women. These findings

Table 4-6

Signs and Symptoms of 41 Cases of Malignant Disease that Mimicked TMD

Symptom	Patients (%)
Swelling	54
Trismus	34
Auditory changes	34
Paresis or parathesia	27
Occlusal change	10

After Bavitz JB, Chewning LC. Malignant disease as temporomandibular joint dysfunction: review of the literature and report of case. J Am Dent Assoc 1990;120:163.

indicate that previously asymptomatic individuals 50 years or older should be examined carefully for malignancy if TMD-like symptoms suddenly appear.

Significance: Subjects should be questioned about the possibility of previous malignancy.

Uncommon Causes

NEURALGIAS. Neuralgias, including trigeminal, glossopharyngeal, or atypical (vascular) neuralgias, contribute little to TMD symptoms. No mention was made of concomitant TMD symptoms in a review of 689 cases of trigeminal neuralgia[81] or in 6 cases of glossopharyngeal neuralgia.[82] The quality of pain for most neuralgias differs so sharply from the pain of TMD that they are not easily confused.[83] Well-defined jabs of pain characterize these neuralgias, whereas the quality of muscular pain is more constant. The severity of neuralgia may lead secondarily to increased muscular complaints. Other clinical findings, such as tenderness or limitation on opening, may be present simultaneously. They are not primarily related to the neuralgia.

A case of acute inflammation of the TMJ has been proposed as causing the onset of trigeminal neuralgia.[84] The authors concluded that this distant focus of inflammation represented a peripheral mechanism triggering the onset of neuralgia by increased afferent stimulation.

Significance: Neuralgias should be ruled out during the diagnostic phase. No firm relation has been established between TMD and neuralgias.

VASCULAR DISORDERS. Reports of TMD-like pain from cardiac origin are rare. An episode of mandibular pain appeared a few hours preceding an acute myocardial infarction in a white woman with coronary insufficiency.[85] Four other cases of mandibular pain were attributed to myocardial infarction and 1 case to angina pectoris.[86] The 2 male patients with infarcts had right mandibular pain, and the 2 women had bilateral mandibular pain. Another case of left jaw pain or toothache present in a white woman was attributed to left atrial hypertrophy and right bundle branch block.[87] Simultaneous presence of jaw pain and vascular pain was explained by overlap of cervical nerve C_3–spinal nerve T_1 with the trigeminal nerve. These examples

Table 4-7

Final Diagnosis of 42 Cases of Malignant Disease That Mimicked TMD

Malignant Disease	No. of Cases
Women (21 Patients)	
Metastatic breast	6
Pharyngeal	4
Nasopharyngeal (3)	
Oropharyngeal (1)	
Parotid	3
Mucoepidermoid (2)	
Adenocystic (1)	
Maxillofacial squamous cell	2
Hypophyseal	1
Transitional cell	1
Undifferentiated	1
Schwannoma	1
Fibrous histiocytoma	1
Metastatic adenocarcinoma	1
Men (21 Patients)	
Maxillofacial squamous cell	5
Prostatic adenocarcinoma	3
Adenocarcinoma	3
Sarcoma	3
Synovial cell (1)	
Synovial fibrosarcoma (1)	
Chondrosarcoma of TMJ (1)	
Nasopharyngeal	2
Multiple myeloma	1
Adenoid cystic	1
Metastatic lung	1
Schwannoma	1
Intercranial metastatic melanoma	1

Data from Bavitz JB, Chewning LC. Malignant disease as temporomandibular joint dysfunction: review of the literature and report of case. J Am Dent Assoc 1990;120:163, and Boyczuk EM, Solomon MP, Gold BD. Unremitting pain to the mandible secondary to metastatic breast cancer: a case report. Compend Contin Educ Dent 1991;12:104.

of myocardial pain referred to the jaw or teeth were identified by historical relation with vascular disease.

Significance: Vascular disorders, exclusive of headache, generally contribute little to TMD symptoms.

RESPIRATORY DISORDERS. Other bizarre causes of orofacial pain have been described. Hyperventilation, or overbreathing, has been documented as a cause of orofacial pain. Light-headedness, dizziness, and shortness of breath were described as classic symptoms of hyperventilation.[88] The authors examined a patient with recurring episodes of sharp, burning pain on the left side of the face, radiating from the top of the scalp to the midline of the mandible. The pain was accompanied by dizziness, sweating, and a tingling sensation over the affected area. Deep breathing for 1 minute initiated severe orofacial pain. Blood pressure and heart rate rose dramatically. Psychometric evaluation found elevated levels for hypochondriasis, depression, and hysteria.

Significance: Hysteria leading to hyperventilation may mimic some TMD symptoms. Fortunately, this is not a common occurrence.

CONNECTIVE TISSUE DISORDERS. Few patients with TMD symptoms have connective tissue disease. In systemic lupus erythematosus, muscle pains occur in up to one third of these patients and appear unrelated to the degree of disease.[48] Some patients may develop a painless form of myositis.

Significance: Individuals with suspicious recurrent skin or circulatory complaints should be referred for laboratory testing.

Precipitating Factors

Trauma

Trauma as a potential precipitating factor in TMD has created much interest and speculation. Aside from the pain and discomfort experienced by the injured person, the potential for litigation may be considerable. A blow to the head or whiplash of the neck, especially during a motor vehicle accident, has been and continues to be a reason for litigation.

Retrospective studies have implicated many kinds of physical trauma in the etiology of TMD symptoms.[89–91] An analysis of different investigations revealed that the prevalence of trauma ranges from 9% to 43% in large clinical populations with TMD symptoms (Table 4-8). A history of trauma was found in 68% of 75 patients.[92] The sample was limited, however, to patients with secondary osteoarthritis of the TMJ.

Trauma was considered the precipitating factor in 43% of TMD cases in a large private practice. Two percent of the accident victims had no immediate or residual complaints from the head or neck injuries.[93] Attempts have been made to divide cases of precipitating from predisposing trauma. Evaluation of a large TMD clinic population showed that 30% had a history of trauma (see Table 4-8). Precipitating trauma was identified as the major factor in causing TMD pain. Percentages were not significantly different for precipitating and predisposing trauma.

Trauma to the jaw was considered etiologically important in only 16.8% of 246 patients consecutively admitted to a TMD clinic.[94]

Significantly greater TMD symptoms have been found in patients with a trauma history compared with nontrauma subjects (see Table 4-8). Examination of patients after road traffic accidents showed significantly higher levels of orofacial pain, abnormal joint sounds, and restricted jaw opening when compared with other TMD cases.[95] Trauma figured in the difference between TM symptomatic patients and asymptomatic normals and between symptomatic women and asymptomatic normal dental students and hygienists.[96]

Table 4-8
Reports of Trauma Associated With TMD

Sample	No. of Patients	Gender F/M	Trauma	TMD Symptoms (%)	Reference
TMD clinic	227	—	Accident	11	89
			Oral surgery	11	
			Prosthetic tx	16	
			Unknown	52	
			Miscellaneous	10	
Hospital clinic	401	1/1	Road accident	9	95
TMD clinic and	90	8/1	Joint injury	21	90
			Dental tx	24	
Private practice	48	2.7/1	Emotional stress	26	
			Unknown	36	
Clinic	75	—	Orofacial	68	92
TMD clinic	224	3/1	Accident—		91
			Predisposing	13	
			Precipitating	11	
			Both	6	
Private practice	729	8/1	Accident—		93
			Blow to head or neck, vehicle, fall, fight	22	
			Whiplash	19	
			Oral surgery	1	
			Intubation	<1	
TMD clinic	152	2/1	Head or neck		96
			Women	35	
			Men	58	
			Ortho tx		
			Women	50	
			Men	42	
			Oral surgery		
			Women	71	
			Men	57	
Dental and hygiene students		1.3/1			96
Symptomatic	215		Head or neck		
			Women	21	
			Men	17	
			Ortho tx		
			Women	48	
			Men	37	
			Oral Surgery		
			Women	49	
			Men	56	
Asymptomatic	116		Head or neck		96
			Women	8	
			Men	12	
			Ortho tx		
			Women	32	
			Men	38	
			Oral surgery		
			Women	47	
			Men	44	
Hospital clinic	540		Head or neck		34
		7/1	Primary	33	
			Secondary	9	
TMD clinic	—	—	Jaw	17	94
Hospital clinic	40		Cervical trauma		103
	75		Radiologic pos.	0	
			Radiologic neg.	<1	

tx, treatment

Trauma may cause specific disturbances of the TMJ area. Direct injury to the joint has been proposed as a cause of TMJ osteoarthritis.[97] Several authors have proposed it as the etiology for anterior dislocation of the disk.[34,42,92,98] Statistical analysis showed a positive relation between trauma and internal derangement (Fig. 4-7).[96]

Extensive damage to the joint has been documented after injury. In a study of 30 patients who sustained TM joint injuries, direct blows to the mandible accounted for 20 of the injuries, and 10 cases were whiplash injuries.[42] Various symptoms were found. Of the 30 patients, 27 denied that they had previously bothersome TMD symptoms. Eight patients had mandibular fractures. Radiologic imaging performed on the joints 2 days to 2 years after the injuries showed evidence of disk derangement, degenerative condylar remodeling, osteoarthritis, osteochondritis dissecans, avascular necrosis, swelling of retrodiskal tissue, joint effusion, musculotendinous injuries, and atrophy of masticatory muscles.

If injury is sufficient to alter normal mechanics of the mandible, then internal derangement might account for the dental occlusal discomfort experienced by traumatized individuals (see Fig. 4-7).[96] Sudden changes in the vertical dimension, caused by disk derangement, have been suggested as capable of altering the occlusion.[99,100] A little trauma may be sufficient to promote the appearance of symptoms.[34] Primary trauma was differentiated from secondary trauma. Secondary trauma was designated when there was an obvious, preexisting derangement.

Significance: The clinician must document any serious trauma experienced by the patient. The chief problem in most cases will be to determine whether the joint was struck directly by a blow or whether the injury occurred indirectly when another part of the head, jaw, face, or neck was injured.

Whiplash

Anecdotal remarks imply a direct relation between whiplash and TMD symptoms. Judged from complaints of subjects injured in vehicular mishaps, whiplash may precipitate TMD symptoms. Because reports of whiplash are obtained retrospectively, pretrauma objective data are usually lacking. Some information may be obtained from preexisting dental or medical records.

The similarity of whiplash symptoms in so many patients under different circumstances points to pathophysiologic changes. A review of the literature indicates that whiplash accounted for 19% of the accident-related TMD symptoms in a large clinic population (see Table 4-8).[93] Although TMD pain was not related specifically to whiplash, its onset was reported to be related to motor vehicular accidents in 17.7% of 164 cases of myofascial pain.[28]

One study predicted that nearly 60% of 37 whiplash victims or subjects sustaining blows to the face or neck and developing myofascial pain or headache would remain symptomatic for the remainder of their lives.[47]

Whiplash may produce disturbances at specific anatomic sites of the head, TMJs, and cervical musculature. Ten of 14 patients treated for whiplash obtained relief from

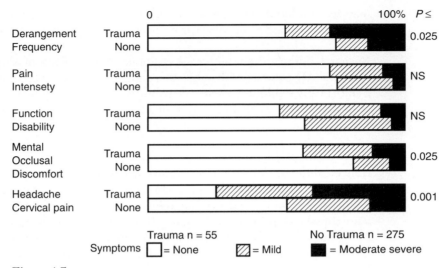

Figure 4-7.
Five symptoms of non-TMD patients with or without a history of moderate to severe head trauma. Significant relations were found for internal derangement, headache–cervical pain, and occlusal discomfort. (After Pullinger AG, Monteiro AA. History factors associated with symptoms of temporomandibular disorders. J Oral Rehabil 1988;15:117.)

head pain and 8 from cervical pain.[101] Assessment of 28 patients injured by whiplash showed that 22 of 25 suffered arthrographically evident internal derangement.[37] Arthrograms of the inferior joint space confirmed varying degrees of derangement. On average, the patients were examined 126 days after the accident.

Ten patients symptomatic for TMJ pain were examined for internal derangement 2 days to 2 years after the whiplash event.[100] Imaging studies showed the joints of 3 patients to be normal. Six patients had build-up of intra-articular fluid. Of 3 patients with painful, clicking joints, 2 showed early stages of disk derangement and 1 was normal. These variable findings confirm the possibility of internal derangement in certain patients. A complete radiographic and imaging study of the joints may be necessary to rule out derangement.

The literature on the effects of whiplash on the cervical spine is large. There is popular support for and against the argument that whiplash produces cervical dysfunction and TMD-like symptoms. Whiplash may alter normal craniovertebral posture (see Fig. 4-3). Mechanoreceptors present in the upper cervical spine are quite sensitive to slight changes in normal posture of the head, neck, and mandible. Postconcussional syndrome, including headache, may occur in the absence of cranial injury when the subject has experienced acceleration–deceleration forces.[63] Post-traumatic craniovertebral symptoms mimic many symptoms of TMD. Superficial structures of the head and face posterior to the trigeminal area and extending to the angle of the mandible are innervated by C_1 to C_3 nerves (see Table 4-4). The ear surface and surfaces posteriorly, and the sternocleidomastoid and trapezius muscles, are innervated by these sensory fibers. Irritation, compression, or entrapment of these nerves may lead to localized pains of the orbit, occiput, and angle of the mandible. Post-traumatic headache may occur from occipital and posterior cervical pain.[63]

Research findings differ with respect to the adverse effects of whiplash. A comparison of non-TMD patients with subjects having a history of head or neck trauma showed a statistically significant greater distribution of mild and moderately severe symptoms of headache-cervical pain in the traumatized group than in the nontrauma group (see Fig. 4-7).[96]

Many similarities and few differences have been found between subjects who experienced different kinds of overt injury and whiplash. A comparison of patients (31 with overt head trauma, 35 with whiplash without overt head trauma, and 34 with whiplash and overt head trauma) found no consistent differences in muscle pressure pain threshold, prior pain duration, time before pain onset, or scores obtained on psychological tests between groups.[102] Whiplash subjects with overt trauma reported the greatest pain on presentation. Subjects without overt trauma were more likely to be in litigation and to have more sleep disturbances, painful sites on palpation, and neck pain than subjects of the other groups.

In contrast, another study presents contradictory evidence of adverse effects. Patients with cervical musculoskeletal injury were interviewed, examined, and divided into those with radiologic and those without radiologic evidence of injury (see Table 4-8).[103] Just 1 patient without radiologic damage reported new TMJ symptoms. Follow-up conducted 1 month later revealed that just 2 patients with radiologic pathology had TMJ pain. No patient without radiologic pathology had new TMJ symptoms. The follow-up interview was made by telephone.

Significance: Whatever role whiplash plays in precipitating TMD symptoms, its effects vary widely between individuals and situations. Differences between studies confirm the need for thorough neuromuscular examination of the cervical spine in subjects with TMD symptoms who have experienced whiplash.

Dental Treatment

Patients often ask if a particular dental treatment causes adverse effects or improves a preexisting TMD condition. Loss of teeth, orthodontics, prosthetic treatment, or root canal therapy are the most frequently asked about procedures.

Loss of Teeth

Many clinicians consider that the loss of teeth and subsequent loss of vertical dimension produces overclosure. The overclosure causes the mandible to be malaligned, resulting in joint disturbances. This malalignment alters the position of the condyle in the fossa, which tends to "overload" the joint. Although collapse after loss of posterior teeth has been suggested as a contributing factor in TMD, doubt remains about any positive relation.[15]

There is evidence to contradict the argument that joint disturbances occur with tooth loss. No significant difference between tooth loss and joint disturbances was found in one study,[104] but opposite findings were presented in two other studies. Unilateral tooth loss was common on the side opposite the dysfunction[105] but was identified with the same side in another study.[106] The latter study involved 326 patients admitted to a hospital dental clinic. Three fourths of the patients had missing teeth. The author concluded that occlusal support was important in the etiology of TMD, reaching a maximal relation with 3 to 5 teeth missing and declining thereafter. Differences were found between patients when compared with individuals of the general population, but the data were not analyzed statistically. Finally, no statistically significant correlation was found between loss of molar support and crepitation or tenderness to palpation of the TMJ.[107]

Studies on muscle tenderness to palpation showed that equal and unequal tooth loss occurred in 20 of 22 patients with myofascial pain.[108] Tooth loss and dysfunction were not correlated among 406 Swedish patients diagnosed as having various TM disorders.[109] Eighty-two percent of the patients had myofascial complaints. An investigation of 72 Egyptian men found that 50% with premolar and molar support had muscles tender to palpation.[110] No similar occlusal support was found in 33% of the subjects with painful muscles. These findings suggest that complete occlusal support is not a preventive measure for controlling muscle tenderness because the number of subjects with complete and incomplete posterior teeth was almost equal.

One might expect the loss of teeth to have a significant effect on joints undergoing degeneration. According to one author, the status of the dentition appears to have no direct effect on the production of TMJ osteoarthritis.[41]

Extraction of Teeth

Overmanipulation of the mandible during the extraction of molars has been considered a factor in producing TMD problems. Oral surgery and other surgical procedures were associated with TMD pain in 17.7% of 164 patients diagnosed with myofascial pain.[28] The findings in another study muddle the picture because a history of molar extractions in the general population was considered marginal.[96] A history of molar extractions was more common in patients with TMD at 66%, compared with students who were either symptomatic at 53% or asymptomatic at 46%. Women TMD patients had the highest history, but no difference was found between asymptomatic and symptomatic students.

A slight increase in TMD symptoms has been reported after third molar surgery.[111] The effects proved transient. Symptoms diminished within the first week after surgery. They disappeared after 4 to 6 weeks or remained at the level found before surgery.

Significance: Although the loss of tooth support or overmanipulation of the mandible might be detrimental to the health of the TMJs and surrounding soft tissues, evidence is lacking on any long-term adverse effect.

Restoration of the Occlusion

If occlusal support is necessary to avoid TMD, then restoration of the occlusion should reduce or eliminate symptoms. If dysfunction is present, restoration should help lessen the severity. Although this thinking may be correct, information on denture patients fails to support it completely.

Although transient symptoms were present in 2000 male hospital patients, none was classified as having TMD.[11] About 26% had complete dentures, 16% had mutilated dentitions, and most suffered from overclosure. Another study of 93 TMD patients showed mixed patterns of dentition. Nearly 20% had complete dentures, 20% had an upper denture opposing either restored or unrestored dentitions, and 34% had natural dentitions.[112] Just 15% of 160 complete denture patients demonstrated TMJ disturbances. Joint pain was not always present with muscular tenderness, joint sounds, or restricted movements.[113]

A survey of 43 Swedish patients fitted with unsatisfactory complete dentures found that the frequency of dysfunction was 63% for men and 83% for women.[68] Most dysfunction was attributed to myogenic pain. The investigator concluded that tolerance to dysfunction appeared greater in complete denture wearers than in groups not wearing them.

The restoration of occlusion by fixed partial dentures does not necessarily eliminate symptoms. In 50 subjects, who had fixed partial dentures placed in all posterior quadrants, the frequency of symptoms was 68%.[114] Most dysfunction was classified as slight (38%), but some was moderate (20%) and severe (10%).

Significance: A summary of these results complements the previous findings of no well-defined relation between occlusal support and TMD. Restoration of the occlusion has not been demonstrated to improve a preexisting TMD condition.

Orthodontics

Numerous anecdotal remarks have been made about orthodontics and TMD. Some clinicians suspect that there is a greater prevalence of TMD in people treated by conventional orthodontics. Others believe that orthodontic treatment causes changes in occlusal function that lead to TMD. Still others believe that orthodontic treatment can be used successfully to avoid TMD.[115] Recent literature noted that shortened orthodontic treatment time and an improved occlusion can reduce potential TM problems.[116] The different opinions make a review of the literature worthwhile.

Cross-sectional survey of 347 patients examined for TMJ sounds before, during, and after orthodontic treatment showed significant associations between joint sound, age, and treatment.[117] It was unclear whether joints sounds increased from orthodontic treatment, age, or both. The status of sounds was unrelated to functional occlusal factors, dental wear, and chewing of gum. The authors recognized that joint sounds represent one sign of TMD and that other dysfunctions are possible.

No major long-term effects of orthodontic treatment were found after evaluation of dental and dysfunctional parameters in another study.[118] The analyses made between 82 orthodontically treated patients 52 months postretention and 28 untreated controls were of extraction patterns, self-reports of symptoms, presence of a slide between retruded contact and intercuspal positions, occlusal stability, posterior inter-ferences, tenderness on palpation, joint noises, and number of restorations. Among these parameters, soft clicks and number of restorations were slightly higher in the post-treatment group than in the untreated group.

Neither orthodontic nor other dental treatments figured as significant etiologic fac-tors based on self-reported symptoms obtained by questionnaire among 343 women.[119] A total of 451 asymptomatic patients undergoing orthodontic treatment were evaluated for TMD symptoms.[120] No significant relation was found between symptoms and the course of orthodontic treatment 18 months later. Eleven subjects with preexisting symptoms were not worsened by treatment.

Correlational studies showed that significantly more TMD patients had prior orth-odontic treatment than non-TMD individuals.[96] In particular, women with TMD symptoms had a greater history of orthodontics than asymptomatic women. Accord-ing to the authors, the relation of specific symptoms to the orthodontic treatment was very weak.

Other information weighs against detrimental effects of orthodontics on factors often associated with TMD. Test of null hypothesis that a slide from retruded contact po-sition to intercuspal position was not different in postretention orthodontic patients than in an untreated population showed that slides or orthodontically treated patients were comparable to slides of untreated controls and measurements of slides of the general population reported in the literature.[121]

Self-reports of the onset of myofascial pain and a history of orthodontic treatment were extremely low among 164 patients admitted to a TMJ–Facial Pain clinic.[28] Just 2.4% of the patients mentioned orthodontics as an event related to the pain. TMD symptoms, excluding joint sounds, were considered rare in 1180 patients seeking orthodontic treatment.[122]

Evaluations of condyle position and vertical overlap of anterior teeth were made in patients who had the premolars extracted for orthodontic purposes and in patients without extractions. No statistically significant differences were found in joint space, condyle position, or vertical overlap of anterior teeth between 30 patients after ex-traction and 37 patients without extractions.[123]

Significance: Although some authors argue that orthodontic treatment superim-posed on preexisting subclinical symptoms may lead to a full blown TMD condi-tion, evidence is lacking to confirm or to deny how much or how little orthodontics produces or improves TMD conditions. Thus, despite the personal impressions that clinicians might form about orthodontically treated cases, the literature refutes hypotheses of cause.

Root Canal Therapy

Tooth pain may be eliminated by root canal therapy. Because these procedures re-quire that the mouth remains open under a rubber dam for long periods, it is gen-erally agreed that prolonged mandibular hyperextension may elicit new or aggravate preexisting TMD symptoms. One can never rule out the possibility that additional suffering may incur if there is a preexisting TMD condition.

Significance: Although prolonged hyperextension during root canal therapy may be considered significant as an etiologic factor, evidence is lacking in the literature that shows the genesis of new symptoms. Subjects should be examined for tenderness of muscles before treatment.

Perpetuating Factors

Bruxism

There are many who feel that excessive clenching or grinding of the teeth produces unhealthy symptoms of the masticatory system. Some bruxers may complain of pain or other symptoms of the jaw, head, or neck. The simultaneous presence of these complaints does not necessarily mean that the symptoms resulted from the bruxing. Both may occur at the same time and be independent of one another. Arguments for and against this relation are addressed.

Support for the concept that bruxing contributes to dysfunction appears widespread. Complaints about the masticatory muscles have received the most attention.[133,134,139] The words used to express these complaints are similar (Table 4-9). This suggests that different investigators have observed similar complaints or different stages of the same complaint but have used different words to express them.[110,124–137] The same conclusion can be drawn from complaints of the jaw, face, head, and neck.[138–142] Pain was the dominant complaint regardless of the anatomy.

Table 4-9

Location of Symptoms Associated With Bruxism

Location	Symptom	Reference
Masticatory muscle	Tenderness	133–135, 138, 139
	Soreness	130
	Spontaneous contraction	131, 132
	Spasm	124
	Trismus	136, 140
	Hyperactivity	131
	Hypertrophy	126, 148
	Pain	110, 127–129
Jaw	TM joint pain	127–129
	Limited opening	139
	Tiredness	142, 145, 146
	Aching	138, 141
Face	Pain	116, 128, 129, 147, 148
Head	Headache	68, 128, 129, 133, 147–150
Neck	Cervical dysfunction	131, 154
	Pain	128, 129
TMD symptoms	Positive association	
	Children	144, 151–153
	Adults	68, 138, 143

TMD symptoms have been reported among adult bruxers.[68,138,143] Positive associations have been found between bruxing and TMD symptoms in children.[144–153] Equating adult symptoms with children symptoms may be questionable.[154]

An association between muscle-related complaints and bruxing remains controversial. One study found little association between bruxing and myofascial symptoms. Among 899 dentists who attended a dental convention, 16% bruxed only, 3.7% had muscle symptoms only, and 4.6% bruxed with muscle symptoms.[127]

In a group of college students, nocturnal tooth contacts, tenderness of the superficial masseter muscles, and limited mouth opening were significantly related.[139] Still, the investigators concluded that nocturnal tooth grinding was not a major controlling factor in dysfunction. This conclusion was supported by a study of 410 students that found no association between bruxism and facial pain.[155] The literature reveals an exception to this conclusion. Tenderness of the masticatory muscles was found in 39% of 219 male Siwian desert dwellers.[110] The prevalence of incisal or occlusal abrasion was 39%. Two thirds of the dwellers with incisal abrasion had muscle tenderness. Muscle tenderness was present among 30% with generalized occlusal abrasion. The author concluded that bruxing habits involving protrusive movements were more harmful than posterior occlusal habits.

If bruxism causes muscular changes, the damage should be obvious from biochemical analysis of this tissue. In fact, assay of an enzyme has been used to assess the degree of muscle damage in bruxers. No statistically significant differences were found in the levels of serum creatinine kinase activity between bruxers and individuals with TMD and normal, nonbruxer, non-TMD individuals.[156]

Significance: Research has provided little direct support for a link between most TM symptoms and bruxism. Muscle tenderness may be a prominent symptom in certain bruxers. It does not appear to be reflected in major enzymatic changes in the muscle.

Other Oral Behavioral Patterns

Different kinds of oral behavior patterns have been related to head pain, orofacial pain, or increased masticatory muscle activity. A few incidental remarks have been made about chronic chewing of gum and TMD symptoms. No positive association was found in two studies.[28,55] Jutting of the mandible forward or prolonged lip biting induced pain in the anterior temporalis muscle.[128] The pain was moderate, lasting from 30 minutes to 2½ hours. Active motions, such as retruding the mandible or biting the tongue, lips, or cheeks of the oral cavity significantly increased the electromyographic (EMG) level in the anterior temporalis muscle.[70] Facial posturing, such as cupping the chin in the hand or resting the hand on the side of the face, produced similar effects. Most of the symptoms are transient in nature.

Interesting associations have been found between oral habits, muscular changes, facial pain, and different kinds of headache.[157] The study involved three groups. Group 1 included subjects with a history of facial pain, migraine, and combined headache. Group 2 subjects had tensional (muscular) headaches, and Group 3 subjects had no similar pains. Clenching was significantly more frequent among group 1 subjects than subjects of the other groups. Resting the hand under the chin was more frequent for group 1 than for group 3, and thrusting the mandible forward was more common for group 1 than for groups 2 and 3. Reclassification of groups into subjects with TMJ pain, TMJ and muscle pain, or no facial pain showed that nocturnal bruxism was more frequent in the combined TMJ and muscle pain subjects than in other subjects. Ongoing assessment for 28 days revealed that migraineurs had significantly higher frequencies of clenching and putting their hands on the face than nonheadache subjects.[158] Additional study showed subjects with common migraine reported significantly more oral habits than subjects with tensional headaches.[159] No statistically significant differences were found between a nonheadache group and either of the other groups. The authors concluded that high frequencies of oral habits can be expected in migraineurs but that not all cases of common migraine headaches are related to daily clenching or resting the chin on the hand. The number of subjects studied in these groups was small. Replicate studies are needed to confirm these findings.

Significance: It is unclear whether even the most noxious of these habits leads to chronic, painful syndromes. In some cases, they may simply reflect expressions of behavior symbolic of preexisting painful conditions.

Emotional Factors

Research on psychological and social factors has shown that patients with generalized chronic pain may differ from subjects without chronic pain. Emotional factors have been suggested as being involved in the genesis of TMD pain. Whether any particular social or psychological factors can be found, however, to predict which individuals will become susceptible or prone to TMD is problematic. So many potential trigger factors exist that causal associations in relation to TMD symptoms are likely to be complex and involve multiple competing mechanisms. It is unclear to what degree these relations are mediated by neurotic and hypochondriacal tendencies that would influence somatic focus and symptom report in general.

Successful identification of the trigger factors is difficult because of the complex psychological somatic interrelations of any chronic pain syndrome. Recent information on the United States population shows the magnitude of this problem. About 15% of the population between the ages of 25 and 74 years suffer with definite chronic pain related to the joints and musculoskeletal system.[160] Another 7.4% have pain of uncertain origin. Eighteen percent of the definite pain group and 8% without pain suffer from depression. Many attempts have been made to determine the causes of depression and the relation with pain. The number of painful conditions reported has proved a better predictor of major depression than other measures of the pain experience, including pain severity and persistence.[161] Studies of different populations have not consistently related TMD syndrome to depression.

The psychophysiologic concept of the etiology of myofascial pain syndrome relies on emotional tension or stress as the initiating factor (see Fig. 4-5).[32] A stressful event was reported by just one fourth of 164 MPD patients with the onset of pain.[28] Subjective reports, including the general history of 170 clinic patients, showed no sig-

Table 4-10
Events Associated With Onset of Chief Complaint

Report	Reversible Disk (%)	Permanent Disk (%)	Myogenic Complaints (%)
Hyperextension from chewing or yawning	33	35	5*
Dental treatment	7	12	16
Blow to jaw	4	4	6
Stressful period	4	11	18
Unknown	52	38	55

*Reversible disk and myogenic complaints and permanent disk and myogenic complaints were significantly different, but reversible disk and permanent disk complaints were not.

After Isacsson G, Linde C, Isberg A. Subjective symptoms in patients with temporomandibular joint disk displacement versus patients with craniomandibular disorders. J Prosthet Dent 1989;61:70.

nificant relation between stressful periods and kind of TMD dysfunction (Table 4-10). Self-reports of stressful working or stressful private lives were similar in patients with either reversible disk displacement, permanent disk displacement, or myogenic disorders.[162] A higher percentage of patients diagnosed with myogenic complaints had histories of somatic or psychiatric disease than patients of the other groups. The findings associated with psychological and social predictors must be interpreted with caution because of significant methodologic shortcomings in many of these reports.

Evaluation of 356 chronic pain patients found that problems in concentration and memory were related to emotional stress, poor family support, and interference with daily activities.[163] Both concentration and memory were unrelated to pain intensity, pain duration, and demographic factors. Analysis of 93 chronic pain patients showed that most patients tended to overestimate their pain intensity levels.[164] Patients with headache, facial pain, or abdominal pain were less accurate in remembering their pain than patients with cervical and low back pain. Individuals who had histories of emotional stress or home conflicts, who were less active, and who relied on medication were most inaccurate in remembering their pain.

Significance: Many factors besides pain quality and quantity influence the discomfort and suffering associated with recurrent pain. The emotional response to pain is influenced by factors such as ethnic background, socioeconomic status, current environment, and the meaning of pain to the individual. It is unclear whether emotional factors, including individual personality traits such as neuroticism, vulnerability to stress, and anxiety, predispose to TMD.

References

1. Moss RA, Garrett JC. Temporomandibular joint dysfunction syndrome and myofascial pain dysfunction syndrome: a critical review. J Oral Rehabil 1984;11:3.
2. Nelson SJ, Narendran S, Barghi R, Ash MM. Potential factors in temporomandibular disorders (TMD). J Dent Res 1990;69(special issue):194. Abstract 685.

3. Keith DA. Etiology and diagnosis of temporomandibular pain and dysfunction: organic pathology (other than arthritis). In Laskin DM, et al (eds). The President's Conference on the Examination, Diagnosis and Management of Temporomandibular Disorders. Chicago: American Dental Association, 1983:118.

4. Sarnat GG. Developmental facial abnormalities and the temporomandibular joint. Dent Clin North Am 1966;66:587.

5. Solberg WK, Hansson TL, Nordstrom B. The temporomandibular joint in young adults at autopsy: a morphologic classification and evaluation. J Oral Rehabil 1985;12:303.

6. Graber TM. Orthodontics: principles and practice, 3rd ed. Philadelphia: WB Saunders, 1972:480.

7. Ingervall B, Thilander B. Activity of temporal and masseter muscles in children with a lateral bite force. Angle Orthod 1975;45:249.

8. McLaughlin RP. Malocclusion and the temporomandibular joint: an historical perspective. Angle Orthod 1988;58:185.

9. American Association of Oral and Maxillofacial Surgeons. AAOMS Surgical Update. 1991;Winter:4.

10. Perry HT. Relation of occlusion to temporomandibular joint dysfunction: the orthodontic viewpoint. J Am Dent Assoc 1969;79:137.

11. Loiselle RJ. Relation of occlusion to temporomandibular joint dysfunction: the prosthodontic viewpoint. J Am Dent Assoc 1969;79:145.

12. Egermark-Eriksson I, Ingervall B, Carlsson GE. The dependence of mandibular dysfunction in children on function and morphological malocclusion. Am J Orthod 1983;83:187.

13. Stringert HG, Worms FW. Variations in skeletal and dental patterns in patients with structural and functional alterations of the temporomandibular joint: a preliminary report. Am J Orthod Dentofacial Orthop 1986;89:285.

14. Solberg WK, Bibb CA, Nordstrom BB, Hansson TL. Malocclusion association with temporomandibular joint changes in young adults at autopsy. Am J Orthod 1986;89:326.

15. Bush FM. Occlusal etiology of myofascial pain dysfunction syndrome. In Laskin DM, et al (eds). The President's Conference on the Examination, Diagnosis and Management of Temporomandibular Disorders. Chicago: American Dental Association, 1983:95.

16. McNeill C (ed). Craniomandibular disorders: guidelines for evaluation, diagnosis, and management. The American Academy of Craniomandibular Disorders. Chicago: Quintessence, 1990.

17. De Laat A, van Steenberghe D, Lesaffre E. Occlusal relationships and temporomandibular joint dysfunction. Correlations between occlusal and articular parameters and symptoms of TMJ dysfunction by means of stepwise logistic regression. J Prosthet Dent 1986;55(pt 2):116.

18. Mongini F, Capurso U, Ventricelli F. Aetiopathogenetic factors in stomatognathic dysfunctions. J Oral Rehabil 1988;15:204. Abstract.

19. Schiffman E, Fricton J, Haley D. Association between etiological agents and mandibular dysfunction. J Dent Res 1990;69(special issue):194. Abstract 685.

20. Moss RA, Garrett J, Chiodo JF. Temporomandibular joint dysfunction and myofascial pain dysfunction syndromes: parameters, etiology, and treatment. Psychol Bulletin 1982;92:331.

21. Vincelli J. Letter to the editor. J Prosthet Dent 1986;55:149.

22. Hodges JM. Managing temporomandibular joint syndrome. Laryngoscope 1990;100:60.

23. Costen JB. Syndrome of ear and sinus symptoms dependent upon disturbed function of the temporomandibular joint. Ann Otol Rhinol Laryngol 1934;43:1.

24. Greene CS. Temporomandibular joint disorders. In Clark JW (ed). Clinical dentistry, vol 2. Philadelphia: Harper & Row, 1984;37:1.

25. Pullinger AG, Hollender L, Solberg WK, Petersson A. A tomographic study of mandibular condyle position in an asymptomatic population. J Prosthet Dent 1985;53:185.

26. Vandenberghe LJ, De Boever JA, Adriaens PA. The interpretation of condyle position on radiographs: inter-examiner reliability and relationship with clinical parameters. J Oral Rehabil 1988;15:211.

27. Zenker W. Researchers elucidate causes of neck pain in physiology. Pain Topics 1990;4:3.

28. Fricton JR, Kroening R, Haley D, Siegert R. Myofascial pain syndrome of the head and neck: a review of clinical characteristics of 164 patients. Oral Surg Oral Med Oral Pathol 1985;60:615.

29. Weiner G. Heading, Letter to editor. J Craniomandib Pract 1989;7:184.

30. Dolwick, MF. Diagnosis and etiology of internal derangements of the temporomandibular joint. In Laskin DM, et al (eds). The President's Conference on the Examination, Diagnosis and Management of Temporomandibular Disorders. Chicago: American Dental Association, 1983:112.

31. Greenberg SA, Jacobs JS, Bessette RW. Temporomandibular joint dysfunction: evaluation and treatment. Clin Plast Surg 1989;16:707.

32. Laskin DM. Etiology of the pain-dysfunction syndrome. J Am Dent Assoc 1969;79:147.

33. Farrar WB. Craniomandibular practice: the state of the art—definition and diagnosis. J Craniomandib Pract 1982;1:4.

34. Wilkes CH. Internal derangement of the temporomandibular joint: pathological variations. Arch Otolaryngol Head Neck Surg 1989;115:469.

35. Westesson PL, Rohlin M. Internal derangement related to osteoarthrosis in temporomandibular joint autopsy specimens. Oral Surg 1984;57:17.

36. Eversole LR, Machado L. Temporomandibular joint internal derangements and associated neuromuscular disorders. J Am Dent Assoc 1985;110:69.

37. Weinberg S, Lapointe H. Cervical extension-flexion injury (whiplash) and internal derangement of the temporomandibular joint. J Oral Maxillofac Surg 1987;45:653.

38. Wilkinson TM. The relationship between the disk and the lateral pterygoid muscle in the human temporomandibular joint. J Prosthet Dent 1988;60:715.

39. Meyenberg K, Kubik S, Palla S. Relationships of the muscles of mastication to the articular disc of the temporomandibular joint. Helv Odont Acta 1986;30:815.

40. Tegelberg A. Temporomandibular joint involvement in rheumatoid arthritis: a clinical study. Swed Dent J 1987;49(suppl):1.

41. Alling CS. The diagnosis of chronic maxillofacial pain. J Prosthet Dent 1981;45:300.

42. Schellhas KP, Piper MA, Omlie MR. Facial skeletal remodeling due to tem-

poromandibular joint degeneration: an imaging study of 100 patients. AJR Am J Roentgenol 1990;155:373.

43. Blackwood HJJ. Adaptive changes in the mandibular joints with function. Dent Clin North Am 1966;66:559.

44. Helmy ES, Bays RA, Offenbacher S. Internal derangement: is it a primary inflammatory disorder? J Dent Res 1990;69(special issue):217. Abstract 866.

45. De Bont LGM, Boering G, Liem RSB, et al. Osteoarthrosis and internal derangement of the temporomandibular joint: a light microscopic study. J Oral Maxillofac Surg 1986;44:634.

46. Stegenga B, Lambert GM, de Bont, Boering G. Ostoarthritis as the cause of craniomandibular pain and dysfunction: a unifying concept. J Oral Maxillofac Surg 1989;47:249.

47. Brooke RI, Stenn PG, Mothersill KJ. The diagnosis and conservative treatment of myofascial pain dysfunction syndrome. Oral Surg Oral Med Oral Pathol 1977;44:844.

48. Andreoli TE, Carpenter CC, Plum F, Smith LH Jr (eds). Cecil's essentials of medicine, 2nd ed. Philadelphia: WB Saunders, 1990:640.

49. McCarty W. Diagnosis and treatment of internal derangements of the articular disk and mandibular condyle. In Solberg WK, Clark GT (eds). Temporomandibular joint problems. Chicago: Quintessence, 1980:145.

50. Yemm R. Temporomandibular dysfunction and masseter muscle response to experimental stress. Br Dent J 1969;127:508.

51. Haber JD, Moss RA, Kuczmierczk RA, Garrett JC. Assessment and treatment of stress in myofascial pain-dysfunction syndrome: a model for analysis. J Oral Rehabil 1983;10:187.

52. Nishioka GJ, Montgomery MT. Masticatory muscle hyperactivity in temporomandibular disorders: is it an extrapyramidally expressed disorders? J Am Dent Assoc 1988;116:514.

53. Baker GE, Dolwick MF, Rugh JR, Steed DL. Post-operative muscle pain in internal derangement patients: with and without MPD. In press, 1983. (Quoted in Dolwick MF. The President's Conference on the Examination, Diagnosis and Management of Temporomandibular Disorders. Chicago: American Dental Association, 1983:116.

54. Lundeen TF, George JM, Sturdevant JR. Stress in patients with pain of the muscles of mastication and the temporomandibular joints. J Oral Rehabil 1983;15:631.

55. Wänman A, Agerberg G. Subjective reports of fatigue in the jaws—an indication of dysfunction. J Oral Rehabil 1988;15:212.

56. Travell J. Myofascial trigger points: a clinical view. In Bonica J, Albe-Fessard D (eds): Advances in pain research and therapy. New York: Raven Press, 1976:919.

57. Awad EA. Pathological changes in fibromyalgia. First International Symposium on Myofascial Pain and Fibromyalgia. Minneapolis: University of Minnesota, 1989:24, 89. Abstract.

58. Simons DG, Travell J. Myofascial trigger points, a possible explanation (correspondence). Pain 1981;10:106.

59. Smyth HA. "Fibrositis" as a disorder of pain modulation. Clin Rheum Dis 1979;5:823.

60. McCain GA, Scudds RA. The concept of primary fibromyalgia (fibrositis): clin-

ical value, relation and significance to other chronic musculoskeletal pain syndromes. Pain 1988;33:273.

61. Bennett RM. Etiology of the fibromyalgia syndrome: a contemporary hypothesis. Intern Med 1990;11:48.

62. Bland JH. Disorders of the cervical spine: diagnosis and medical management. Philadelphia: WB Saunders, 1987.

63. Campbell JK. Headache in adults: an overview. J Craniomandib Disord Fac Oral Pain 1987;1:11.

64. Bland JH. Pain in the head and neck: where does it come from? J Craniomandib Pract 1989;7:167.

65. De Jong JMBV, Bles W. Cervical dizziness and ataxia. In Bles W, Brandt Th (ed). Disorders of posture and gait. New York: Elsevier, 1986.

66. Guide to dental health, temporomandibular joint disorders: a dental problem in disguise. J Am Dent Assoc 1985;110:49.

67. Magnusson T. Prevalence of recurrent headache and mandibular dysfunction with unsatisfactory complete dentures. Community Dent Oral Epidemiol 1980;8:159.

68. Magnusson T, Carlsson GE. Recurrent headaches in relation to temporomandibular joint pain-dysfunction. Acta Odontol Scand 1978;36:333.

69. Lous I, Olesen J. Evaluation of pericranial tenderness and oral function in patients with common migraine, muscle contraction headache and "combination headache." Pain 1982;12:385.

70. Ruff GA, Moss RH, Lombardo TW. Common migraine: a review and proposal for a non-vascular etiology. J Oral Rehabil 1986;13:499.

71. Schokker RP, Hansson TL, Ansink BJJ. Craniomandibular disorders in patients with different kinds of headache. J Craniomandib Disord Fac Oral Pain 1990; 1:47.

72. Forssell H. Mandibular dysfunction and headache. Proc Finn Dent Soc 1985; 81:1.

73. Sjaastad O, Saunte C, Hovdahl H, Breivik H, Groenbaek E. "Cervicogenic headache": an hypothesis. Cephalalgia 1983;3:249.

74. Pfaffenrath V, Dandekar R, Pollman W. Cervicogenic headache: the clinical picture, radiological findings and hypotheses on its pathophysiology. Headache 1987;27:495.

75. Mark BM. Cervicogenic headache differential diagnosis and clinical management: literature review. J Craniomandib Pract 1990;8:332.

76. Jansen J, Bardosi A, Hildebrant J, Lucke A. Cervicogenic headache attacks associated with vascular irritation or compression of the nerve root C2. Clinical manifestations and morphological findings. Pain 1989;39:203.

77. Jaeger B. Are "cervicogenic" headaches due to myofascial pain and cervical spine dysfunction? Cephalalgia 1989;9:157.

78. Amery WK, Vandenbergh V. What can precipitating factors teach us about the pathogenesis of migraine? Headache 1987;27:146.

79. Bavitz JB, Chewning LC. Malignant disease as temporomandibular joint dysfunction: review of the literature and report of case. J Am Dent Assoc 1990; 120:163.

80. Boyczuk EM, Solomon MP, Gold BD. Unremitting pain to the mandible secondary to metastatic breast concern: a case report. Compend Contin Educ Dent 1991;12:104.

81. Peet MM, Schnieder RC. Trigeminal neuralgia: a review of six hundred and eighty-nine cases with a follow-up study on sixty-five per cent of the group. J Neurosurg 1952;9:367.

82. Giorgi C, Broggi G. Surgical treatment of glossopharyngeal neuralgia and pain from cancer of the nasopharynx: J Neurosurg 1984;61:952.

83. Stevens JC. Cranial neuralgias. J Craniomandib Disord Fac Oral Pain 1987; 1:51.

84. Turkewitz L, Levin M. Acute inflammation of the TMJ presenting as classical trigeminal neuralgia: case report and hypothesis. Headache 1987;27:24.

85. Matson MS. Pain in the orofacial region associated with coronary insufficiency. Oral Surg 1963;16:284.

86. Norman JE De B. Facial pain and vascular disease. Br J Oral Maxillofac Surg 1970;8:138.

87. Graham LL, Schinbeckler GA. Orofacial pain of cardiac origin. J Am Dent Assoc 1982;104:47.

88. Grace EG, Malinow KL. Hyperventilation and facial pain. J Am Dent Assoc 1982;104:52.

89. Greene CS, Lerman MD, Sutcher HD, Laskin DM. The TMJ-pain dysfunction syndrome: heterogeneity of the patient population. J Am Dent Assoc 1969; 79:1168.

90. Weinberg LA, Lager LA. Clinical report on the etiology and diagnosis of TMJ dysfunction-pain syndrome. J Prosthet Dent 1980;44:642.

91. Truelove E, Burgess J, Dworkin S, Lawton L, Sommers E, Shubert M. Incidence of trauma associated with temporomandibular disorders. J Dent Res 1985;64(special issue):329. Abstract 1482.

92. Hohmann A, Wilson K, Nelms RC. Surgical treatment in temporomandibular joint trauma: symposium on trauma to the head and neck. Otolaryngol Clin North Am 1983;16:549.

93. Harkins SJ, Marteney JL. Extrinsic trauma: a significant precipitating factor in temporomandibular dysfunction. J Prosthet Dent 1985;54:271.

94. Dornan R, Clark GT. Incidence of trauma induced disease in a TMD clinic population. J Dent Res 1991;70(special issue):1401. Abstract 1401.

95. Brooke RI, Stenn PG. Postinjury myofascial dysfunction syndrome, its etiology and prognosis. Oral Surg 1978;45:846.

96. Pullinger AG, Monteiro AA. History factors associated with symptoms of temporomandibular disorders. J Oral Rehabil 1988;15:117.

97. Kopp S. Pain and functional disturbances of the masticatory system: a review of etiology and principles of treatment. Swed Dent J 1982;6:49.

98. Wakeley C. The mandibular joint. Ann R Coll Surg Engl 1947;2:111.

99. Juniper RP. Temporomandibular joint dysfunction: a theory based upon electromyographic studies of the lateral pterygoid muscle. Br J Oral Maxillofac Surg 1984;22:1.

100. Schellhas KP. Temporomandibular joint injuries. Radiology 1989;193:211.

101. Roydhouse RH. Whiplash and temporomandibular dysfunction. Lancet 1973; 1:1394.

102. Burgess JA. Symptom characteristics in post-trauma facial pain and temporomandibular disorders (TMD). J Dent Res 1991;70(special issue):371. Abstract 844.

103. Heise A, Laskin D, Gervin A. Temporomandibular joint pain secondary to cervical musculoskeletal injury. J Dent Res 1990;69(special issue)296. Abstract 1503.

104. Thomson H. The mandibular dysfunction syndrome. Br Dent J 1971;130:187.

105. Boering G. Arthrosis deformans van het. In Toller P. Nonsurgical treatment of dysfunction of the temporomandibular joint. Oral Sciences Review 1976;7:53.

106. Franks AST. The dental health of patients presenting with TMJ dysfunction. Br J Oral Maxillofac Surg 1967;5:157.

107. Kopp S. Clinical findings in temporomandibular joint osteoarthritis. Scand J Dent Res 1977;85:434.

108. Winter AA, Yavelow AA. Oral considerations of the myofascial pain dysfunction syndrome. Oral Surg Oral Med Oral Pathol 1975;40:720.

109. Helöe B, Helöe LA. Characteristics of a group of patients with temporomandibular joint disorders. Community Dent Oral Epidemiol 1975;3:72.

110. Abdel-Harkim AM. Stomatognathic dysfunction in the western desert of Egypt: an epidemiological survey. J Oral Rehabil 1981;10:461.

111. Moser BV, Kremenak CR, Zeitler DP, Seydel SK. TMD and third molar surgery: one-year follow-up of relationships. J Dent Res 1991;70(special issue):466. Abstract 1599.

112. Zarb GA, Thompson GW. The treatment of patients with temporomandibular joint pain dysfunction syndrome. J Can Dent Assoc 1975;41:410.

113. Choy E, Smith DE. The prevalence of temporomandibular joint disturbances in complete denture patients. J Oral Rehabil 1980;7:331.

114. Lederman KH, Clayton JA. Restored occlusions: the relationship of clinical and subject symptoms to varying degrees of TMJ dysfunction. J Prosthet Dent 1982;47(pt 2):303.

115. Ingervall B, Ronnerman A. Index for need of orthodontic treatment. Odont Rev 1975;26:59.

116. Sinclair PM, Proffit WR. How patients benefit from surgical-orthodontic care. J Am Dent Assoc 1991;122:94.

117. Sadowsky C, Muhl ZF, Sakols ET, Sommerville JM. Temporomandibular joint sounds related to orthodontic therapy. J Dent Res 1985;64:1392.

118. Smith A, Freer TJ. Post-orthodontic occlusion function. Aust Dent J 1989; 34:301.

119. Andrikopulu MA, Gleason MJ. Etiological factors in temporomandibular disorders in women. J Dent Res 1991;70(special issue):329. Abstract 508.

120. Rendell J, Norton L, Gay T. Relation between orthodontic treatment and TMJ disorders. J Dent Res 1991;70(special issue):441. Abstract 1404.

121. Johnston LE (EICO Orthodontic Study Group of Ohio). Gnathologic assessment of centric slides in postretention orthodontic patients. J Prosthet Dent 1988;60:712.

122. Lundeen T, Phillips C, Tulloch C. Prevalence of TMD symptoms in orthodontic patients. J Dent Res 1990;69(special issue):218. Abstract 874.

123. Gianelli AA, Hughes HM, Wohrgemuth P, Gildea G. Condylar position and extraction treatment. Am J Orthod Dentofacial Orthop 1988;93:201.

124. Kraus S. Cervical spine influences on the craniomandibular region. In Kraus S. Craniomandibular complex: physical therapy and dental treatment. New York: Churchill Livingstone, 1987.

125. Nadler SC. Bruxism, a classification: critical review. J Am Dent Assoc 1957; 54:615.

126. Ramfjord SP. Bruxism: a clinical and EMG study. J Am Dent Assoc 1961;62:21.

127. Ayer WA, Machen JB, Getter L. Survey of neurofacial pain dysfunction syndrome and pathologic bruxing among dentists. J Am Dent Assoc 1977;94:730.

128. Villarosa GA, Moss RA. Oral behavioral patterns as factors contributing to the development of head and facial pain. J Prosthet Dent 1985;54:427.

129. Yemm RA. A neurophysiological approach to the pathology and aetiology of temporomandibular dysfunction. J Oral Rehabil 1985;12:343.

130. Bolero RP. The physiology of splint therapy: a literature review. Angle Orthod 1990;59:165.

131. Ingle JI. Alveolar osteoporosis and pulpal death associated with compulsive bruxism. Oral Surg 1960;13:1371.

132. Thaller JL. Bruxism: a factor in periodontal disease. New York State Dental Journal 1965;31:17.

133. Ingerslev H. Functional disturbances of the masticatory system in school children. J Dent Child 1983;50:455.

134. Lindquist B. Bruxism in children. Odontol Rev 1971;22:413.

135. Kampe T, Hannerz H. Three year longitudinal study of mandibular dysfunction in young adults with intact and restored dentitions: a comparative study. Acta Odontol Scand 1987;45:31.

136. Marbach JJ, Lipton JA, Lund PB, Delahanty F, Blank RT. Facial pains and anxiety levels: considerations for treatment. J Prosthet Dent 1978;40:434.

137. Moore DS. Bruxism, diagnosis and treatment. J Periodont Res 1956;27:277.

138. Ramfjord SP. Diagnosis of bruxism. Les Paradontophaties (Paris Annual) 1963;53.

139. Solberg WK, Woo MW, Houston JB. Prevalence of mandibular dysfunction in young adults. J Am Dent Assoc 1979;98:25.

140. Molin C, Levi K. Psycho-odontological investigations of patients with bruxism. Acta Odontol Scand 1966;24:373.

141. Strother EW, Mitchell GE. Bruxism: a review and a case report. J Dent Med 1954;9:189.

142. Bell DG. Bruxism. J Periodontol 1947;18:46.

143. Osterberg T, Carlsson GE. Symptoms and signs of mandibular dysfunction in 70-year old men and women in Gothenberg, Sweden. Community Dent Oral Epidemiol 1979;7:315.

144. Egermark-Eriksson I, Ingervall B, Carlsson GE. Prevalence of mandibular dysfunction and orofacial parafunction in 7-, 11- and 15-year-old Swedish children. Eur J Orthod 1981;43:163.

145. Helkimo M. Studies on function and dysfunction of the masticatory system: an epidemiological investigation of symptoms of dysfunction in Lapps in the North of Finland. Proc Finn Dent Soc 1974;70(pt 1):37.

146. Reding GR, Rubright WC, Zimmerman SO. Incidence of bruxism. J Dent Res 1966;45:1198.

147. Monica WS. Headaches caused by bruxism. Annals of Otorhinolaryngology 1959;68:1159.

148. Nadler SC. The effects of bruxism. J Periodont Res 1966;37:311.

149. Berlin R, Dessner L. Bruxism and chronic headache. Dental Digest 1961;67:32.

150. Nilner M. Functional disturbances of the stomatognathic system among 7- to 18-year-olds. J Craniomandib Pract 1985;3:358.

151. Ingervall B. Tooth contacts on the functional and non-functional side in children and young adults. Arch Oral Biol 1972;17:191.

152. Lindquist B. Bruxism in twins. Acta Odontol Scand 1974;32:177.

153. Wigdorowicz-Makowerowa N, Grodzki C, Panek H, Maslanka T, Plonka K, Palacha A. Epidemiological studies on prevalence and etiology of functional disturbances of the masticatory system. J Prosthet Dent 1979;41:76.

154. Cash RC. Bruxism in children: review of the literature. Journal of Pedodontics 1990;12:107.

155. Moss RA, Sult S, Garrett JC. Factors related to craniomandibular pain in a college population. J Craniomandib Pract 1984;2:364.

156. Cox PJ, Rothwell PS. Serum creatine kinase studies in mandibular pain dysfunction. J Oral Rehabil 1984;11:45.

157. Moss RA, Ruff MH, Sturgis ET. Oral behavioral patterns in facial pain, headache and non-headache populations. Behav Res Ther 1984;22:683.

158. Moss RA, Lombardo TW, Villarosa GA, Hodgson JM, O'Carroll MK, Cooley JE, Smith P. Ongoing assessment of oral habits in common migraine and non-headache populations. J Craniomandib Pract 1988;6:352.

159. Moss RA, Lombardo TW, Hodgson JM, O'Carroll MK. Oral habits in common between tension headache and non-headache populations. J Oral Rehabil 1989;16:71.

160. Magni G, Caldieron C, Rigatti-Luchini S, Merskey H. Chronic musculoskeletal pain and depressive symptoms in the general population: an analysis of the First National Heart and Nutrition Examination Survey Data. Pain 1990;43:299.

161. Dworkin SF, Von Korff M, LeResche L. Multiple pains and psychiatric disturbance: an epidemiological investigation. Arch Gen Psychiatry 1990;47:239.

162. Isacsson G, Linde C, Isberg A. Subjective symptoms in patients with temporomandibular joint disk displacement versus patients with myogenic craniomandibular disorders. J Prosthet Dent 1989;61:75.

163. Jamison RN, Sbrocco T, Parris WCV. The influence of problems with concentration and memory on emotional distress and daily activities in chronic pain patients. Int J Psychiatry Med 1988;18:183.

164. Jamison RN, Sbrocco T, Parris WCV. The influence of psychic and psychosocial factors on accuracy of memory for pain in chronic pain patients. Pain 1989;37:289.

The Temporomandibular Joint and Related Orofacial Disorders,
by Francis M. Bush and M. Franklin Dolwick.
J.B. Lippincott Company, Philadelphia, © 1995.

5

Epidemiology

Epidemiology is the field of science dealing with the relations of the various factors that determine the frequencies and distributions of a disease in the human community. It is the study of distribution and determinants of diseases and injuries in human populations.[1] The goals of epidemiology are multifold: classifying and understanding development of disease, determining etiology, and recognizing factors leading to prevention.[1a] The goals of clinical epidemiology focus on success of treatment or cure of disease.

Rationale

Clinicians have been concerned with epidemiology of TMD for at least 20 years. Practically, why would a clinician need to be concerned with the epidemiology of TMD? One answer is that the difference between healthy and unhealthy conditions is not always obvious. Normal anatomy and physiology vary widely between and among individuals of different populations. Because dentists have acquired the major responsibility for diagnosis and treatment of TMD, this information affects dental clinicians and individuals of the general population who are treated or advised to undergo treatment by these practitioners.

Questions frequently asked by patients include the following: How common is this disorder? What do my symptoms mean? If one of my parents has it, can I get it too? Is there a test or examination for it? What risks are involved in this condition? What is the prognosis?

Attempts to provide satisfactory answers are fraught with problems. Many clinicians and patients are obsessed with deriving a specific percentage for a given disorder. A projection of future outcome is expected from this percentage. Although such figures sound impressive, some questions have answers and some do not. The present level of information may be too low to explain the disorder.

131

Recently, multidisciplinary clinics have evolved in major health centers to consolidate clinical efforts and research on major health problems. Information about health problems is often biased because conclusions are drawn from patient referral to the clinics. It is not known whether these clinics reflect a representative sample of persons in the community who suffer from complaints. Lack of information about clinic populations versus the population at large often limits general understanding of disorders. Thus, false associations are made about diagnosis and treatment outcome.

Types of Studies

Epidemiologic studies may be characterized as observational or experimental. Observational studies are subgrouped as either descriptive or analytic.[2] Analytic studies involve interpretation and evaluation of an observed pattern of disease. Descriptive studies concern descriptions of occurrence and determinants of disease. Interventive studies describe the effect of environmental changes or effect of treatment on the occurrence of disease in selected risk groups.[3]

Descriptive studies deal with prevalence. Prevalence denotes the frequency of a disease or condition in a population at a given time. Period prevalence refers to the frequency of accumulated cases of a disease in a population during a certain period. Analytic studies deal with incidence. Incidence denotes the frequency of new cases of a disease or conditions diagnosed for the first time during a certain period (usually 1 year).

Most research on the epidemiology of TMD has involved the prevalence in cross-sectional studies of single populations. Little information is available on the incidence of TMD. Typically, incidence focuses on longitudinal studies, mostly prospective in nature. A few have been conducted on children and young adults.

Assessment

It is not easy to study the epidemiology of TMD. Consider the problem of estimating the prevalence of serious, chronic musculoskeletal disorders. Such disorders have complex organic and psychological variables. Drawing conclusions about them from individuals in the United States is complicated. There are so many diverse races and ethnic groups that declaring a sample as representative is difficult. A smaller percentage of these individuals would be expected to suffer from chronic head and neck complaints. A lesser percentage would suffer from orofacial TMD.

In epidemiology, the definition of what is and what is not a case of the disease is critical. Opinions differ about which symptoms and signs should be considered important in TMD and which complaints or clinical findings should be judged dysfunctional. Lack of consistency across studies makes comparison of prevalence rates difficult. Estimates are complicated by the absence of universally accepted classification for these disorders. Various clinicians have applied different criteria for diagnosis.

Conclusions drawn about rates of TMD in the population at large contrast with judgments made from rates on populations perceiving themselves in need of treatment.

Information about the natural course of development of TMD is limited. It is unclear whether individuals with mild symptoms develop serious, chronic conditions. This paucity of information is understandable because the field is virtually in a stage of infancy compared with what is known about many other musculoskeletal disorders.

Several other factors confound understanding the epidemiology of TMD. These variables are age, gender, ethnic group, occupation, social factors, and educational level.

The existing epidemiologic studies of TMD have been criticized by investigators.[4] The major criticisms are poor research design, selection of different methodologic criteria, and lack of or inappropriate statistical analyses. Summarily, most of the inherent bias in these studies may relate to asking individuals the wrong kinds of questions.

Critical problems include differences in the manner of collecting and processing data. Information may include anamnestic data and data collected subjectively from individual self-report by questionnaire, interview, or both. Objective data are obtained by clinical evaluation. Collection of anamnestic and objective data simultaneously provides the most comprehensive picture of the disorder.

Reliability

The criteria for evaluation of population-based studies need to be reliable.[1] Reliability means that results can be repeated under the same conditions. Although sampling of a population once may be significant, greater reliability can be implied if the population is sampled again with the same findings.

Validity

Although opinions and clinical judgments are important, appropriately designed studies need validity. A screening test should give some indication of which individuals have the disease and which do not.[1] This validity should include the testing of an hypothesis, objective measures, and appropriate controls.

Often, questionnaires employed in collection of data are not standardized and thus are not reliable instruments. Validity can be enhanced by an understanding of its components, namely sensitivity and specificity. An ideal test or questionnaire would be 100% sensitive and 100% specific.[1]

Sensitivity

Sensitivity is the ability to correctly detect the presence of a condition in individuals with confirmed disease (true-positive results). Failure to detect disease is called a false-negative result. It is the conditional probability of a positive response to a question given the presence of a clinical sign. The higher the value for sensitivity, the greater the correspondence. The lower the value, the lesser the correspondence. Generally, little correspondence exists if values fall below 0.7 (70%).

Specificity

Specificity is the ability to correctly detect the absence of disease in individuals without the disorder. This is a true-negative result. Detection of disease in individuals without the disorder is a false-positive result. It is the probability of correctly identifying (negative response to a question) an asymptomatic person given the absence of a sign (questionnaire). Like sensitivity, little association exists if values fall below 0.7 (70%).

Measurements of sensitivity and specificity allow the clinician to determine the correspondence between information obtained about symptoms from the questionnaire or interview with data obtained about signs from the clinical examination. Ideally, findings of the clinical examination should reveal associations or coincide with symptoms reported by the individual. Hence, there would be a high correspondence. Poor correspondence would be reflected by low sensitivity (inability of questions to detect clinical signs) and high false-positive rates.[5]

Unfortunately, few extant studies use these criteria. A study conducted on Michigan children used these criteria and found low sensitivity (5% to 40%) and high false-positive rates (52% to 77%) for complaints of pain, pain on opening wide, joint sounds, headache, and grinding of the teeth compared with the clinical signs of joint clicking and tenderness on palpation of the masticatory muscles and the TMJs.[5] The authors concluded that the correspondence was poor; they challenged the findings of several other researchers who ignored these criteria while working with children and adults.

Comparative study showed that headache frequency, masticatory muscle tenderness, cervical muscle tenderness, and maximal opening differed between adults with and without TMD.[6] Only tenderness of masticatory muscles proved highly sensitive and specific. Maximal opening and cervical muscle tenderness showed high specificity but low sensitivity. Both specificity and sensitivity were low for headache. The authors claimed that the relevance of headaches was questionable because of 37% false-negative and 33% false-positive findings.

Indices and Scales

Other means of assessment combine symptoms with signs and provide an overall estimate of the extent of dysfunction of individuals. A widely used assessment instrument has been the Helkimo index.[7-8] The index has an anamnestic component (A_i) and a clinical component (D_i). The A_i questionnaire combines pain complaints with other symptoms, such as joint sounds, locking, and fatigue. The D_i assesses range of jaw movement, detection of joint sounds, deviation on opening–closing movements, tenderness on palpation of masticatory muscles, tenderness on palpation of TMJs, and pain on movement of the mandible. Although scores on this questionnaire correlate fairly well with clinical ratings, it is unclear whether this scale is an index of dysfunction due to TMD or simply represents some subset of symptoms often associated with facial pain disorders.[9]

A modification of the Helkimo D_i index has proved useful in clinical assessment of the functional status of the masticatory system in children.[10] Numerous signs were evaluated at two examinations. Findings were judged on whether they were positive or negative at both examinations, or were different at the first and second examinations. From these findings, a constancy index was obtained to evaluate the reproducibility of single signs. The reproducibility of single signs was high when including both positive and negative findings, but the reproducibility of positive findings was lower. The authors concluded that the greatest value of this index was to differentiate between children with no moderate signs and children with severe signs.

Another instrument useful for screening of symptoms is the validated Orofacial Pain Symptom Checklist (OPSC). The series of 14 questions indicated that TMD symptoms could be described by four indices: joint movement symptoms (JMI), parafunction (PI), pain symptoms of daily living (PSI), and other vague circumoral complaints (CI) around the ears, temporal area, or cheeks.[11] Only the PSI index was related to clinical pain and illness behavior, most likely reflecting individuals with a "somatic focus" to their complaints. Two of the indices were influenced by diagnosis. Individuals primarily having joint complaints scored higher on the JMI and lower on the PI than individuals primarily having myofascial pain. The OPSC was unrelated to personality and appears to be a simple index useful for screening orofacial pain patients and evaluating treatment outcome.

Significance: Future studies on TMD should rely on the criteria of reliability, validity, sensitivity, and specificity. Adherence to these criteria would establish standards against which signs and symptoms could be tested.[12]

Given the multifactorial etiology of chronic orofacial pain disorders and the lack of knowledge concerning etiology, it is unlikely that even the best questionnaire would be more than supportive in the diagnostic process. Based on the heterogeneity of signs found after clinical examination of individuals in populations at large and among symptomatic individuals reporting to health care centers, the need is to validate a scale for nonevident patients.[9] A given scale must be validated and capable of detecting patients correctly. Nondysfunctional individuals must be classified, thus reducing false-positive and false-negative results.

Aside from obvious shortcomings, the findings from the extant literature on epidemiology have some face validity, set a baseline for estimating signs and symptoms, establish a source for discussion with colleagues and patients, and provide reference for future studies of this disorder.

Prevalence

Numerous surveys describe the prevalence of orofacial complaints in populations around the world (Table 5-1).[6–191] Because of heterogeneity about descriptions of in-

(text continues on page 142)

Table 5-1

Epidemiologic Studies of Asymptomatic Individuals and Patients With One or More Symptoms or Signs of TMD

Location	Population Sampled	No. of Patients	Female/ Male (%)	Age (y)	Investigation	References
Argentina	TMD clinic cases	763	80/20	1–80	Carraro et al 1969 (A)	168
Australia	TMD cases	222	80/20	32–63	Bezuur et al 1989 (Au)	137
	TMD cases	136	?	40 ± 18	Gerke et al 1988 (Au1)	46
	Citizens	55	?	40 ± 17		
	Citizens, edentulous	201	76/24	47–89	Mercado & Faulkner 1991 (Au2)	71
Belgium	Dental students	121	42/58	23	de Laat & van Steenberghe 1985 (B)	123
Brazil	Citizens	90	62/38	22	Fonseca et al 1991 (Br)	119
Canada	TMD cases	56	88/12	36–41	Zarb & Thompson 1970 (Ca)	167
	TMD cases	93	88/12	36–41	Zarb & Thompson 1975 (Ca1)	99
	Citizens, institutionalized	488	66/34	31–85	MacEntee et al 1987 (Ca2)	91
	Citizens	148	62/38	18–82	Locker & Slade 1989 (Ca3)	39
	TMD cases	246	80/20	11–72	Blasberg & Chambers 1989 (Ca4)	172
Denmark	Children	92	—	14–16	Nielsen et al 1988 (D) (D)	10
	Children	705	50/50	14–16	Nielsen et al 1989 (D1)	98
	Citizens	216	—	67	Petersen & Moller 1991 (D2)	30
	Citizens			60–75	Budtz-Jorgensen et al 1985 (D3)	95
	Dentate	91	48/52			
	Edentate	55	38/63			
Egypt	Desert dwellers	215	0/100	17–65	Abdel-Hakim 1983 (E)	105
England	TMD cases	100	74/26	12–75	Thomson 1959 (En)	60
	Citizens	100	65/35			
	TMD cases	186	79/21	21–50	Copeland 1960 (En1)	136
	Citizens	19	51/49	17–36	Wood & Branco 1979 (En2)	122
	TMD cases	400	82/18	?	Rothwell 1987 (En3)	173
Finland	Children	200	50/50	6–25	Nevakari 1960 (F)	143
	Lapps	321	52/48	15–65	Helkimo 1974 (F1)	7a
	Lapps—same patients as F1				Helkimo 1974 (F2)	7b
	Lapps—same patients as F1, F2				Helkimo 1974 (F3)	7
	Dental nurses	58	100/0	18–28	Helkimo 1979 (F4)	8
	Workers	583	61/39	18–64	Swanljung & Ratanen 1979 (F5)	44
	Workers	853	0/100	18–57	Alanen & Kirveskari 1982 (F6)	97
	Children	156	57/43	10–16	Könönen et al 1987 (F7)	75

(continued)

Table 5-1 *(Continued)*

Location	Population Sampled	No. of Patients	Female/Male (%)	Age (y)	Investigation	References
	Citizens	1600	50/50	25–65	Tervonen & Knuuttila 1988 (F8)	61
	Children	167	50/50	12–15	Heikinheimo et al 1989 (F9)	76
	Children, rural	1008	43/57	5–15	Pahkala & Laine 1991 (F10)	104
Germany	Children	212	—	12–16	Seibert 1975 (G)	33
	Citizens	2000	0/100	19–29	Pöllmann 1980 (G1)	162
Greece	Citizens	1160	57/43	18–70	Mezitis et al 1989 (G4)	124
	TMD cases	195	76/24	16–70	Koidis et al 1993 (Gr1)	177
Hungary	Citizens, urban	600	53/47	12–85	Szentpetery et al 1986 (Hu)	106
India	Citizens, rural	1187	67/33	16–56	Rao & Rao 1981 (In)	31
Iraq	College students	600	48/52	18–22	Al-Hadi 1993 (Ir)	151
Israel	Children	369	50/50	10–18	Gazit et al 1984 (I)	103
	Elderly	110	68/32	61–90	Serfaty et al 1989 (Il)	47
Japan	Children	2198	50/50	10–18	Ogura et al 1985 (J)	56
	Children	2198	50/50	10–18	Ohno et al 1988 (J1)	28
	TMD cases	71	80/20	?	Ozaki et al 1990 (J2)	29
Mexico	Dental students	217	75/25	19 29	Martinez & Barghi 1981 (Mx)	96
New Zealand	TMD cases	182	82/18	1–79	Crooks et al 1991 (NZ)	18
Norway	Children	264	—	8–14	Seyffart & Steen-Johnsen 1956 (N)	32
	TMD cases	406	75/25	10–70+	Helöe & Helöe 1975 (N1)	169
	Citizens	241	53/47	65–79	Helöe & Helöe 1977 (N2)	52
	TMD cases	333	75/25	10–60+	Helöe et al 1977 (N3)	111
	Citizens	332	51/49	20–69	Norheim & Dahl 1978 (N4)	82
	TMD cases	49	86/14	14–74	Helöe 1979 (N5)	183
	Citizens, rural	246	49/51	25	Helöe & Helöe 1979 (N6)	85
	Dental patients	872	54/46	20–79	Gustavsen et al 1991 (N7)	45
Poland	Children	2100	—	10–15	Wigdorowicz et al 1979 (P)	13
	Soldiers, young	1000	0/100	20–23		
	Soldiers, old	1000	0/100	39–43		
	Medical students	429	—	—		
	Military students	400	—	—		
	Children	250	50/50	6–8	Grosfeld & Czarnecka 1977 (P1)	86
	Adolescents	250	50/50	13–15		
	Adolescents	400	49/51	15–18	Grosfeld et al 1985 (P2)	81
	Young adults	400	49/51	19–22		
South Africa	Citizens	51	67/33	31–67	Wilding & Owen 1987 (SA)	36
Sweden	Children, young adults	273	61/39	6–25	Ingervall 1970 (S)	23
	Dental nurses	269	100/0	19–22	Posselt 1971 (S1)	120
	TMD cases	40	78/22	?	Werndahl et al 1971 (S2)	174

(continued)

Table 5-1 *(Continued)*

Location	Population Sampled	No. of Patients	Female/Male (%)	Age (y)	Investigation	References
	Citizens, retired	62	40/60	67	Hansson & Oberg 1971 (S3)	49
	Clinic cases	299	66/34	40	Carlsson & Svardstrum 1974 (S4)	121
	Citizens, urban	1106	52/48	15–74	Agerberg & Carlsson 1972 (S5)	40
	Citizens, urban	1106	52/48	15–74	Agerberg & Carlsson 1973 (S6)	72
	Citizens, retired	194	56/44	70	Agerberg & Osterberg 1974 (S7)	50
	Children	33	50/50	1–3	Agerberg 1974 (S8)	138
		150	50/50	6		
	Naval cadets, dental and nursing students	205	50/50	20	Agerberg 1974a (S9)	15
	Conscripts	287	0/100	18–20	Ingervall & Hedegaard 1974 (S10)	150a
	Children	228	—	10–14	Lindquist 1974 (S11)	26
	TMD cases	82	80/20	15–74	Agerberg & Carlsson 1975 (S12)	41
	Citizens	94	48/52			
	Citizens	628	—	Adults	Lignell & Ransjök 1967 (S13)	14
	Shipworkers	1069	8/92	20–65	Hansson & Nilner 1975 (S14)	92
	Draftees	253	0/100	18–20	Molin et al 1976 (S15)	145
	Conscripts	248	0/100	18–25	Carlsson et al 1982 (S16)	141
	TMD cases	10	70/30	19–55	Helkimo & Ingervall 1977 (S17)	175
	TMJ crepitation	20	74/26	16–88	Kopp 1977a (S18)	25
	TMJ tenderness	20				
	Non-TMD cases	20				
	TMD-headache cases	80	—	15–74	Magnusson & Carlsson 1978 (S19)	89
	Dental cases	80	—	20–82		
	Citizens, retired	1148	51/49	70	Osterberg & Carlsson 1979 (S20)	79
	Soldiers	389	0/100	21–54	Ingervall et al 1980 (S21)	107
	Adolescents, young adults	309	53/47	15–18	Nilner 1981 (S22)	114
	Children	440	50/50	7–14	Nilner & Lassing 1981 (S23)	109
	Children	402	50/50	7–15	Egermark-Eriksson et al 1981 (S24)	88
	TMD cases	350	68/32	—	Carlsson et al 1982 (S25)	141
	Children	136	54/46	7	Egermark-Eriksson et al 1983 (S26)	144
		131	47/53	11		
		135	44/56	15		
	TMD cases	132	100/0	18–60	Mejersjö & Carlsson 1983 (S27)	185
	Dental students	48	49/51	25	Droukas et al 1984 (S28)	150
	Citizens	129	—	67	Lysell 1984 (S29)	115

(continued)

Table 5-1 *(Continued)*

Location	Population Sampled	No. of Patients	Female/Male (%)	Age (y)	Investigation	References
	TMD cases	282	72/28	20–39	Magnusson 1984 (S30)	129
	Citizens	20				
	Children, young adults	440	49/51	7–18	Nilner 1985 (S31)	65
	Adolescents, young adults	119	46/54	15–20	Magnusson 1986 (S32)	66
	Adolescents, young adults	121	46/54	15–20	Magnusson et al 1986 (S33)	68
	Adolescents	285	49/51	17	Wänman & Agerberg 1986 (S34)	73
	Adolescents, young adults	285	49/51	17–19	Wänman & Agerberg 1986 (S35)	110
	Adolescents, young adults	285	49/51	17–19	Wänman & Agerberg 1986 (S36)	74
	Adolescents	285	49/51	17	Wänman & Agerberg 1986 (S37)	35
	Adolescents, young adults	258	49/51	17–19	Wänman & Agerberg 1986 (S38)	87
	Adolescents	93 (ID) 129 (RD)	—	13–15	Kampe et al 1986 (S39)	67
	Young adults	67	36/64	18–23	Agerberg 1987 (S40)	125
	Adolescents	13 (D)	—	16–18	Kampe et al 1987 (S41)	24
	Young adults	16 (RD)				
	TMD cases	331	69/31	11–84	Agerberg & Helkimo 1987 (S42)	178
	Arthritic cases	40	70/30	9–28	Forsberg et al 1988 (S43)	80
	Nonarthritics	40	70/30	9–28		
	Citizens, random	1992	50/50	25–65	Agerberg & Bergenholtz 1989 (S44)	64
	TMD cases	158	—	15–76	Isacsson et al 1989 (S45)	180
	TMD cases	106	39/61	15–84	Rubinstein et al 1990 (S46)	176
	Citizens, urban	637	51/49	18–64	Agerberg & Inkapool 1990 (S47)	53
	Citizens, random	967	51/49	20–80+	Salonen et al 1990 (S48)	42
	Adolescents, young adults	285	49/51	17–19	Wänman & Agerberg 1990 (S49)	94
	Needing TMD tx	32	46/54	20	Magnusson et al 1991 (S50)	130
	Non-TMD cases	87				
	Adolescents, young adults	153	50/50	15–20	Kampe et al 1991 (S51)	69
Switzerland	Children	238	—	8–14	Geering-Gaerny & Rakosi 1971 (Sw)	20
	Children	64	50/50	5	Landtwing 1978 (Swl)	139
		70	60/40	12		
		70	20/80	19		
Taiwan	Univ. students	2033	43/57	17–32	Shiau & Chang 1992 (T)	153
Tanzania	Citizens	100	39/61	35–74	Mazengo & Kirveskari 1991 (Ta)	102
The Netherlands	Children	112	—	8–17	Dibbets 1977 (TN)	19
	TMD cases	58	86/14	<20–50+	Hijzen & Slangen 1985 (TN1)	140
	Non-TMD cases	64	86/14			

(continued)

Table 5-1 *(Continued)*

Location	Population Sampled	No. of Patients	Female/Male (%)	Age (y)	Investigation	References
	Headache cases	100	66/34	34–49	Schokker et al 1990 (TN2)	142
	Citizens	3468	52/48	15–74	De Kanter et al 1993 (TN3)	186
United States (US)						
California	Dental clinic cases	153	58/42	10–79	Rieder 1976 (C)	158
	Dental clinic cases	323	58/42	10–79	Rieder 1977 (C1)	187
	Dental clinic cases	226	55/45	20–70	Rieder 1978 (C2)	118
	TMD cases	95	70/30			
	Univ. students	739	50/50	19–25	Solberg et al 1979 (C3)	34
	Dental cases	1049	63/37	13–86	Rieder et al 1983 (C4)	156
	Dental cases	1040	63/37	13–86	Rieder & Martinoff 1983 (C5)	160
	TMD clinic cases	152	67/33	18–35	Pullinger & Monteiro 1988 (C6)	149
	Dental students, hygienists	331				
	Dental students, hygienists	222	46/54	19–40	Pullinger et al 1988 (C7)	131
	Dental students	40	46/54	19–40	Cacchiotti et al 1991 (C8)	7
	TMD cases	41	65/35			
Georgia	TMD cases	236	84/16	20–70	Kaye et al 1979 (Ga)	135
	Dental students	569	17/83	20–43	Allen et al 1990 (Ga1)	16
Hawaii	Random	148	—	3–70	Sheppard & Sheppard 1965 (H)	117
	Military enlistees	100	0/100	18–30		
	Dental patients	100	—	31–40		
	TMD cases	124	—	6–70		
Illinois	TMD cases	467	—	40–50	Perry 1968 (Il)	163
	TMD cases	277	?	?	Greene et al 1968 (Ill)	22
Iowa	Dental patients	1000	?	16–74	Vincent & Lilly 1988 (Io)	161
Kentucky	Citizens	562	?	71 (median)	Marciani et al 1984 (K)	27
Maryland	Dental students	123	10/90	25	Graham et al 1982 (M)	128
	TMD cases	48	85/15	41	Heft 1984 (M1)	38
	Citizens	144	43/57	19–86		
	Citizens	434	50/50	18–76	Huber & Hall 1990 (M2)	133
Michigan	Children	1342	50/50	6–17	Riolo et al 1987 (Mi)	70
	Children, migrant	151	56/44	6–18	Gunn et al 1988 (Mi1)	93
	Children	1342	50/50	6–17	Riolo et al 1988 (Mi2)	6
Minnesota	Children	50	—	10–14	Brussel 1949 (Mn)	17
	TMD cases	56	84/16	16–73	Butler et al 1975 (Mn1)	127
	TMD cases	164	82/18	17–89	Fricton et al 1985 (Mn2)	101
	Nursing students	269	100/0	22–25	Schiffman et al 1990 (Mn3)	112
	Nuns	117	100/0	75–94	Harriman et al 1990 (Mn4)	48
Missouri	Citizens	149	50/50	21–65 +	Duckro et al 1990 (Mo)	51

(continued)

Table 5-1 *(Continued)*

Location	Population Sampled	No. of Patients	Female/ Male (%)	Age (y)	Investigation	References
	Citizens	534	59/41	8–65 +	Glass et al 1993 (Mo1)	21
New York	Children	10	—	7–11	Travell 1960 (Ny)	116
	Young adults	150	54/46	19–21		
	TMD cases	153	69/31	Adults		
	Citizens	—	—	45–65		
	TMD clinic cases	742	84/16	10–180	Gelb et al 1967 (Ny1)	165
	TMD clinic cases	90	89/11	16–71	Weinberg & Lager 1980 (Ny2)	154
	and dental cases	48	77/23			
	Dental cases	943	59/41	3–89	Gross & Gale 1983 (Ny3)	126
	TMD clinic cases	837	79/21	7–76	Cooper et al 1986 (Ny4)	164
	Dental cases	1109	58/42	3–89	Gross et al 1988 (Ny5)	157
Ohio	Children	304	58/42	6–16	Williamson 1977 (O)	108
Pennsylvania	Citizens	700	?/50	19–30	Markowitz & Gerry 1949 (Pa)	155
	Children	50	—	10–14		
	Clinic patients (calm group, children)	250	57/43	6–10	Vanderas 1988 (Pa1)	77
	Clinic patients (not-calm group, children)	105	57/43	6–10	Vanderas 1989 (Pa2)	78
	Clinic patients (dentofacial injuries)	25				
Tennessee	TMD cases	448	87/13	<10–50>	Hodges 1990 (Tn)	171
Texas	Dental clinic patients	279	1/99	18–87	Rosenbaum 1975 (Tx)	159
Virginia	Dental cases	1016	53/47	11–77	Bush et al 1982 (V)	37
	Citizens, urban	178	54/46	24–70	(Vo)	
	Dental students, hygienists	105	10/90	22–31	(Vs)	
	Dental students	324	83/17	22–37	Bush et al 1985 (V2)	100
	Dental students	298	81/19	22–37	Bush et al 1983 (V1)	152
	TMD clinic cases	85	85/15	37	Bush et al 1989 (V3)	166
	TMD clinic cases	112	90/10	11–72	Abbott et al 1991 (V4)	170
	TMD clinic cases	79	82/18	18–69	Harkins et al 1991 (V5)	11
Washington	Citizens, urban	1106	—	18–75	Von Korff et al 1988 (W)	63
	COCL cases	121	—	18–75	Dworkin et al 1988 (W1)	83
	COCO controls	210				
	CLCA cases	261				
	Same patients as W1				Dworkin et al 1990 (W2)	84
Regions	Northeast Midwest South West	42,370	56/44	18–75 +	Lipton et al 1993 (X)	58

?, gender unknown; *ID*, intact dentition; *CLCA*, TMD clinic cases; *COCL*, TMD community cases; *COCO*, community controls; *RD*, restored dentition.

dividuals (eg, age), studies have been divided arbitrarily into categories. Minor overlap occurs between assignments, but most investigations fit one of the following:

1. *Nonclinical settings*: Children, adolescents, and young adults (18 years or younger) and adults (18 years or older) surveyed randomly from the population at large
2. *Selected groups*: Adults of similar age or gender and usually from different localities (dental or medical students, nurses, military personnel)
3. Patients presenting to *private clinicians* or *clinics* for routine dental care
4. TMD cases presenting to *diagnostic or treatment clinics for TMD*, usually at large dental and medical centers.

Table 5-1 alphabetizes assignments of populations according to country of origin. Specific symptoms and signs are reviewed because they most likely represent useful predictors of TMD.

Symptoms include the following: general complaint of orofacial pain, pain or difficulty on opening the jaws wide, pain on chewing, pain on mandibular movement, headache, feeling of fatigue or tiredness in the jaws, complaint of joint sounds, and report of joint locking.

Signs include the following: tenderness on palpation of the masticatory muscles, tenderness of specific muscle groups, tenderness on palpation of the TMJs, limitation on opening wide, deviation of the mandible on opening, and detection of joint sounds during mandibular movement.

The effects of age and gender as related to signs and symptoms are reviewed. Clinician estimates of need for treatment, demand by subjects for treatment, and the frequency of advice or treatment sought by subjects are considered.

Morphologic and functional malocclusions are excluded because of inconsistent agreement on the meanings of terms and data on occlusal studies suggest that the teeth should be considered minor contributing factors in dysfunction.

Nonclinical Settings

Signs and Symptoms in Adults

A summary of 25 different studies of adults across America, Europe, Taiwan, and Tanzania indicates that symptoms ranged from 12% to 64% and that signs ranged from 27% to 88% (Table 5-2). With little exception, more signs were found after examination by investigators than symptoms reported by individuals. The broad diversity of populations severely limits comparison between populations.

Age and Symptoms

The relation between symptoms and age is controversial. Some symptoms have been reported as stable with increasing age, whereas others have been reported to increase or decrease with age. This difference depends partly on the way in which the

Table 5-2

Percentage of Adults With at Least One Symptom and at Least One Sign of TMD

Symptom (%)	Sign (%)	Population Sampled	Method	Investigation	Reference
40	72	Belgium, dental students	Quest/Exam	de Laat & van Steenberghe 1985 (B)	123
13	27	Canada, elderly institutionalized	Quest/Exam	MacEntee et al 1987 (Ca2)	91
64	88	Canada, citizens, urban	Interview/Exam	Locker & Slade 1989 (Ca3)	39
57	88	Finland, Lapps	Interview/Exam	Helkimo 1974 (F1)	7a
45	60	Finland, dental training nurses	Quest/	Helkimo 1979 (F4)	8
58	86	Finland, workers	Interview/Exam	Swanljung & Ratanen 1979 (F5)	44
—	50	Iraq, college students	Exam	Al-Hadi 1993 (Ir)	151
—	76	Norway, citizens, rural	Quest/	Helöe & Helöe 1979 (N6)	85
57	41	Sweden, citizens urban	Quest/	Agerberg & Carlsson 1972 (S5)	40
23	74	Sweden, citizens retired	Quest/Exam	Agerberg & Osterberg 1974 (S7)	50
12	—	Sweden, conscripts	Quest/	Ingervall & Hedegaard 1974 (S10)	150a
>23	70	Sweden, shipworkers	Quest/Exam	Hansson & Nilner 1975 (S14)	92
12	28	Sweden, draftees	Quest/Exam	Molin et al 1976 (S15)	145
59	—	Sweden, citizens retired	Quest/	Osterberg & Carlsson 1979 (S20)	79
—	60	Sweden, military draftees	Quest/	Ingervall et al 1980 (S21)	107
32	64	Sweden, dental students	Quest/Exam	Droukas et al 1984 (S28)	150
20	88	Sweden, urban	Quest/Interview/Exam	Agerberg & Inkapööl 1990 (S47)	53
21	44	The Netherlands, citizens	Quest/Exam	De Kanter et al 1993 (Tn3)	186
25	—	California, dental patients	Quest/	Rieder 1976 (C)	158
26	79	California, Univ. students	Quest/Exam	Solberg et al 1979 (C3)	34
14	—	Missouri citizens	Telephone survey	Glass et al 1993 (Mo1)	21
—	28	Pennsylvania, citizens, random	Exam	Markowitz & Gerry 1949 (Pa)	155

Exam, examination; *Quest*, questionnaire.

data are expressed. The change may be expressed as two or more symptoms lumped together rather than being reported as a single symptom.

Generally speaking, no major relations have been found between age and the total complex of TMD symptoms in populations at large from the same localities, including Virginia,[37] Maryland,[38] Canada,[39] Sweden,[40–42] Finland,[7,43,44] Norway[45], and Australia.[46] In these and the remaining populations, changes within a few symptoms have been associated with age. Unless the data of two or more symptoms have been grouped, each change is discussed under a specific heading described below.

A study among Israeli elderly persons from 61 to 90 years of age showed fewer dysfunctions than were present in many young individuals sampled at random from other countries.[47] This same relation was found in a comparison of a group of elderly nuns in Minnesota (75 to 94 years of age)[48] with younger individuals.

Age and Signs

Although certain signs have been found to change with age, few changes have proved statistically different in populations at large. The findings indicate that the number of individuals free of signs markedly decreased with age.[42,49,50] To put it another way, more signs appear with advancing age.

Gender and Symptoms

Many investigators have ignored possible differences in gender and grouped the gender data for an entire population. In a study conducted in North America that considered gender, the findings were minimal for the total complex of symptoms.[51] In Scandinavia, Norwegian women reported twice as many symptoms of general bodily rheumatic and joint pain as men.[52] Swedish women reported more frequent symptoms (18 versus 10%) than men.[53]

Gender and Signs

Generally, few differences exist between older subjects. Slightly higher frequencies for some signs have been reported in women more often than in men.

Significance: Generally speaking, one third of the adults sampled from non-clinical settings have one or more symptoms. One half to nearly three fourths have at least one sign. These estimates would put the prevalence of one or more TMD symptoms at roughly 80 million and the signs at 185 million in individuals in the United States. These figures are higher than mentioned in a general statement about TMD reported in one reputable journal.

According to the *Guide to Dental Health*, published by the American Dental Association, roughly 20% of the adults of the United States suffer from overlooked, misdiagnosed, and complex dental conditions known as TMD.[54] Considering the diversity of total symptoms (eg, TMJ sounds, limited opening, deviation on opening, pain), fewer than 20% would be expected to suffer from orofacial pain. This estimate conflicts with a report issued by the National Institute of Dental Research in

1990, which stated that some 25% of the population in the United States suffers from orofacial pain.[55]

Signs and Symptoms in Children and Young Adults

A summary of 15 studies conducted in 10 countries showed that the prevalence of TMD symptoms ranged from 7% to 74% and the prevalence of signs from 33% to 80% (Table 5-3). In older adults, signs proved more common than symptoms. The wide variation in symptoms results partly from inclusion of data on bruxism and malocclusion in some studies and not in others. Several studies focused on the need for orthodontic treatment. Sampling for malocclusion and bruxism might be expected in these reports. In contrast to most studies conducted on older adults, percentages were nearly equal for gender and age groups. This equality allows greater uniformity when comparing signs and symptoms across populations.

Few gender differences have been reported in young children. None existed in a gender-equal sample of 2198 Japanese children.[56] The findings have been lumped in most other studies. Fluctuations have been observed in certain signs of adolescents and young adults.

Table 5-3
Percentage of Children and Young Adults With at Least One Symptom and at Least One Sign of TMD

Symptom (%)	Sign (%)	Population Sampled	Age (y)	Method	Investigation	Reference
64 67	—	Finland	12–15	Quest/	Heikinheimo et al 1989 (F9)	76
	62–80	Germany	12–16	Exam/	Siebert 1975 (G)	33
56	—	Israel	10–18	Quest/	Gazit et al 1984 (I)	103
7		Japan	10–18	Exam/	Ogura et al 1985 (J)	56
10		Japan	10–18	Exam/	Ohno et al 1988 (J1)	28
—	54	Norway	8–14	Exam/	Seyffart & Steen-Johnsen 1956 (N)	32
—	56	Poland	6–18	Exam/	Grosfeld &	86
—	68		13–15		Czarnecka 1977 (P1)	
23	68	Poland	15–22	Quest/Exam	Grosfeld et al 1985 (P2)	81
41	77	Sweden	15–18	Interview/Exam	Nilner 1981 (S22)	114
36	72	Sweden	7–14	Interview/Exam	Nilner & Lassing 1981 (S23)	109
16(39)*	33	Sweden	7	Interview/Exam	Egermark-Eriksson et al 1981 (S24)	88
17(67)*	46		11			
25(74)*	61		15			
20	56	Sweden	17	Quest/Exam	Wänman & Agerberg 1986 (S34)	73
—	41	Switzerland	8–14	Exam/	Gerring-Gaerny & Rokosi 1971 (Sw)	20
	46	The Netherlands	8–17	Quest/	Dibbets 1977 (TN)	19
—	36	Minnesota	10–14	Exam/	Brussel 1949 (Mn)	17

*Symptoms in parentheses include TMJ sounds, jaw tiredness, difficult opening, and pain/tiredness of jaw on chewing. Symptoms not in parentheses exclude chewing pain.

Significance: The prevalence of symptoms and signs in children and young adults is lower than in older people. Comparison between studies suggests that about one half of white children could present with signs, although less than one half would be expected to complain. Complaints are more likely to be important than are signs because young people often lack understanding of signs, particularly when questioned about palpation of muscles or joints or how to perform jaw movements. Further study is required to determine which signs and symptoms are important.

Report of Orofacial Pain

Subjective pain of the orofacial region has been reported as a common complaint in TMD. The meaning of this broad expression is not clear. Much ambiguity exists because of the diverse questions asked. If specific anatomic regions of pain, such as the angle of the mandible, cheek, or TMJ, have been designated, improved interpretation follows. If the location is ignored, uncertainty remains.

Comparison across cultures shows that generalized orofacial pain varies widely (Table 5-4). Evaluation of most nonclinical studies confirms that many individuals are either asymptomatic or cope effectively with the pain.

The 1989 National Health Interview Survey (NHIS) conducted on 42,370 individuals within the United States should be considered the "gold standard" on orofacial and dental pains. The number of adults with an acute episode of pain around the jaw joint was 9.495 million, a prevalence of 5.3% (US Public Health Service, Hanes II Epidemiological Survey).[57,58] For facial or cheek pain, the numbers were 2.541 million and 1.4%, respectively. The prevalence of combined joint and facial pains was 6.4%. Within this group, 67% reported that the pain became chronic, which was defined as lasting longer than 6 months.

Similar findings have been reported for other populations from North America. A telephone survey conducted among 897 French Canadians in Quebec revealed clinically significant jaw pain of frequent to moderate intensity in 5% of the population.[59] One third of adults 18 years or older reported the presence of jaw pain, and 27% had frequent episodes of pain. Within the group with episodic pain, 69% had moderate to severe pain. Of the one fourth with frequent jaw pain, 9% had accompanying joint sounds, and 4% had difficulty opening the mouth widely.

Large percentages have been cited in other reviews for pain localized to the jaw region. Reviewers have discussed this pain based on tenderness to palpation of the face or TMJs or based on the presence of static jaw pain occurring without mandibular movement. Still others have grouped pains of the head, face, or ear with pain of the jaw. Although these pains may be of the same etiology, they should be differentiated from one another until this issue is resolved.

Complaint of generalized orofacial pain was almost nonexistent in citizens randomly sampled from England.[60] Pain localized to the face or head was found in less than 1% to 5% of a group of Swedish citizens.[42] However, face-ache was reported as occurring in 38% and neckache in 52% of a Finnish population.[61] An extremely low

(text continues on page 150)

Table 5-4

Percentages for Adults with Orofacial (Jaw/Face) Pain, Other Pain, Pain on Chewing, Headache, Pain on Opening the Mouth Wide, and Pain on Mandibular Movement. References are Coded According to Country and Investigation (see Table 5-1).

Orofacial (y)	Other Pain	Chewing	Headache	Opening	Movement	Reference
Nonclinical Settings						
20	25 neck	—	16	—	6	Au2
	16 shoulder					
16	—	13	—	11	16	Ca1
—	0 dentate	34	—	—	—	D3
—	2 edentate	23	—	—	—	
24 ear	—	—	29	10	—	E
—	—	—	—	—	—	En
15 face—jaw	9	—	21	—	30	F1
18(15–24)	5 neck/	—	60	—	—	F2
22(25–34)	25 shoulder	—	29	—	—	
40(35–44)	42	—	35	—	—	
29(45–54)	52	—	19	—	—	
32(55–65)	51	—	20	—	—	
—	—	—	—	14	4	F4
38(25)	48 neck/	—	8	2	—	F8
—(35)	— shoulder	—	—	3	—	
—(50)	—	—	—	6	—	
—(65)	—	—	—	3	—	
6 face/neck/ears	—	—	23	20	3	Hu
10	—	—	18	—	—	I1
4(16–25)	—	—	—	—	—	In
4(26–35)	—	—	—	—	—	
4(36–45)	—	—	—	—	—	
7(46–55)	—	—	—	—	—	
5(56+)	—	—	—	—	—	
4 TMJ	—	2	—	—	—	K
—	—	8b	26	—	—	N1
—	—	3	—	<1	—	N3
—	—	6	—	—	—	SA
—	—	—	—	—	—	S2
24*	—	7	—	6	12	S4
—	—	—	—	—	4–7	S6
10	—	—	5	—	11	S11
7	—	—	18	3	—	S14
—	—	15	—	3	—	S20
5 A	—	0	13	5	3	S43
2(25) cheek	3 ear, 24 neck	—	8†	—	—	S44
1(35)	3 35	—	6	—	—	
<1(50)	3 47	—	6	—	—	
1(65)	7 52	—	7	—	—	
21	8 ear	<1	16	3	—	S47
9(20–29)‡	—	8	—	—	7	S48
3(30–39)	—	4	—	—	5	
6(40–49)	—	12	—	—	10	
5(50–59)	—	8	—	—	4	
5(60–69)	—	8	—	—	2	
3(70–79)	—	12	—	—	3	
1(>80)	—	10	—	—	1	
—	—	—	—	—	7	Ta
—	—	4	—	7	6	TN3
20(<56)§	—	—	—	—	—	M1
27(>56)	—	—	—	—	—	
6	—	—	35	1	—	Mo
10 jaw, teeth	—	—	—	—	—	Mo1

(continued)

Table 5-4 *(Continued)*

Orofacial (y)	Other Pain	Chewing	Headache	Opening	Movement	Reference
9	10 ear	3	24	4	—	Vo
—, COCO	—	1	—	—	7–10	W1, W2

Selected Groups

Orofacial (y)	Other Pain	Chewing	Headache	Opening	Movement	Reference
15 TMJ	—	—	—	—	—	B
36 ear symptoms	—	5	20	—	—	F6
—	—	2	27	8	—	N6
<1 medical student	—	—	—	—	—	P
1 military student						
3 (20–23)						
5 (39–45)						
4 ear	—	—	15	—	5	S
5 face/TMJ	—	—	8	—	3	S9
5	7 TMJ	—	—	—	—	S15
—	—	—	11	—	—	S16
5 ‖	—	—	8	—	—	S21
2	—	—	18	—	4	S28
—	—	75 tx	91	—	3	S50
—	—	51 no tx	78	—	—	
9 jaw	<1 TMJ	—	—	0	—	T
9	—	—	13	—	4	C3
0	<1 cervical	—	33	—	—	C8
12 #	—	—	—	—	—	Ga1
5 orofacial	—	—	55	—	—	M
5 face	22 jaw	—	—	—	—	Mn3
	18 temples					
6 jaw	—	—	—	—	—	Mn4
3 jaw	8 ear	4	12	—	—	Vs

Private/Clinic Dental Patients

Orofacial (y)	Other Pain	Chewing	Headache	Opening	Movement	Reference
2 jaw						Ca2
25 mild-jaw	6 mild TMJ	—	34	—	5 mild	S19
31 severe	3 severe				0 severe	
12 face	17 jaw/TMJ	—	43	—	—	Tn1
5 ear, 34 neck						
19 face/ear	—	—	43	—	—	C
19 face/ear(<30)		—	25	22	—	C1, C4
21 (31–39)		—	22	13	—	
22 (41–49)		—	24	14	—	
16 (51–59)		—	13	10	—	
15 (>60)		—	15	11	—	
18			19	—	5	C5
—	—	—	—	—	—	Ny3
6 ear (day)	11 neck	—	—	—	—	Ny5
3 (night)	4	—	—	—	—	
11 jaw	—	—	—	—	—	Pa
—	—	—	34	—	4	Tx
14 face/neck	—	9	25	6	—	Vd

TMD Clinic Cases

Orofacial (y)	Other Pain	Chewing	Headache	Opening	Movement	Reference
—	60 TMJ	—	—	—	—	A
36 face My	—	—	21	—	—	Au
58 face Ar	—	—	11	—	—	
46 face Ps	—	—	—	—	—	
59	—	41	—	46	—	En
82	—	—	—	—	—	En1
76	—	—	—	—	64	En3

(continued)

Table 5-4 *(Continued)*

Orofacial (y)	Other Pain	Chewing	Headache	Opening	Movement	Reference
—	—	—	61(<30)	—	—	Gr1
			54(<50)	—		
77	—	—	—	—	—	J2
78	—	—	—	—	44	N3
70	—	—	—	—	53	N5
90	15 cheek	32	—	—	48	NZ
—	—	—	—	—	88	S1
75 C	—	—	40	—	—	S17
84 T	—	—	42	—	—	
68 N	—	—	31	—	—	
91 jaw/muscle	29 TMJ	—	—	—	13	S18
—	—	—	75	—	14 mild	S19
					9 severe	
38 face/jaw	—	18	—	—	18	S25
69 IE	—	—	—	—	49	S27
22 FE	—	—	—	—	8	
23 My	—	—	17	—	—	S30
63 Ar	—	—	—	—	—	
4 Ad	—	—	—	—	—	
40	—	—	49	—	37	S42
8 face/jaw	—	0	13	23	10	S43
—	—	—	30	—	7	S46
—	—	—	—	—	3	S50
12 face	83 jaw/TMJ 5	—	59	—	—	TN1
	ear, 34 neck					
57 Te	—	—	100	49	33	TN2
45 Mig	—	—	100	—	10	
62 Co	—	—	100	—	15	
—	—	—	63	—	—	C8
33 face, 29 jaw	16 ear,* 79 TMJ	—	36	—	—	Ga
98	—	—	—	—	—	I1
87	—	—	—	—	—	I11
90 face/head/ear	—	—	—	—	42	M1
66 face	61 ear	61	50	46	—	Mn1
63 jaw	42 ear, 55 TMJ	—	6V,1Cl	—	—	Mn2
1 face(10–20)	4 TMJ	—	<1	—	<1	Ny1
1 face(21–30)	8 TMJ, 1 neck	—	3	—	<1	
2 face(31–40)	10 TMJ, 1 neck	—	6	—	<1	
2 face(41–50)	9 TMJ, 2 neck	—	4	—	<1	
3 face(51–60)	7 TMJ, 1 neck	—	4	—	<1	
1 face(61–70)	3 TMJ, 1 neck	—	2	—	<1	
1 face(71–80)	1 TMJ, 1 neck	—	<1	—	<1	
91 head/neck	76 TMJ	59	—	39	26–33	Ny2
40 face	50 ear, 47 TMJ	21	76	—	—	Ny4
	45 cervical					
11 jaw	48 ear, 6 neck	—	23	—	—	Tn
94 jaw My	—	81	76	78	—	V3
78 jaw Ar	—	68	72	79	—	
79 face	58 ear	54	61	—	—	V5
12	—	13	26	—	50	W, W1, W2
CLCA + COCA		CLCA				
—	—	8	—	—	21	
		COCA				

*Face/head 1–2 times/wk.

†Once/wk.

‡Face/head/ear.

‖ Face/TMJ/ear.

#Stiff or sore jaw, sore teeth, cracking/locking TMJ, headache.

A, asymptomatic; *Ad*, articular dysfunction; *Ar*, arthrogenous; *C*, ; *Cl*, cluster headache; *CLCA*, TMD clinic cases;
Co, combination tension and migraine headache; *COCA*, community TMD cases; *COCO*, community controls;
FE, final examination 7 y later; *IE*, initial examination; *Mig*, migraine; *My*, myogenous; *N*, ; *Ps*, psychogenous; *Te*,
tension headache; *tx*, treatment group; *no tx*, no treatment group; *V*, vascular headache; (y), age in years.

percentage of 0.47 was described for various symptoms among 5142 citizens visiting dental centers in Zimbabwe.[62]

Age

Based on cumulative probability of onset, TMD pain has been predicted to increase steadily between 20 and 70 years of age (Fig. 5-1).[63] This prediction was made from information obtained by standardized questionnaire through a mail survey of enrollees (mainly white) of the Group Health Cooperative of Puget Sound. Although making such predictions is interesting, the clinical relevance appears diffuse, considering the uncertainty of what is meant by TMD pain. It contrasts with findings reported for nonclinical settings across the world.

Specific anatomic regions with localized pain have been reported to increase with age. Based on the NHIS for the adult civilian population, the incidence of jaw joint pain decreased from 6,500 per 100,000 at 18 to 34 years to 3,873 per 100,000 at 75 years and older.[58] Facial pain remained constant between these ages.

In a sample from Virginia, only pain associated with the ear region (not jaw, head, facial, or chewing pains) increased significantly with age.[37] The highest frequency of ear pain was found in citizens 70 years and older. Still, the percentage was low, as was found in a study of very elderly nuns in Minnesota.[48]

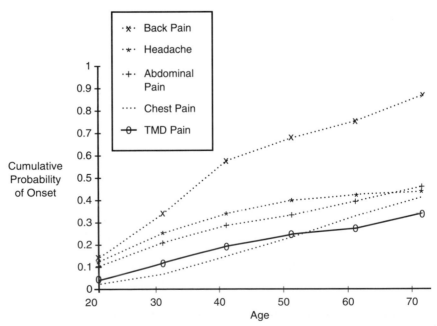

Figure 5-1.
Life-table estimate of the cumulative probability of developing selected pain conditions by age. (Von Korff M, Dworkin S, LeResche L, Kruger A. Epidemiology of temporomandibular disorders. II. TMD pain compared to other pain sites. In Dubner R, Bebhart FG, Bond MR [eds]. Pain research and clinical management. New York: Elsevier, 1988:506.)

Studies conducted in Scandinavia support the above findings that changes in pain with age are generally minimal. Some exceptions exist. Unfortunately, some data have been lumped together. For instance, face, ear, temple, head, and neck and shoulder pains increased from 61% to 77% between the ages of 25 and 65 in Finnish citizens.[61] Pain in or near the ear increased from 3% to 6% and throat pain from 7% to 27% between 25 and 65 years of age in Swedish citizens.[64] The greatest prevalence of facial pain and headache occurred in Swedish women between 20 and 59 years of age.[42] Mild to severe symptoms occurred between the ages of 20 and 39. In men, moderate to severe symptoms appeared at 80 years of age and older. These differences imply lower prevalence in women younger than 20 and older than 39, and less occurrence in men under 80 years.

An analysis of several Swedish populations showed variability in young subjects (Table 5-5). No significant difference in orofacial pain was found between 7 and 14 year olds.[65] The percentage was low and remained so for young adults.[66] A prevalence of about 1% was reported in populations of 13 to 15 year olds[67] and 15 to 20 year olds.[68] Twenty-one percent (17 occasional; 4 frequent) was reported for 15 to 20 year olds.[69] The highest recorded percentage of orofacial pain was facial or jaw pain in adolescents and young adults whose dentitions had been restored. A comparison with adolescents and young adults of the same age and with intact dentitions showed only occasional pain in 2% of this group. The authors concluded that dental filling therapy was etiologically important in producing the pain.

Gender

Among civilians of the United States, both jaw joint (6,885 women versus 3,524 men per 100,000) and facial pain (1,874 women versus 908 men per 100,000) were nearly twice as prevalent in women as in men.[58] In a random sample from Virginia, no significant gender difference was found for pain of the face, eyes, neck, or throat.[37]

No specific reference was found in the literature that described the frequency of static orofacial pain in children from the United States. In Michigan children, an association was made between TMJ pain and status of the occlusion. TMJ pain correlated with excessive overjet and negative overjet.[70] The authors concluded that adolescent and young adult males with class II and cusp-to-cusp relation and females younger than 11 years with class II and cusp-to-cusp relation appeared to be at greater risk of TMJ pain than their class I cohorts.

In Australia, jaw pain and fatigue, head, neck, and shoulder pains were generally more frequent in women than in men.[71]

In Sweden, women reported more frequent head and facial pain than men.[72] In other adults, no gender differences were found for pain of the face, ear region, eyes, throat, or neck.[53] In young subjects, pain in the temples was significantly more frequent in females than males.[73] No pain was found in the face or jaw (mostly around the ears) or cheeks. Nonetheless, face/jaw pain was more prevalent in 19-year-old women than in men of the same age, but not in 17 and 18 year olds.[74]

Table 5-5

Percentages of Orofacial (Jaw/Face) Pain, Pain on Chewing, Headache, Pain on Opening Wide, and Pain on Mandibular Movement in Children, Adolescents, and Young Adults of Different Populations. References are Coded According to Country and Investigation (see Table 5-1).

Orofacial (y)	Chewing	Headache	Opening	Movement	Reference
0–4 face	—	8–13	1–8	1	F7
10–14 temporal					
19(12)	—	—	—	—	F9
13(15)	—	—	—	—	
3(10–18)	—	—	—	3	I
—(6–8)	—	—	—	6	P1
—(13–15)	—	—	—	10	
—(15–18 A)	4	—	3	27	P2
—(19–22 A)	2	—	3	20	
—(15–18 S)	5	—	4	39	
—(19–22 S)	3	—	5	29	
—	—	—	—	—	S11
—	—	16	—	—	S22
3	2	14	6	—	S23
—(7)	32	13	—	2	S24
—(11)	65	22	—	2	
—(15)	62	36	—	1	
3(7–14)	2	13	6	—	S31
4(15–18)	5	15	5	—	
1(15)	66	18	—	1	S32
1(20)	59	—	—	3	
—(15)	12f	14w	2	1	S33
	54o	35m			
—(20)	16f	9w	10	3	
	43o	44m			
3 face/jaw	—	—	—	—	S34
5 temporal	—	—	—	—	
14 cheek					
4	2	18	—	4	S36
1(13–15 ID)	13	27	—	0	S39
6(13–15 RD)	16	46	—	2	
5(A)	0	13	—	3	S43
8(S)	0	13	—	10	
2(15–20 ID)	25	21	—	5	S51
21(15–20 RD)	29	26	—	8	
—	29	28	—	—	Mi, Mi2
—	23	9*	<1	—	Mi1
—	—	—	—	—	O
—(6)	4	7	17	—	Pa1
—(7)	6	7	15	—	
—(8)	6	9	15	—	
—(9)	10	14	25	—	
—(10)	11	17	15	—	
—(6)	5	0	24	—	Pa2
—(7)	5	15	5	—	
—(8)	4	13	—	—	
—(9)	17	25	21	—	
—(10)	—	0	6	—	

*Combination of jaw/ear/head pain. f, frequent; o, occasional; w, weekly; m, monthly; *A*, asymptomatic; *ID*, intact dentition; *RD*, restored dentition; *S*, symptomatic; (y), age in years.

In other parts of northern Europe, no gender difference was found in face/jaw pain of Finnish Lapps.[7b] Pain at more distant sites showed differences. Neck/shoulder pain was significantly greater in women than men.

In Finnish children, no gender difference was found in the frequency of orofacial pain.[75] Pain prevalence ranged from 0% to 4%, whereas temporal pain was slightly increased at a second examination (16% versus 10%) in girls but not in boys.

Pain of the TMJ region decreased significantly (19% versus 13%) in both sexes of Finnish children sampled initially at 12 years of age and then again at 15 years.[76] No gender difference was found during that period. Overall symptoms did not change much from 12 to 15 years of age in either sex.

TMJ pain in either gender was less than 2% of 2198 Japanese children between 10 and 18 years of age.[56]

Significance: Generalized orofacial pain is an uncommon complaint in older adults and is of minimal importance in young children and adolescents from populations at large. Little clinical data exist to differentiate individuals suffering orofacial pain of musculoskeletal origin from individuals suffering dental pains caused by eruption or decay of teeth or by periodontal problems.

The site of the pain must be determined. A quantitative estimate should be made of the intensity and unpleasantness of the pain.

Report of Pain on Chewing

Fewer individuals complain of pain on chewing, compared with people suffering orofacial pain of nonchewing origin (see Tables 5-4 and 5-5). Difficulty exists in interpreting findings because some clinicians do not always differentiate pain caused by chewing from other generalized orofacial discomfort.

Age

Information is scant about the relation of age to chewing pain. No age effect was found in a random adult population from Virginia.[37] A slight increase was observed in two populations of Pennsylvania children between 6 and 10 years of age.[77,78] The children were divided into "calm" and "non-calm" groups based on parental opinion of the activities of the children. Frequencies for the youngest children were similar between the groups and were lower than reported for older children and adults sampled from Virginia.[37]

Findings of Scandinavian populations are conflicting. Less than 1% of a random sample of urban Swedish citizens complained of problems with chewing,[53] whereas 15% of retired Swedish citizens experienced these problems.[79] In children and young adults, no difference was found in a small sample.[80] None was found in another population of adolescents and young adults.[69] However, in adolescents and young adults sampled by questionnaire at age 15 and again at 20 years, pain or tiredness of the jaws or face during chewing was reported initially as 66% (12 frequent; 54 occasional) and later as 59% (16 frequent; 43 occasional).[66] Inclusion of tiredness with painful symptoms inflated the percentage. Clearly, the frequency for pain precipitated by chewing would have been less.

A difference might be expected between elderly and younger adults because the elderly tend to lose teeth more readily and likely experience discomfort associated with dental prostheses. A general dissatisfaction with chewing ability was reported more often by older than younger adults in a Swedish population.[64]

Support for this logic is found in other studies. Greater difficulty in chewing was reported more frequently in older than in younger Lapps from Finland.[7b] Furthermore, children with erupting permanent teeth would be more likely complain of greater pain on chewing. These fluctuations have been reported. Pain on chewing increased significantly (5% to 10%) in Finnish boys, but not girls, from 12 to 15 years of age.[76]

In Poland, no significant difference was found between subjects 15 to 22 years old.[81]

Gender

In a community-based population in Virginia, significantly more women reported pain on chewing than men.[37]

In Sweden, no gender difference was found in individuals of the general population,[40] in elderly women and men,[79] or in adults of another population.[53]

Significance: Taken together, pain caused by chewing relates more to dental and periodontal problems than to joint and muscle complaints. Dental problems must be ruled out during the screening and interview.

Report of Pain on Opening Wide

Overall, few individuals across populations complain of pain on opening wide (see Tables 5-4 and 5-5). Samples from Virginia[37] and Missouri[51] showed that frequencies were low.

In northern Europe, just one of 358 Norwegian citizens[82] sampled by questionnaire had this problem. A prevalence of 11% was reported by Finnish workers,[44] but the data are inflated by inclusion of pain on chewing.

Age

Prevalence ranged from 1% to 6% in most populations of children (see Table 5-5). An exception was in Pennsylvania, where the overall frequency was 17% and reached 25% in 9 year olds.[77] Still, no significant difference was found between 6 to 10 year olds.[77,78]

The absence of age as a factor was confirmed in Swedish children and young adults between 7 and 18 years of age.[65] Impaired mobility, identified as difficulty on opening wide and joint sounds, was significantly greater in Swedish citizens aged 55 to 75 years than in younger individuals.[72]

No significant difference was found in an adult Finnish population.[61] Citizens were sampled at 25, 35, 50 and 65 years.

No difference was found between adolescents and young adults from a Polish sample.[81]

Gender

In Swedish populations, significantly more women than men complained of difficult opening, but no difference was found in report of pain on opening wide.[40] When difficulty opening wide was lumped with joint sounds as impaired mobility, significantly more women than men had impairment.[72] But findings differ between populations. No significant difference occurred among the elderly,[79] younger adults,[53] or adolescents.[73]

In Finnish populations, no significant gender difference was found among 10 to 16 year olds[75] or among 12 to 15 year olds.[76]

Significance: Although difficult opening is considered important, it is unclear whether the pain that accompanies it is the same as that reported when the mandible is in the static position.

Difficulty opening may be caused by muscle, joint, or combined muscle/joint problems. Clinicians must determine the origin to make a definitive diagnosis.

Report of Pain on Mandibular Movement

Review of the literature shows large discrepancies in the report of pain on mandibular movement. Typically, percentages were low across populations (see Tables 5-4 and 5-5). About 10% or less of citizens in Washington complained of this problem.[83,84]

In Sweden, just 1% of elderly 80 years or older and 10% between 40 and 49 years complained of this pain.[42]

Exceptionally larger percentages were probably related to discomfort from loss of teeth, dental pain, or fatigue on chewing. For example, 30% of Finnish Lapps reported this pain.[7b] Apparently, chewing dissatisfaction from loss of teeth contributed to this high percentage in Lapps. Variation in age accounted for some divergence.

Age

Functional pain was significantly greater in young Swedish adults than in older subjects.[72] Functional pain was interpreted as pain on chewing, difficulty opening, and making mandibular movements. No pain was reported on mandibular movement by 13- to 15-year-old Swedes.[67]

A study of three different groups from Norway showed little age effect involved with TMJ pain on function.[85] Prevalence was 9% for a random sample of 1740 subjects from the population at large and was the same in 25 year olds, but it decreased slightly to 6% in 65 to 79 year olds. Frequencies were generally low overall for the population, but women reported pain more frequently than men at each age group.

In Poland, 39% of 15 to 18 year olds experienced this pain.[81] Lower frequencies were found in younger and older individuals of this same population. A major increase was found from 6 to 22 years.[81,86]

Gender

In Swedish populations, no significant difference was found in citizens of various ages.[40,72] None was found for pain on gaping[40] or for pain on mandibular movement between 17 and 19 years of age.[74,87]

None was found in Finnish children between the ages of 10 and 16 years.[75]

In Norway, women reported significantly more frequent pain on movement than men at 25 years and at 65 to 79 years.[85]

Significance: Pain associated with joint movement must be differentiated from static pain and dental pain on chewing.

Report of Headache

Whether headache should be viewed as part of TMD symptomatology is debatable, but this symptom is considered because some individuals are unable to differentiate headache from TMJ or from other facial pains.

Much variation exists between populations (see Tables 5-4 and 5-5). The manner in which data are expressed accounts for some of the confusion. Some findings are expressed as generalized headache, others as headache occurring daily, once or more per week, once or more per month, or even once or more over the last 6 months.

In North America, about one fourth to one third of adult populations from Virginia[37] and Missouri[51] reported generalized headache.

This percentage compares favorably with samples from northern Europe. Twenty-one percent of Finnish Lapps reported headache.[7b] Recurrent headache (once or more per week) occurred in 8% of citizens randomly sampled from Sweden.[64] About 70% never complained of this symptom. Put another way, 30% probably suffered headache at some previous time.

Age

Most information about adult headache derives from studies conducted in Finland and Sweden (see Tables 5-4 and 5-5). In Finnish Lapps, generalized headache reached a peak of 60% in 15 to 24 year olds and decreased significantly to 20% by 55 to 65 years of age.[7b] Unlike headache, neck and shoulder pain increased from 5% to 51% during that period.

In Sweden, headache increased little between 25 and 65 years of age;[64] prevalence was one tenth that reported in Lapps.[7b] When adjusted for age, neck and shoulder pain increased by the same ratio as found in the population of Lapps.

In young children and young adults, variation is wide within and between populations. The mean was about 15% across populations. In Swedish children, the findings varied. No difference was found between 7 and 18 year olds.[65] None was found between adolescents and young adults questioned at 15 years and then questioned again 5 years later.[66] On the other hand, headache increased from 13% at 7 years to 36% at 15 years.[88]

Among children from Pennsylvania belonging to the "calm" group, headache was twice as frequent in 10 year olds as in 6 year olds.[77] Within children belonging to the "non-calm" group, no difference was found between 6 and 10 year olds, although the frequency was 25% in 9 year olds.[78] Dissimilarities in the number of subjects sampled probably affected these findings.

Gender

Significant differences occur across all populations. Females suffered from headache more often than males. For example, headache was significantly more frequent (29% versus 17%) in women than in men of an urban Virginia population.[37]

This trend was consistent across Scandinavian populations. In Sweden, the occurrence of daily headache was low but was more prevalent in women than in men.[40,89] Recurrent headache was more prevalent in women (28% versus 15%) than men.[53] Women reported headache in the afternoon and on waking in the morning more frequently than men.

At 20 years of age, significantly more young women reported headache than young men.[66] Adolescent girls reported significantly more frequent headache (18%) than adolescent boys (1% to 6%).[74]

In Finland, women reported more frequent headache than men.[7b] The findings on children differ slightly. No difference was found between girls and boys of 10 to 16 years in headache once or more weekly.[75] At 15 years of age, girls reported significantly more recurrent headache (2 to 3 times per month) than boys.[76] No difference was found at 12 years. The difference at 15 years resulted from a significant decrease in headache for boys (19% versus 10%).

Headache occurred more often in Norwegian women (31% versus 24%) than men.[85]

Significance: Because headache may occur simultaneously with major symptoms of TMD, its presence should be recorded in the charts of patients. Reasons for the reporting of headache more frequently in females than males need investigation. Efforts should be directed towards diagnosing the kind of headaches.

Report of Jaw Fatigue and Tiredness

A feeling of fatigue, tiredness, or stiffness of the jaw is a fairly common complaint across populations. For individuals of early to middle age, the variation ranges from 12% to 40% (Tables 5-6 and 5-7). Slightly less than one third of citizens randomly sampled from Canada had this symptom.[39]

Age

This symptom was age related in Scandinavian populations. In Sweden, prevalence of fatigue was 2% in the elderly but was 22% in 20 to 29 year olds.[42] Only 4% to 8% of children between 7 and 15 years of age had this symptom.[88] The frequency in adolescents and young adults was 26%.[69] In another population, the frequency was the same at 15 years as it was at 20 years for the same subjects.[66,68] At both 17 and 19 years, fatigue related to facial pain, difficulty opening wide, and recurrent headache.[90] The authors suggested that fatigue may mean impending dysfunction.

In Finnish Lapps, the prevalence was 40% within 35 to 44 year olds, but was only 18% in 15 to 24 year olds.[7b] No change was found in the same children questioned at 12 years and again at 15 years.[76]

Gender

Significantly more elderly Canadian women than men reported jaw fatigue or ache.[91] The prevalence of this feeling was 2% to 9% and was lower than observed for most other populations. These same women complained of generalized arthritic pain.

Among Swedish populations, women had significantly greater stiffness in the face and jaws on waking in the morning than men.[53] Significantly more women than men reported jaw tiredness at 17 and 18 years, but not at 19 years.[73,74] The authors concluded that for most individuals the symptoms were mild and fluctuated longitudinally. Fifty-six percent with fatigue had four or more areas tender to palpation.

Fatigue was reported more frequently in Finnish women than in men.[7b] But reports of stiffness and tiredness did not differ between girls and boys.[75]

   Significance: Reported jaw fatigue in adolescents may represent dysfunction or imply impending dysfunction. Fatigue should be noted in the charts on admission. Reasons for gender differences require further study.

Report of Difficulty on Opening Wide

Information about the frequency of difficulty in opening wide is low in most populations (see Tables 5-6 and 5-7). The prevalence ranged from 6% in Swedish shipworkers[92] to 13% in heavy metal workers from Finland.[44]

Age

No significant effect was found in a large Swedish population.[40] A slightly lower frequency (2%) was reported in 7 to 14 year olds[65] than in 15 to 20 years olds (11%).[69] Difficult opening occurred in 23% of children.[80]

Table 5-6

Percentage of Adults With Masticatory Muscles and TMJs Tender to Palpation, Fatigue (Tiredness) of the Jaws, and Difficult Opening in Different Populations. References are Coded According to Country and Investigation (see Table 5-1).

Muscle (y)	TMJ	Fatigue	Difficult Opening	Reference
Nonclinical Settings				
69 LP	19	—	—	Au2
44	16	29	11	Ca3
32 dentate	—	—	—	D3
55 edentate	—	—	—	
39	20L,10P	—	8	E
66	32	—	—	F1
43(15–24)	—	18	—	F2
63(25–34)	—	22	—	
68(35–44)	—	40	—	
67(45–54)	—	29	—	
68(55–65)	—	32	—	
67	45	—	—	F3
—	2	19	13	F5
3–16	5L	—	—	F8
17	3L&P	13	—	Hu
36	10	—	—	I1
20	—	—	—	IN
18–23	4–21	—	—	Ir
8	10	—	—	SA
35	10	—	—	S3
37	7L,4P	—	6	S14
33M,49LP	4L,5P	—	12	S20
24(25)	2L	—	—	S44
23(35)	1L	—	—	
24(50)	1L	—	—	
33(65)	2L	—	—	
17	21L,8P	4	—	S47
18(20–29)	2L,<1P	22	—	S48
17(30–39)	—	12	—	
16(40–49)	—	14	—	
19(50–59)	—	5	—	
20(60–69)	—	2	—	
27(70–79)	—	2	—	
14(>80)	—	3	—	
15LP	4L,4P	13	4	Ta
74	—	—	—	M1
—	—	—	2	Mn4
—	—	21(<25)	—	Mo1
		39(25–35)		
		16(36–45)		
		18(46–54)		
		4(55–65)		
		2(>65)		
10–15, COCO	9L,3P	—	—	W1,W2
Selected Groups				
29	15	—	—	B
29	14	9	—	F6
—	2	—	—	S1
24	—	—	—	S10
13	7	—	—	S15
17	1	—	—	S21

(continued)

Table 5-6 *(Continued)*

Muscle (y)	TMJ	Fatigue	Difficult Opening	Reference
40	—	—	—	S28
24	2	2	9	S50
16	—	—	—	T
34	5	—	—	C3
48	14	—	—	C6,C7
10	—	—	—	C8
40	—	—	—	M
24	25L,18P4	—	—	Mn3
12	3L,1P	—	—	Vs,V2

Private/Clinic Dental Patients

Muscle (y)	TMJ	Fatigue	Difficult Opening	Reference
<1	2	9	—	Ca2
33	11	—	—	N7
21 mild	6	—	—	S19
31 severe	3	—	—	
16	32	38	14	C
15	45	—	—	C4
15	4L,<1P	—	—	Ny3
27	—	25	—	Tx

TMD Clinic Cases

Muscle (y)	TMJ	Fatigue	Difficult Opening	Reference
—	45	—	—	Au
—	63L	17	—	En
73(<30)	—	—	26	Gr1
55(>50)			30	
66	—	—	—	J2
90	—	41	—	N1,N3
95	—	49	—	N5
71	63	12	35	NZ
—	—	32	—	S2
45	21L,15P	—	60 C	S18
			58 Ten	
			50 N	
23 mild	15	—	—	S19
63 severe	14	—	—	
84, IE	52	29	35	S27
59, FE	17	44	13	
78 My	23	—	16	S30
33 Ar	63	—		
15 Ad	4	—		
—	—	40	32	S42
67	10	23	10	S46
78 (Tx)	6	9	9	S50
54	—	—	—	TN1
55M,48T, Te	—	48	—	TN2
38M,41T, Mg	—	21	—	
73M,73T, Co	—	38	—	
75	—	—	—	C8
73	—	—	—	Ga
81,MC	—	—	—	IL1
96	—	—	—	M1
62	39	—	—	Mn1
56–64	—	—	—	Mn2
81	—	—	—	Ny1
89	31L,12P	—	—	Ny2
69,I	61L,61P	—	21	Ny4

(continued)

Table 5-6   *(Continued)*

Muscle (y)	TMJ	Fatigue	Difficult Opening	Reference
49,E	49	—		
64	92	—	—	Tn
—	—	56 My	—	V3
		51 Ar		
78	45	495	—	V4
40–69, CLCA	57L,10P	—	—	W2
35–45, COCA	35L,6P	—	—	

A, asymptomatic; *Ad*, articular dysfunction; *Ar*, arthrogenous; *C*, crepitus; *CLCA*, TMD clinic cases; *Co*, combined headache; *COCA*, community TMD cases; *COCO*, community controls; *E*, extraoral palpation; *FE*, final examination 7 years later; *I*, intraoral palpation; *IE*, initial examination; *L*, lateral pole of condyle; *L&P*, lateral pole and meatus; *LP*, lateral pterygoid; *M*, masseter; *MC*, masticatory and cervical tenderness; *Mg*, migraine headache; *My*, myogenous; *N*, neither crepitus nor tenderness; *P*, intrameatus of TMJ; *T*, temporalis; *Te*, tension headache; *Ten*, tenderness; *Tx*, needing treatment; (y), age in years.

Limited opening was found in less than 1% of 2198 Japanese adolescents.[56]

Gender

Analysis of gender reflects the ambiguity between populations. This difference was notable in Swedish people. Difficulty in opening wide proved greater in women than in men.[40,72] But no significant gender difference was found on taking a large bite.[10] In other populations, more women reported problems opening wide[41,53] and complained more of locking of the TMJs than men.[41] But no difference was found in another adult population,[79] or between 17 and 19 year olds in opening the jaws wide or taking a big bite.[74]

Significance: There is scant information to explain possible reasons for difficult openings. Examination should follow these reports to determine whether the complaint is joint, muscle, or joint and muscle related.

Report of Locking

Little information exists about locking of the TMJs (Tables 5-8 and 5-9). A prevalence of 10% was found in Canadian citizens sampled by telephone questionnaire.[39] Examination of certain subjects showed 1% experienced locking and 17% had problems with luxation.

A prevalence of less than 1% was reported in Swedish citizens of various ages.[42] Locking was virtually absent in most studies on children and occurred in only 3% of 15 year olds.[68]

Age

Locking increased significantly (4% versus 7%) in Finnish boys at 12 years and when they were questioned again at 15 years.[76] No change was observed in girls during the same time.

(text continues on p. 166)

Table 5-7
Percentage of Tenderness on Palpation of the Masticatory Muscles and TMJ Jaw Fatigue (Tiredness), and Difficult Opening in Young Children, Adolescents and Young Adults of Different Populations. References are Coded by Country and Investigation (see Table 5-1).

Muscle (y)	TMJ	Fatigue	Difficult Opening	Reference
67* (14–16)	16L,7P	—	—	D1
17 (10–16)	<1	4–19	—	F7
— (12)	—	13	—	F9
— (15)	—	16	—	
30 (5–8)	—	—	—	F10
34 (9–12)	—	—	—	
13 (13–15)	—	—	—	
21 (10–13)	28	—	—	I
21 (13–16)	29	—	—	
18 (16–18)	35	—	—	
—	2	—	—	J
15 (6–8)	—	—	—	P1
26 (13–15)	—	—	—	
16LA (15–18 A)	1L,<1P	—	—	P2
10LA (19–22 A)	2L,1P	—	—	
24LA (15–18 S)	4L,1P	—	—	
14LA (19–22 S)	2L,<1P	—	—	
27LA (10–14)	—	—	—	S11
55 (15–18)	34	—	10	S22
64 (7–14)	39	—	3	S23
20 (7)	5L,1P	4	8	S24
37 (11)	5L,2P	8	6	
43 (15)	6L,4P	4	5	
23M, 30T (7–14)	31L,20P	—	3	S31
17M, 19T (15–18)	20L,20P	—	2	
41 (15)	10,1	5	6	S32,S33
39 (20)	3,2	4	9	
— (17)	—	6	2	S34
41 (17)	10L,3P	—	—	S35
—	—	12	4	S36
29 (13–15 ID)	11L,0P	5	—	S39
80 (13–15 RD)	47L,9P	16	—	
6 (9–28 A)	5L,0P	8	5	S43
19 (9–28 S)	8L,15P	8	23	
12 (15–20 ID)	7L,0P	18	2	S51
85 (15–20 RD)	20L,26P	26	11	
41LA (8–14)	—	—	—	Sw
19 (6–17)	9	—	5	Mi,Mi2
34 (6–18)	5	—	10	Mi1
21 (6–16)	—	—	—	O
46 (6 calm)	7	—	—	Pa1
41 (7)	7	—	—	
44 (8)	6	—	—	
51 (9)	6	—	—	
54 (10)	11	—	—	
76 (6 non-calm)	29	—	—	Pa2
65 (7)	20	—	—	
74 (8)	9	—	—	
67 (9)	17	—	—	
59 (10)	24	—	—	

*Probably nearer to 20% if calculated differently.
A, asymptomatic; *ID*, intact dentition; *L*, lateral pole of TMJ; *LA*, lateral pterygoid; *M*, masseter; *P*, intrameatus of TMJ; *RD*, restored dentition; *S*, symptomatic with juvenile rheumatoid arthritis; *T*, temporalis; (y), age in years.

Table 5-8

Percentage of Joint Sounds, Limitation on Opening the Mouth Wide, Deviation on Opening, and Locking of the Jaws in Different Populations of Adults. References are Coded by Country and Investigation (see Table 5-1).

Clinical Sounds (y)	Self-Reported Sounds (y)	Limited Opening (y)	Deviation on Opening	Locking	Reference
Nonclinical Settings					
30,26*	—	—	29	—	Au2
48	—	12	17	—	Ca3
60 dentate	29	12	17	—	D3
50 edentate	7	15	11	—	
31	19	4	23	—	E
—	—	—	54	—	En
31,17*	—	13	—	—	F2
13,11*(15–24)	26	—	—	—	F2
20,10*(25–34)	31	—	—	—	
26,12*(35–44)	39	—	—	—	
28,13*(45–54)	25	—	—	—	
24,19*(55–65)	32	—	—	—	
48,21*	35	—	60–63	—	F3
38	23	6	18	5	F5
19 (25)	—	2	—	—	F8
21 (35)	—	3	—	—	
23 (50)	—	5	—	—	
17 (65)	—	14	—	—	
46,22*	9	4	<1	<1	Hu
26,7*	—	16	21	3	I1
17(16–25)	—	<1	—	8	In
17(26–35)	—	<1	—	—	
30(36–45)	—	0	—	—	
30(46–55)	—	2	—	—	
15(56D)	—	0	0	0	
22,4*	14	1	—	—	N2
	6	—	—	—	N4
14	—	—	—	—	SA
60†	—	—	—	—	S3
—	39	—	—	7	S5,S6,S12
—	23	12	—	—	S13
42,23*	—	2	—	—	S14
25	6	—	40	—	S20
16,3*(25)	—	3	—	—	S44
23,4*(35)	—	5	—	—	
22,2*(50)	—	11	—	—	
23,7*(65)	—	16	—	—	
25,33*	—	—	—	—	S47
12	14(20–29)	0	17D	<1	S48
	9(30–39)	0	26	0	
	17(40–49)	0	36	0	
	6(50–59)	0	35	0	
	5(60–69)	0	34	0	
	2(70–79)	1	29	0	
	3(>80)	1	34	0	
16,3*	18	—	14	1	Ta
14	16	6	34	<1	TN3
—	13	—	—	2	K
—	—	5(<56)	36	—	M1
—	—	13(>56)	38	—	
52	—	6(<37)	47	—	M2
—	19	—	—	—	Mn4
—	18(<25)	—	—	—	Mo

(continued)

Table 5-8 *(Continued)*

Clinical Sounds (y)	Self-Reported Sounds (y)	Limited Opening (y)	Deviation on Opening	Locking	Reference
—	38(25–35)	—	—	—	
—	26(36–45)	—	—	—	
—	5(46–54)	—	—	—	
—	4(55–65)	—	—	—	
—	9(>65)	—	—	—	
—	11(<25)	—	—	—	Mo1
—	40(25–35)	—	—	—	
—	30(36–45)	—	—	—	
—	11(46–54)	—	—	—	
—	13(55–65)	—	—	—	
—	5(>65)	—	—	—	
—	12	—	—	—	Vo
5[‡]	34	2	13	1	W1
23,6*,1G,COCO	6,2*	2	13	1	W2

Selected Groups

30	—	2	34	—	B
20	—	—	—	—	Br
25,10*	22,6*	—	—	7	F6
2–23	—	—	2–4	—	Ir
24	—	—	—	—	Mx
10 medical students	—	—	—	—	P
22 military students					
17 (20–23)					
25 (39–45)					
41	—	—	—	—	S1
—	—	—	—	—	S9
23	—	—	—	—	S13
14	—	—	9	—	S15
—	—	—	—	—	S16
16,<0.1*	—	—	—	—	S21
35	—	—	—	—	S28
18p	27	16 (tx)	50	—	S50
6a	—	8 (no tx)	15	—	
14	29	13	—	—	T
17,12*	—	4	18	—	C3
—	29	—	—	—	C6
29,3*	—	1	22	—	C7
72	—	—	—	—	C8
30	—	—	—	—	M
—	—	8	3	8	Mn3
—	15,6[‡]	—	—	—	Vs
34	—	—	—	—	V1
34	—	—	—	—	V2

Private/Clinic Dental Patients

1	12	2	7	—	Ca2
10,1*	20	—	—	—	G1
(3 clicking, 7 clicking,* 78 auscultation, 94 phonograms)					
27 moderate	13 mild	26 mild	66	—	S19
		9 severe	3		
35	—	—	38	—	C
41(<30)	45,13*	5	30	—	C1,C4,C5
52(30–39)	35,11*	4	28	—	
51(40–49)	33,16*	5	24	—	
49(50–59)	29,15*	5	21	—	

(continued)

Table 5-8 *(Continued)*

Clinical Sounds (y)	Self-Reported Sounds (y)	Limited Opening (y)	Deviation on Opening	Locking	Reference
56(>60)	23,17*	8	21	—	
13,<1*	—	13	—	—	Io
0(0–9)	—	7	28	—	Ny3
26(10–19)	—	—	—	—	
32(20–29)	—	—	—	—	
38(30–39)	—	—	—	—	
44(40–49)	—	—	—	—	
30(50–59)	—	—	—	—	
31(60–69)	—	—	—	—	
45(70–79)	—	—	—	—	
32(80–89)	—	—	—	—	
—	21,6 ‖	—	—	—	Ny5
16	—	—	—	—	Pa
60*	—	7	—	—	Tx
—	6	—	—	—	V

TMD Clinic Cases

—	38	—	—	—	A
45,17*My	—	49	21	4	Au
48,18*Ar	—	—	—	—	
32,35*Ps	—	—	—	—	
—	—	35	79	—	En
—	12	—	—	—	En1
—	75	64	—	—	En3
82(<30)	—	46	—	10	Gr1
64(>50)	—	18	—	6	
66,17*	—	—	—	—	J2
—	53	38–50	60	—	N3,N5
—	61	50	53	—	N5
—	39	—	—	—	N6
69,21*	19	16	68	—	NZ
65*	—	—	—	—	S2
—	79	—	—	—	S12
—	30,55*C	—	—	—	S17
—	63,5*T	—	—	—	
—	62,7*N	—	—	—	
49 moderate	20 mild	25 mild	73	—	S19
		3 severe	10	—	
40,8*	—	—	—	15	S25
81,IE	56	—	53	20	S27
47,FE	42	—	22	11	
31,9*My	—	8	—	—	S30
69,4*Ad	—	40	—	—	
13,33*Ar	—	27	—	—	
—	—	—	—	—	S42
—	23,13* JRA	—	—	—	S43
32	—	20 mild	49 mild	—	S46
		2 severe			
31p	—	16	50	—	S50
22a					
—	—	—	19 Te	7	TN2
—	—	—	14 Mig	0	
—	—	—	15 Co	8	
—	79	—	—	—	C6
82	—	—	—	—	C8
70	20	40	—	1	Ga
92	—	—	56	—	I1
—	66	63	—	—	I11
—	65	33	38	—	M1

(continued)

Table 5-8   *(Continued)*

Clinical Sounds (y)	Self-Reported Sounds (y)	Limited Opening (y)	Deviation on Opening	Locking	Reference
48,34*	—	38	—	—	Mn1
—	—	—	—	—	Mn2
—	<1,<1*(10–20)	6	—	—	Ny1
—	4,2*(20–30)	4	—	—	
—	3,2*(31–40)	6	—	—	
—	5,4*(41–50)	4	—	—	
—	4,3*(51–60)	5	—	—	
—	<1,<1*(61–70)	1	—	—	
—	<1,<1*(71–80)	3	—	—	
68,†18*	—	40	17	—	Ny2
43	37,19	28	29	—	Ny4
8	13	4	—	—	Tn
—	58 My	—	—	66	V3
—	85 Ar	—	—	76	
46,†10*	—	—	—	—	V4
—	58	—	—	—	V5
42,8,*5G,CLCA	20,10*	22	29	9	W2
32,3,*4G,COCA	27,12*	10	26	5	

*Crepitus.
†Clicking/popping.
‡Clinic patients.
‖Night sounds.

a, evidently audible; *Ad*, articular dysfunction; *Ar*, arthrogenous; *C*, TMJ crepitus; *CLCA*, TMD clinic cases; *Co*, combination tension and migraine headache; *COCA*, community TMD cases; *COCO*, community controls; *D*, deviation on opening and TMJ sounds; *FE*, final examination 7 y later; *G*, ; *IE*, initial examination; *JRA*, juvenile rheumatoid arthritis; *Mig*, migraine; *My*, myogenous; *N*, neither tenderness nor crepi; *P*, palpable; *Ps*, psychogenous; *tx*, treatment group; *no tx*, no treatment group; *Te*, tension headache; *T*, TMJ tenderness; (y), age in years.

Gender

Locking was not significantly different between women and men in a Swedish population.[40] No locking or luxation was found in adolescents.[73] Results on adolescents and young adults fluctuated because a difference occurred at 18 years of age but not at 17 and 19 years.[74]

Unusual ear symptoms, including locking, feeling of water, and ringing in the ear were more than twice as common in Finnish girls as boys at 12 years, and were higher, but not significantly higher, at 15 years.[76] Luxation was more common in men than women in another Finnish population.[7b]

Significance: More information is needed about locking, particularly in children from populations of the United States. Reports of locking need confirmation by examination to determine possible long-term outcomes of these restrictions.

Report of Joint Sounds

Joint sounds varied extensively across populations and within the same population (see Tables 5-8 and 5-9). In populations with the highest frequencies, the reporting was consistent for each age level. This suggests differences in the questions asked by investigators. The occurrence of crepitus was low, but this low percentage may relate to pooling of findings under the heading of "joint sounds." Another possibility is that the subjects were unable to differentiate one kind of sound from another.

Table 5-9
Percentages of Joint Sounds, Joint Locking, Deviation on Opening, and Limited Opening in Children, Adolescents, and Young Adults of Different Populations. References are Coded by Country and Investigation (see Table 5-1).

Clinical Clicking (y)	Self-Reported Clicking	Limited Opening	Deviation on Opening	Locking	Reference
20	—	—	—	—	Br
6,0*	—	—	0	—	D
9,1*	—	—	0.5–3	—	D1
12	—	<1	24	—	F7
—(12)	19,3*	—	4	—	F9
—(15)	25,5*	—	7	—	
7(5–8)	—	<1	12	—	F10
7(9–12)	—	<1	15	—	
4(13–15)	—	<1	16	—	
28(10–13)	—	<2	—	—	I
34(13–16)	—	—	—	—	
44(16–18)	—	—	—	—	
9	—	<1	—	—	J
14	—	—	—	—	P
10(6–8)	32	3	30A / 39S	—	P1
20(13–15)	26	—	19A / 25S	—	
—(15–18A)	32	3	6	—	P2
—(19–22A)	29	2	1	—	
15(15–18S)	68	4	9	—	
13(19–22S)	78	3	1	—	
14	17	—	—	—	S22
8,1*(7–14)	13	<1	32	—	S23
11(7)	7	2	7	0	S24
13(11)	11	1	6	0	
29(15)	21	0	10	1	
6(7–14)	13	—	—	—	S31
10(15–18)	17	—	—	—	
30,1*(15)	23	2	—	3	S32, S33
32,2*(20)	30	10	—	—	
—	13	—	—	3	S34
—	22	—	—	—	S35
—	24	—	—	—	S36
9(13–15ID)	10	0	16	0	S39
17(13–15RD)	16	2	36	0	
18,0*(A)	15,0*	3	—	—	S43
23,15*(S)	23,13*	28	—	—	
22(17)	13	—	—	—	S49
18(18)	14	—	—	—	
20(19)	16	—	—	—	
7(15–20ID)	19	0	42	0	S51
14(15–20RD)	33	2	55	1	
10	24	5	—	—	Mi, Mi2
4	20	<1	—	—	Mi1
7	—	—	—	—	O
14 (Calm)	—	<1	6	—	Pa1
11(6)	4	—	—	—	
17(7)	2	—	—	—	
13(8)	7	—	—	—	
10(9)	9	—	—	—	
22(10)	11	—	—	—	
— (Non-calm)	—	—	9	—	Pa2
5(6)	5	—	—	—	
15(7)	5	—	—	—	
17(8)	13	—	—	—	
8(9)	13	—	—	—	
17(10)	6	—	—	—	

*Crepitus.
A, asymptomatic; *ID*, intact dentition; *RD*, restored dentition; *S*, symptomatic.

Age

In North America, the prevalence of clicking was about 32% between the ages of 25 to 45 years and was lowest at 9% in elderly from Missouri.[51] Overall lower percentages were found in a sample from Virginia.[37] Age did not prove an important factor, but the highest percentage occurred between 21 and 40 years of age. A similar relation was found among community citizens from Washington.[83] Crepitus proved an infrequent finding. A prevalence of 2% to 13% was reported in 6 to 10 year olds from Pennsylvania.[77,78] The frequency of noise was higher in two populations of children from Michigan than in the children from Pennsylvania. It was 24% in a population younger than 11 years[70] and 20% in a population of 6- to 18-year-old migrant children.[93]

Among Scandinavian populations, sounds were the most frequently found symptom. The highest prevalence occurred at older ages, but no statistically significant differences existed between age groups.[3] Clicking or popping was reported by 2% to 3% of elderly Swedish citizens and by 17% of 40 to 49 year olds.[42] Crepitus occurred in 2% of Swedes.[42]

Sounds were reported three times as frequently by 15-year-old Swedish children as by 7 year olds.[88] The frequency increased slightly from 23% to 30% between 15 and 20 years.[66,68] A 5-year longitudinal study of adolescents and young adults confirmed that the perception of joint sounds increased in frequency from 15 to 20 years.[68] Sounds were the only symptom that changed significantly during this period.

Longitudinal study of adolescents and young adults from Sweden showed that clicking increased with age.[74,94] The increase was more pronounced in girls, increasing from 14% at 17 years to 23% at 19 years.[74] Much fluctuation was found, with only 5.8% of the group consistently reporting sounds.[94]

Crepitus reached 13% in young Swedish adults with juvenile rheumatoid arthritis but was absent in matched, asymptomatic subjects.[80]

Joint noises proved prevalent in the general population of Lapps.[7b] The highest percentage occurred between 35 and 44 years of age, the same ages reported for Swedish adults.[42]

Age differences have been found in groups of subjects from Norway.[85] Comparison showed that clicking was reported by 15% of 1740 subjects from a random sample of the population at large, by 18% of 25 year olds, and by 11% of 65 to 79 year olds. Older women reported sounds more frequently (20% versus 0.9%) than older men.

Significantly fewer edentulous middle-aged and elderly Danish citizens reported sounds than dentate citizens.[95]

The prevalence of sounds ranged from 32% to 78% in adolescent and young Polish adults.[81] Crepitus was negligible in children. No significant difference was found for clicking between 6 to 8 year olds and 13 to 15 year olds[86] or between asymptomatic adolescents and young adults.[81] The frequency of sounds in adolescents and young adults described as symptomatic was twice that of asymptomatic subjects.[81]

In Japan, joint sounds were reported by about 9% of adolescents.[56]

Gender

Gender was not a factor in a samples from Virginia[37] or in adults from Missouri.[51]

The findings varied in Swedish populations. Women reported sounds more often than men.[40] The sounds proved more embarrassing to women than men in another population.[53] No significant difference was found in another population.[79]

No significant difference was found for joint sounds among Swedes at 17 and 18 years, but girls reported significantly more frequent sounds at 19 years than boys.[73,74] Young Swedish women reported significantly higher frequency of joint sounds than men.[94]

In Finland, no effect was found for clicking or crepitus in Lapps.[7b] Gender was not a factor between the ages of 10 to 16 years.[75] But clicking and crepitus increased significantly (13% versus 22%; 1% versus 6%) from 12 to 15 years in boys but not in girls.[76]

Significance: Evidence suggests that detection of sounds by palpation represents the most reliable means of assessment. Studies should focus on longitudinal changes of the same subjects. Information should be focus on possible differences between genders and what this means to the individual. Specific kinds of sounds should be identified.

Tenderness on Palpation of Masticatory Muscles

Palpation of the head and neck muscles is considered useful to differentiate healthy individuals from those with dysfunction. The results of digital palpation have proved highly variable among populations (see Tables 5-6 and 5-7). The lowest percentages (3% to 15%) were found in middle-aged Finnish citizens.[61] The highest (74%) was recorded in Maryland citizens.[38]

Many reasons account for this variation. There has been a lack of standardized procedures in applying pressure. Investigators have palpated to assess the presence of tenderness,[8] to assess reflex response,[97,98] to assess response to pain rather than tension,[99,100] or to assess trigger points.[101] Some investigators make these distinctions, others do not. Others have selected certain masticatory muscles, ignored others, or have lumped findings of masticatory muscles with findings of paraspinal muscles or TMJs.

Another factor includes the number of individuals used to perform the palpations. In some studies, one examiner may have performed palpations, whereas in other studies the palpations may have been performed by several examiners. In the Maryland study,[38] one examiner performed the palpations and the procedure was standardized. Pain was recorded as present if individuals responded "yes" to the pressure of palpation. No pain was recorded if individuals answered "no." Scores were totaled for eight groups of masticatory muscles and six groups of paraspinal muscles. After such a thorough examination, the high percentage result cited in the previous paragraph was not unexpected.

Finally, the composition of most populations varies widely with respect to age and gender.

Age

Certain muscles have proved more tender to palpation than others in different populations (see Tables 5-6 and 5-7). In Maryland, more young individuals (71%) had more than half of the paraspinal muscles tender compared with older individuals (59%), but the difference was not statistically significant.[38] Little difference was found for the masticatory muscles within Pennsylvania children of various ages.[77,78] No difference was found between 6 and 10 year olds belonging to the "calm" group or between 6 and 10 year olds in the "non-calm" group. But tenderness was significantly greater in the "non-calm" group than in the "calm" group.[78]

In Swedish populations, a prevalence of only 6% was found in a sample of Swedish subjects ranging from 9 to 28 years of age.[80] In 15 to 20 year olds, 85% had tenderness.[69] Tenderness of the lateral pterygoids increased from 20% at 7 years to 43% at 15 years.[88]

In Finnish Lapps, the masseter, temporalis, and trapezius muscles were more commonly tender with advancing age.[7b] No tenderness was found for the digastric and sternocleidomastoid muscles. Comparison of adolescents and young adults showed that tenderness was less than one half that found in subjects between 55 and 65 years of age. In another population, tenderness of the masticatory muscles and TMJs increased from 35% at 25 years to 51% at 65 years.[61]

The lateral pterygoids, but not the temporalis tendons, were more tender in 65-year-old Tanzanians compared with 35 to 44 year olds.[102]

Among Israeli children, no significant difference was found between the ages of 10 and 18 years.[103]

In Polish samples, tenderness of the masticatory muscles increased from 15% in 6 to 8 year olds to 26% in 13 to 15 year olds.[86] Prevalence of tenderness of the lateral pterygoids ranged from 16% in asymptomatic 15 to 18 year olds to 10% in 19 to 22 year olds, but it was 24% and 14%, respectively, in symptomatic individuals.[81]

Among asymptomatic Finnish children, tenderness decreased from 30% at 5 to 8 years to 13% at 13 to 15 years.[104]

Gender

Certain masticatory muscles have proved more tender to palpation in one gender than the other. Differences are complicated by age variation. For Michigan children, no significant difference was found for the population.[70] Higher frequencies occurred in male adolescents and young adults with cusp-to-cusp relations than in their class I cohorts.

In Sweden, women exhibited more frequent tenderness of the lateral pterygoids than men.[79,53] The masseters were more tender in elderly women than elderly men.[79]

Of the 18 areas palpated,[53] 12 were more commonly tender in women than in men. Most common were lateral pterygoid (40% women versus 29% men), temporalis (33% versus 22%), and posterior digastric (24% versus 12%). Tenderness was significantly more common in females at 17 and 18 years than males of the same ages, but not so at 19 years.[87] Only palpation of the temporalis tendon proved significantly different between sexes.[73] No major differences were found for lateral pterygoids, superficial and deep heads of the masseter, anterior temporalis, sternocleidomastoid, and trapezius muscles.

In Finnish populations, no significant difference was found between girls and boys from 10 to 16 years of age.[75]

Tenderness of Specific Muscles

Certain muscle groups appear more tender than other groups (Tables 5-10 and 5-11). Generally, the frequency in adolescents and young adults parallels the prevalence found in most adult populations. This relation is consistent in populations from nonclinical settings, selected groups, and private or clinic dental patients.

Where sufficient data were available for comparison between adults, tenderness localized within or near the lateral pterygoid muscle appeared to be the most frequently involved area (see Tables 5-10 and 5-11). This finding was consistent for studies conducted in Australia,[71] Egypt,[105] Finland,[7b,61] Hungary,[106] and Sweden.[53,64,79,92,107] The lateral pterygoid was reported to be tender to pain in more than one half of Canadians found with muscle tenderness.[39] Tenderness was common in 44% of that sample, making the lateral pterygoid tender in at least 22% of the total population. Coupled with the temporalis muscle, it was cited as being the most tender muscle in Finnish Lapps.[7b]

Tenderness of the temporalis, either at the coronoid attachment or the anterior fibers, was next among remaining muscle groups (Table 5-12; see Table 5-11). When simultaneous palpation is done for other muscles, the superficial fibers of the masseter may approximate the temporalis in tenderness. In a few studies in which palpation has been conducted for the digastric muscle, the posterior fibers may be as tender as those of the masseter.[7b,105] Slightly lower percentages have been found for the medial pterygoid[53,92,105] than for other groups.

Age and Specific Muscles

Based on age studies, tenderness was frequently lower in younger adults than older adults (see Tables 5-6 and 5-7). An exceptionally low prevalence of 4% was recorded for combined palpation of masseter, medial pterygoid, temporalis, and sternocleidomastoid in an elderly population of British Columbia.[91]

Specific muscles exhibit tenderness at an early age (see Table 5-11). Tenderness of the lateral pterygoid was found in 6 year olds from Ohio[108] and in 7 year olds from Sweden.[65,88,109]

This tenderness may be widespread, as found for the temporalis attachment at the coronoid[65,109] and the masseter[88] in Swedish children.

(text continues on p. 175)

Table 5-10

Location and Percentage of Muscle Tenderness or Muscle Pain on Palpation in Adults. References are Coded According to Country and Investigation (see Table 5-1).

				Muscle Tenderness or Pain (%)						Age (y)	Reference
LP	MP	M	D	T	TA	S	SC	C	TR		
Nonclinical Setting											
69	12	14	—	10	—	—	—	—	—		Au2
18	11	17	18	20at 7pt	11	—	—	—	—		E
—	—	9*	7	19*	—	5	—	—	6*	15–24	F2
—	—	22	14	51	—	12	—	—	8	25–34	
—	—	26	25	37	—	12	—	—	16	35–44	
—	—	10	21	48	—	8	—	—	18	45–54	
—	—	19	7	32	—	15	—	—	29	55–65	
14	—	3	—	9	—	—	—	—	—	25	F8
15	—	2	—	9	—	—	—	—	—	35	
17	—	8	—	11	—	—	—	—	—	50	
20	—	9	—	16	—	—	—	—	—	65	
12	—	5	—	—	—	—	—	—	—		Hu
5	6	6	—	9	—	—	—	—	—		In
29	6	2	4p	1at	19	—	—	—	—		S14
49	—	33	—	—	—	—	—	—	—		S20
12f†	—	3	—	6†	—	—	—	—	—	25	S44
8m	—	<1	—	3	—	—	—	—	—		
11f	—	3	—	9	—	—	—	—	—	35	
8m	—	2	—	4	—	—	—	—	—		
15f	—	4	—	9	—	—	—	—	—	50	
9m	—	6	—	6	—	—	—	—	—		
15f	—	3	—	13	—	—	—	—	—	65	
12m	—	2	—	9	—	—	—	—	—		
35	17	4s 4d	18p	—	27	4	—	—	2		S47
15	—	—	—	—	8	—	—	—	—		Ta
Selected Groups											
22	—	<1	—	<1	6	—	—	—	—		F6
15	—	—	—	—	13	—	—	—	—		S15
55	—	—	—	—	24	—	—	—	—		S21
53	—	31s 39d	6p	40at	—	6	34	—	31		Mn3
Private Clinic/Dental Patients											
15	3	2s	—	<1at <1pt	—	—	—	—	—		Nu3
7	16	17	—	—	—	—	—	—	—		Tx
TMD Clinic Cases											
47	—	47	—	32	—	—	—	—	—		NZ
73	45	56s 16d	—	46at	49	—	—	—	—		S18
37	2	23s 11d	—	10at 6pt	17	—	—	—	—		C7
75	—	55	—	33	—	—	—	—	18		Ga
84	35	70	—	49	—	—	—	—	—		Il1
32	36	59s 27	9p	36at 9pt	34	18	—	—	9		Mn1

(continued)

Table 5-10 *(Continued)*

				Muscle Tenderness or Pain (%)						Age (y)	Reference
LP	MP	M	D	T	TA	S	SC	C	TR		
93	82	77s 76d	68p	79at 42pt	69	71	86	—	81		Mn2
63	81	36	—	27	—	—	37	—	—		Ny1
64	41	52	—	53	—	—	41	34	—		Ny2
86	78	24	—	49	—	26	—	38	27		Ny4
—	—	75	33	83	—	—	15	—	—		Tn
74my	—	57s	—	—	—	33*	—	—	—		V4
54jt*	—	44s	—	—	—	63	—	—	—		
73c	—	80s*	—	—	—	70	—	—	—		

*Statistically significant age difference.
†Statistically significant gender difference.
Column Headings: C, cervical; D, digastric; LP, lateral pterygoid; M, masseter; MP, medial pterygoid; S, sternocleidomastoid; SC, splenius capitis; T, temporalis; TA, temporalis attachment at coronoid; TR, trapezius.
Table Abbreviations: at, anterior temporalis; c, combination myogenous/joint group; d, deep masseter; f, female; jt, joint group; m, male; my, myogenous group; p, posterior digastric; pt, posterior temporalis; s, superficial masseter.

Table 5-11

Location and Percentage of Muscle Tenderness or Muscle Pain on Palpation in Children and Young Adults. References are Coded by Country and Investigation (see Table 5-1).

				Muscle Tenderness or Pain (%)						Age (y)	Reference
LP	MP	M	D	T	TA	S	SC	C	TR		
34	26	4	—	4at	11	34	—	—	—	14–16	D
28	4	21s 6d	—	3pt	26	—	—	—	—	10–16	F7
16A	—	—	—	—	—	—	—	—	—	15–18	P2
24S*	—	—	—	—	—	—	—	—	—		
10A	—	—	—	—	—	—	—	—	—	19–22	
14S	—	—	—	—	—	—	—	—	—		
18	—	26	35	27at	32	—	—	—	—	7–14	S23
11	—	11	2	5	9	—	—	—	—	7	S24
25	—	20	7	5	21	—	—	—	—	11	
30	—	19	12	2	19	—	—	—	—	15	
—	—	26	—	27at	32	—	—	—	—	7–14	S31
—	—	17	—	17at	20	—	—	—	—	15–18	
45f	—	7s 2	—	3	16	3	—	—	7	17–19	S35
32m	—	5s 0d	—	3	24†	3	—	—	3		
—	—	—	—	—	—	—	—	—	—		
27—38	—	—	—	—	15–25	—	—	—	—	17–19	S38
41	—	—	—	—	—	—	—	—	—	8–14	Sw
19t	—	11	9	—	6	—	—	—	—	6–16	O
54S*	31	25	—	16	—	—	—	—	—		

*Statistically significant difference between symptomatic group versus total group.
†Statistically significant gender difference.
Column Headings: C, cervical; D, digastric; LP, lateral pterygoid; M, masseter; MP, medial pterygoid; S, sternocleidomastoid; SC, splenius capitis; T, temporalis; TA, temporalis attachment at coronoid; TR, trapezius.
Table Abbreviations: A, asymptomatic group; at, anterior temporalis; d, deep masseter; f, female; m, male; pt, posterior temporalis; s, superficial masseter; S, symptomatic group; t, total group.

Table 5-12
The Mean Mouth Opening in Relation to Gender and Age in Adults From Various Populations

Population Sampled	Mean Opening (mm) Women	Men	Both	Age (y)	Reference
Asymptomatic Group					
Belgium			50.3	23	B
Brazil			51.6	22	Br
Egypt		<40.0 (4%)		17–65	E
		40–55(88%)			
		>55.0 (8%)			
England	46.0	52.7		17–36	En2
Finland	45.7	54.4		15–65	F3
		56.1		18–57	F6
Greece	49.8	56.6		18–20	Gr
	51.0	56.1		21–30	
	49.5	52.7		31–40	
	46.9	55.0		41–50	
	48.3	47.6		51–60	
	44.4	49.1		61–70	
Sweden			50.0–60.0	Adults	S1
	39.2	44.8		40	S4
	49.3	52.7		70	S7
			50.2	Adults	S13
	51.8	53.4		30–74	S14
	45.5	47.7		67	S29
	49.0	53.0		70	S39
	51.0	55.0		25	S43
	50.0	52.0		35	
	46.0	47.0		50	
	44.0	45.0		65	
Taiwan	46.5	51.8		17–32	T
The Netherlands			53	34–49	TN2
United States					
California				20–70	C2
	31–40(11.6%)(5.1%)				
	41–45(25.6%)(13.1%)				
	46–50(27.9%)(24.5%)				
	51–55(25.6%)(25.5%)				
	56–60(6.2%)(20.4%)				
	60+ (1.6%)(9.0%)				
			50.9	19–25	C3
			50.4	19–40	C7
			49.8	19–40	C8
Hawaii					
Random			46.9	3–70	H
Military			53.7	18–20	
enlistees			51.6	21–30	
Peridontal			43.4	21–30	
cases			47.0	31–40	
Maryland			58.6	25	M
New York	53.0	59.0		19–21	Ny
			53.0	45–65	
	45.4	47.9		3–89	Ny3
Texas			44.9	Adults	Tx
Washington			47.9	Adults	W1
COCO	49.4	52.9	51.0	18–75	W2
Symptomatic Group					
Sweden			45.8	Adults	S13
	46.8	49.4		Adults	S25

(continued)

Table 5-12 *(Continued)*

Population Sampled	Mean Opening (mm)		Both	Age (y)	Reference
	Women	*Men*			
Taiwan	44.8	50.4		17–32	T
The Netherlands			48.0	34–49	TN2
United States					
California	26–30(3.0%)(3.6%)			20–70	C2
	31–35(4.5%)(−0 − %)				
	36–40(9.1%)(−0 − %)				
	41–45(25.8%)(10.7%)				
	46–50(28.8%)(21.4%)				
	51–55(15.2%)(39.3%)				
	56–60(7.6%)(14.3%)				
	60+ (3.0%)(7.1%)				
			42.9	19–40	C8
Hawaii			26.1	6–70	H
			(range 5–45 mm)		
New York	44.0	46.0		19–21	Ny
			53.0	Adults	
			16.0(2%)	16–71	Nyl
			23.0(14%)		
			31.0(24%)		
			38.5(27%)		
			47.5(23%)		
			54 +(10%)		
Washington					
CLCA	44.2	47.7	44.6	18–75	W2
COCA	47.9	51.8	48.9		

CLCA, TMD clinic cases; COCA, community TMD cases; COCO, community controls.
% = measurement presented for females or males falling into a range (mm) of opening.

Investigations varied within different populations from the same country (see Tables 5-10 and 5-11). In Swedish populations, young adults had significantly less tenderness of the temporalis and lateral pterygoids than older adults.[64] A trend was observed for the masseters. Increased tenderness was found in several muscles between 5 and 15 years in another population.[88] Still, decreased tenderness was noted at 15 to 18 years compared with younger individuals.[65]

The frequency of tenderness of the trapezius muscle in young Lapps was about one-fourth of that in old Lapps.[7b]

Children and young adults of similar ages in the same population differed in degree of tenderness. In a Polish sample, 15 to 18 year olds and 19 to 22 year olds were separated into symptomatic "TMJ" and asymptomatic "non-TMJ" groups.[81] This distinction was based on the presence of more symptoms and signs in the "TMJ" group. In both age groups, the lateral pterygoid muscles were more tender in the "TMJ" group than in "non-TMJ" individuals (see Table 5-7).

Gender and Specific Muscles

The frequency of tenderness in the lateral pterygoid and temporalis muscles was more common in women than in men in a random sample of Swedish citizens (see Table 5-10).[64] On the other hand, no difference was found for the lateral pterygoids (women 51% versus men 46%), but a significant difference was found for the masseters (women 39% versus men 27%) in retired Swedish citizens.[79] In adolescents and young adults, a single difference occurred for tenderness of the temporalis attachment at the coronoid.[110] Of six groups of muscles palpated, males had more frequent tenderness (24% versus 16%) at the coronoid than females.

Significance: Although review of the literature makes one question the reliability and validity of findings in some studies, muscular tenderness on palpation should be judged particularly relevant as a predictor of dysfunction.[111] Tenderness of muscles seems the major factor responsible for genesis of pain. This finding has strong implications for treatment.[112]

Studies show that tenderness on palpation can be used to distinguish asymptomatic individuals from symptomatic TMD patients.[6] Both sensitivity (0.76) and specificity (0.90) proved high for palpations of masticatory muscles.

In a test–retest for agreement, repeated clinical palpations performed 6 weeks apart on muscles of the same TMD patients showed no major systematic variation between the two examinations.[113] Fifty-seven percent of the palpatory findings were the same at both examinations. In a similar study, the same adolescents were palpated with a minimum of 1 week between palpations, and the agreement for palpations of several masticatory muscles was higher, ranging from 68% to 99%.[10] Thus, the difference in percentage between the two studies suggest that the status of some muscles of symptomatic individuals changed during the longer interval between the first and second examinations.

Known amounts of pressure must be applied. Pressure of 2 lbs has been recommended for extraoral and neck sites.[84]

Tenderness on Palpation of TMJs

Investigators differ widely in the manner of recording data on palpation of the TMJs. Some record a total percentage regardless of the area palpated, whereas others differentiate between palpation at the lateral pole of the condyle and posterior palpation by way of the auditory meatus. Combining sites promotes confusion.

In North America, the percentage for an adult population from Canada fell within the range for adult populations around the world (see Tables 5-6 and 5-7). The lowest percentages, 1% to 4% laterally and less than 1% posteriorly, were found in 6 to 10 year olds from Pennsylvania.[78]

In adult Swedish populations, tenderness was found in 2% of palpations at the lateral pole of the condyle and in less than 1% of posterior palpations.[42] For the total TMJ area, a prevalence of 38% was recorded for another population of citizens of differing ages.[40,41]

In Finnish workers, a frequency of 2% was found by palpation of the lateral pole of the condyle.[44] Tenderness of the entire TMJs was found in 32% to 45% of Lapps.[7b]

A prevalence of 10% was reported for adult Egyptian desert dwellers by posterior palpation.[105] When the lateral and posterior palpations were pooled, 30% were tender, a figure not unlike the total percentages found in the Swedish and Finnish citizens described above.

Age

No significant effect was found in Michigan children between 6 and 17 years of age.[70]

No significant effect was found in a study of Swedish adults.[42] The highest percentages occurred in at study of 13 to 15 year olds, in which 47% had lateral tenderness and 9% had posterior tenderness.[67] Percentages of nearly the same magnitude occurred in another group of 15 to 18 year olds.[114] In another population, no difference was found in children between 7 and 15 years.[88]

None was found between 15 and 22 year olds in Poland[81] or in Israeli children of 10 to 18 years.[103]

Gender

Tenderness of the TMJs was not significantly different in female and male Michigan children between 6 and 17 years old.[70]

In elderly Swedish citizens, significantly more women than men had tenderness on palpation of the lateral pole of the condyle and external auditory meatus.[79] In an urban population, women had more lateral tenderness of the TMJs (25% versus 18%) and more posterior tenderness (13% versus 3%) than men.[53] In another adult population, TMJ tenderness was significantly more common in women (4% versus 1%) than in men.[64] On the other hand, no significant effect was observed on palpation at the lateral pole of the condyle or by way of the meatus in adolescents and young adults.[87]

No significant difference was found between middle-aged and elderly Australians.[71]

Significance: Lateral palpation must be differentiated from posterior palpation. Known amounts of pressure must be applied if values are to be considered meaningful. A pressure of 1 lb applied to either site has been recommended.[84]

Limitation on Opening Wide

Several questions need to be addressed regarding the importance of maximal mouth opening. What is the normal range of opening? How reliable are measurements made at one time compared with measurements made at another? What constitutes limitation on opening wide? Are vertical overbite and horizontal overjet important in making judgments? Are there significant differences in opening capacity between asymptomatic and symptomatic individuals? Are age and gender significant factors?

The first question, how wide is normal, remains debatable.[115] Some conclusions are possible. Comparison of localities across North America, South America, and Europe shows remarkable similarity for asymptomatic individuals of similar age and gender (Table 5-13; see Table 5-12). Maximal mouth opening in adults falls nearer the upper limit of values between 40 and 60 mm. The range on each side of these limits may be greater for a given population, but this 40 to 60 mm grouping is consistent for the

Table 5-13
The Mean Mouth Opening in Relation to Gender and Age for Children and Young Adults From Various Populations

Population Sampled	Mean Opening (mm) Female	Male	Both	Age (y)	Reference
Asymptomatic Group					
Denmark	51.5	52.2		14–16	D1
Finland	45.6	46.4		6–8	F
	48.8	49.6		10–12	
	49.3	54.8		14–16	
	54.0	57.5		20–25	
	54.9	56.4		10–16	F7
			47.0	5–8	F10
			52.0	9–12	
			54.0	13–15	
Japan	47.0	52.0	49.5	10–18	J1
Poland			51.8	15–18	P2
			52.1	19–22	
Sweden	46.4	46.4		7	S
	51.2	51.3		10	
		51.3		20	
			38.4	1.5	S8
			44.8	6	
	53.9	56.5		20	S9
		55.1		19	S16
	47.6	46.8		7	S23
	50.4	54.3		11	
	54.0	52.7		14	
			51.0	7	S31
			56.0	15	
			56.7	15–20	S33
	54.8	57.8		17	S37
	55.1	58.0		18	
	55.7	59.4		19	
	53.0	59.0		18–23	S39
Switzerland			43.0	5	Sw1
			49.0	12	
			53.0	19	
United States					
Michigan			39.6	6–8	Mi
			38.4 OJ		
			41.5	9–10	
			39.8 OJ		
			43.8	11–12	
			41.6 OJ		
			45.1	13–14	
			44.6 OJ		
			43.0	15–17	
			39.0 OJ		
New York			45.6	7–11	Ny
	53.0	59.0		19–21	
Symptomatic Group					
Poland			50.8	15–18	P2
			50.8	19–22	

OJ, age groups with overjet.

populations surveyed. These findings are interesting, considering the potential racial variation.

In North America, the mean openings for young adults examined from New York[116] do not differ significantly from mean openings for military enlistees living in Hawaii.[117] They do not differ from means of patients visiting a dental clinic in California[118] or a group of dental patients treated for periodontal disease in Hawaii.[117]

The values on North American populations correspond favorably with asymptomatic individuals randomly sampled from Brazil.[119]

Means for individuals from numerous locations across northern Europe[7b,50,64,92,115,120,121] are within the range of 40 to 60 mm. They differ little from means obtained on samples from England,[122] Belgium,[123] and Greece,[124] if age and gender are excluded.

The second question concerns repeatability of measurements of maximal mouth opening. Study of the normal range among asymptomatic individuals shows that maximal mouth opening is stable from one time to the next. Interincisal openings were not significantly different when measured in women at different occasions (initially, 1 week later, and 4 months later) or in men measured initially and 18 months later.[125] The author concluded that observed differences should be at least 4 mm in vertical mobility if they are to be accepted as a sign of a true effect of treatment for a given patient. Furthermore, no significant difference was found in maximal vertical opening after measuring patients with TMD initially and 6 weeks later.[113] Jaw movement capacity proved a reproducible parameter in children.[10]

Although limitation of jaw opening has been considered a major sign of dysfunction, disagreement exists about what constitutes limitation. The argument has been made that establishing a limit at less than the traditional 40 mm fails to recognize that some individuals may open much wider but be dysfunctional, whereas other individuals may open less and have no evidence of dysfunction.[92,126] A similar opinion has been voiced after study of jaw movement capacity in children.[10] This logic deserves praise.

Most researchers judge the opening to be limited if the interincisal distance is <40 mm.[7,34,38,39,42,52,53,61,64,68,80,92,94,105,112,123,127–131,156,160] Others set the limit at <39 mm,[44] at 38 mm,[132] at <37 mm,[133] and at <35 mm.[52,93,97,134,135] Some investigators consider 30 to 35 mm as a normal range and <30 mm as abnormal,[136] whereas others judge <35 mm for men and <30 mm for women as restricted opening.[84] Still others consider 32 ± 6 mm as limited and 42 ± 5 as within normal limits.[137] Finally, others make this judgment if the patient cannot insert the index and middle fingers interincisally when the hand is turned vertically in the mouth. So much variation causes problems in determining differences between symptomatic and asymptomatic individuals and among individuals of different populations.

In children and young adults, restricted opening has been accepted at <50 mm,[73] at <40 mm for 7 to 14 year olds[65,109] and for adolescents and young adults,[68,69,104] at <38 mm for 9 to 12 year olds, at <36 mm for 6 year olds,[138] and at <35 mm for 5 to 8 year olds.[104] Other accepted measures of restricted opening are <30 mm,[86] 30 to 39 mm (grade 1) and <30 mm (grade 2) limitation,[88] and <31 mm to 42 mm as moderate limitation and <31 mm as severe limitation.[10,98] An argument has been made that limited movement cannot be used as a sole indicator of function in children because they suffer functional disorders of the chewing apparatus even when they have no limits of movement capacity.[10,98]

In a classic paper, 35-mm interincisal distance was set as the limit for 5 to 10 year olds and 38 mm for 11 to 19 year olds.[139] But the author showed that measurements made between the alveolar crests represented more valid indices than measurements of interincisal distance. With this procedure, 44 mm was accepted as the limit for the younger group and 49 mm for the older group. In a recent study conducted in Pennsylvania, 44 mm was accepted as the limit set by the recommendation of Landtwing.[77]

The question of whether vertical overbite should be included during measurements has been studied. An impressive analysis of 1050 subjects showed that determination of normal mandibular opening using the alveolar crest distance proved superior to that of interincisal distance.[139] The author recommended that alveolar crest distance be used routinely in general practice. Unfortunately, most studies on asymptomatic and symptomatic individuals have findings reported as interincisal distance. Inconsistency has been found between maximal opening capacity and overjet in Michigan children.[70]

Whether limitation on opening can be used to distinguish asymptomatic individuals from symptomatic individuals is open to question. Mouth-opening capacity has been considered to have high discriminant power in identifying individuals with and without jaw pain.[140] Because of its constancy, maximal mouth opening was considered to be the most reliable clinical parameter for evaluating treatment.[113] It has been recommended that this variable be routinely recorded because even a moderate reduction of mouth-opening capacity may indicate TMD.[68,73,81] In contrast, the value of limited opening as an indicator of dysfunction was considered small[97] and not highly predictive of TMD.[6] The argument is that restricted opening capacity might be significant if there is severe hypomobility or hypermobility.[97] Although statistically significant difference was found between TMD patients and asymptomatic individuals in maximal opening capacity, the sensitivity score was too low to confirm a relation.[6]

Review of the literature shows reduced opening capacity for many symptomatic TMD cases around the world (see Tables 5-12 and 5-13). Data supporting this belief have been sampled from populations in Hawaii,[117] California,[6] New York,[116] Sweden,[6,141] and The Netherlands.[142] In contrast, no statistically significant differences in opening capacity were found between symptomatic and asymptomatic patients in a large dental clinic sample from California.[118] Further study of a population from Washington supports this conclusion. Although TMD clinic cases showed less maximal opening capacity than asymptomatic individuals, when the clinic cases were assisted in opening their mouths, two thirds achieved an opening of 40 to 54 mm.[84] The authors concluded that clinic cases had adequate vertical opening capability and lacked structural changes preventing a wider opening.

Age and Normal Opening

Variation in mouth opening has been related to age (see Tables 5-12 and 5-13). Differences have proved dependent on both age and body stature.[139] Maximal mouth opening increased with age from a mean of 45 mm at 5 years to 59 mm at 19 years, a 31% increase. During this period, the bodily stature increased 54%, confirming that the change in mouth opening is significantly less than the change in stature. Maximal opening capacity is reached in the early teens.[70,138]

The mean opening capacity differs between populations of similar ages. Children from Michigan[70] have smaller openings than children from Finland.[143] Starting at 6 years, children from Michigan average nearly 6 mm less opening than children from Finland. By about 16 years, the difference is nearly 8 mm.

In a community-dwelling population from Maryland, limitation on opening occurred in 13% of individuals 56 years or older compared with 5% for younger adults.[38]

No limitation was found in 15- to 20-year-old Swedish adolescents and young adults.[67,69,144]

Age and Limited Opening

In Sweden, limited opening was found from 1% to 15% in a random population.[42] This range compared with the 3% to 16% in a similar population.[64] A change in prevalence was observed at 2% in 15 year olds to 10% for the same individuals 5 years later.[66,68] A high occurrence of 28% was found in a small sample of symptomatic juvenile rheumatoid arthritic patients between 9 and 28 years of age.[80]

Limited opening was not significantly different between 6- to 8-year-old Polish children and adolescents and young adults.[81,86]

Little difference was found in Israeli children between 10 and 18 years.[103]

Gender and Normal Opening

On average, males have greater opening capacities than females (see Tables 5-12 and 5-13). When compared within the same population, the results of all the studies confirm this relation. This disparity relates to body stature. Typically, girls have smaller openings compared with boys. This relation remains throughout life.

Gender and Limited Opening

Reduced opening was more common in older Greek women and men than in younger individuals of the same population.[124] The decrease was comparable in both genders. The loss was about 12% between 18 and 20 years and 61 and 70 years.

A similar loss was found in Swedish men and women.[42,53,64] The decrease to <40 mm between 25 and 65 years was about 13%.[64] No significant difference was found between Swedish adolescents and young adults.[74]

In Maryland, no significant difference was recorded in a gender-equal sample of adults.[133]

Significance: Definitions of what constitutes normal opening vary widely, but most adults fall within the 40 to 60 mm range. Measurements are repeatable over time if no dysfunction occurs. Measurements made between the alveolar crests proved more reliable than measurements made interincisally. Universal agreement is needed to establish what is meant by limitation. Whether opening capacity can be used as a significant predictor of TMD remains conjectural. Clearly, setting the limits at 35 mm for men and 30 mm for women recognizes differences in stature not otherwise considered by the traditional interincisal measurement of <40 mm. Individuals 60 years and older can be expected to have less opening capacity than younger individuals.

Measurement of mouth opening has potential clinical value for assessment of mandibular function in children. But allowance must be made for variation in body size, populational difference, deviation from the normal range, age, gender, and the manner in which measurements are taken.

Study across populations shows that age and gender significantly affect findings. Younger children have less limitation than young adults. Girls have smaller opening capacity than boys. Although arbitrary, establishing interincisal restriction on opening at <35 mm for boys and <30 mm for girls in the early teens fits most children. Extrapolation of measurements for interincisal distance yields <39 mm alveolar crest distance for boys and <34 mm for girls. In sum, this modification fits children of most populations.

There is not much value in measuring horizontal mobility unless individuals become symptomatic or have growth anomalies. For example, the mean for horizontal mobility was about 9.5 mm (6 to 13 mm) to each side in 24 asymptomatic women.[125] The mean for protrusion was 8.6 (6 to 12) mm. Agerberg found no significant difference after measuring on different occasions (initially, 1 week later, and 4 months later). He concluded that the observed difference in horizontal mobility should be at least 2 mm if it is accepted as a sign of a true effect of treatment for a given patient.

Deviation on Opening

Most investigators record this percentage if the mandible deviates laterally from straight opening or from the midline by >2mm (see Tables 5-8 and 5-9). Yet 1 mm was accepted as the limit in dental patients examined from New York.[126] Among elderly of Canada, >5 mm was used.[91] The inflated percentages reported in some studies resulted from pooling of data with joint sounds, locking, or luxation.[7,42]

The scattered findings in children are variable (see Table 5-12). Clearly, this parameter depends on interpretation of the investigator. Most studies follow >2 mm lateral deviation on opening, but >5 mm has been used.[81]

Deviation on opening has been correlated with difficult opening, joint clicking, pain on jaw movement, and tenderness of the TMJs.[145] It has been associated with dysfunction based on analysis of tooth contacts[97] and has been used to differentiate patients with orofacial muscle-related or TMJ-related complaints from patients with psychogenous complaints.[137] The prevalence was significantly higher (50% versus 15%) in Swedish young adults judged to need treatment than in Swedish young adults not needing treatment.[130]

Age

Within populations at large, 17% deviated in a sample of Canadian citizens.[39] A high frequency of 60% to 63% was recorded in Finnish Lapps.[7a]

With age as a factor, results are mixed. In North America, deviation was significantly higher among adult Canadians younger than 65 years compared with more elderly individuals.[91] None was found between girls and boys of different ages in a Pennsylvania study.[77,78]

None was found in 14 to 16 year-old Danish adolescents.[10] Deviation on opening was unusually high (50%) in another population.[146] But irregular opening and deviation on opening were low in a comparable Danish sample.[98] The authors attributed the difference to sensitivity.

In Sweden, 55% of 15- to 20-year-old adolescents and young adults had this problem.[69] A higher percentage was found in children with dental restorations than in children with intact dentition.[67] The authors related this difference to symmetrical function of the lateral pterygoid muscle in the intact group.

Among Polish children between 6 and 15 years of age, deviation was unusually high in a group described as having slight dysfunction.[86] These children were divided into those with normal occlusion and those with malocclusions or lack of teeth. In 6 to 8 year olds, deviation occurred in 30% of normals and 38% in abnormals. Deviation was present in only 19% of 13- to 15-year-old normals and in 19% to 25% of abnormals of these ages.

Gender

Irregular opening pattern was not found to differ with respect to gender in several populations[71,79,84,126,133,137] or with respect to laterality.[84,126]

No significant difference was found in Finnish children between 10 and 16 years of age.[75] Yet deviation proved more frequent (22% versus 13%) in adolescent females than in adolescent males.[104] No gender difference was found in younger children.

  Significance: Coupled with radiographic and palpable findings, this sign should be a useful parameter for discerning developmental anomalies, muscular incoordination, internal derangement, or pathologic changes. It is simple to observe and measure. Uniformity would be improved by acceptance of >2 mm as the limit for adults and children who possess anterior teeth.

Detection of Joint Sounds

As found for self-reports of joint sounds, some investigators group these sounds, whereas others differentiate sounds from one another (see Tables 5-8 and 5-9). Most distinguish between clicking and crepitus, whereas few discern between clicking and popping. Other variation is related to the way the sounds are detected. Reports are based on findings by palpation, by auscultation with stethoscope, and by both procedures.

Clicking or popping was found in 5% of community residents of Washington.[84] The frequency was recorded as 48% in Canadian citizens.[39]

In Sweden, joint sounds have been recorded in up to 65% of shipworkers.[92] A division of these sounds showed that 42% had clicking, 21% had crepitus, and 2% had both noises. Crepitus was 2% in 50 year olds[64] and 33% in subjects of an urban population.[53] When examined by stethoscope, 58% of these citizens had sounds.

Age

According to studies conducted on Swedish adults, age was not a significant factor influencing TMJ function, including joint sounds, deviation on opening, luxation, or locking.[42] This broad statement is not supported by findings in other studies.

Crepitation was more frequent (37% versus 7%) in 65- to 74-year-old Tanzanians compared with 35 to 44 year olds.[102] No difference existed in clicking.

Joint sounds are frequent in children and young adults. Usually they are less prevalent than in older adults (see Tables 5-8 and 5-9). Crepitus is uncommon in children and young adults. Even when recorded, values average 2% or less.

In North America, clicking was significantly lower at 6 years of age than at 10 years in Pennsylvania children belonging to "calm" or "non-calm" groups.[77,78] A prevalence of only 4% was recorded for migrant children from Michigan.[93]

Furthermore, regression analysis showed an age effect and clicking in Michigan children.[70] Between 6 to 12 years of age, boys with cusp-to-cusp molar relations had a higher risk for clicking than their class I cohorts. From 11 to 17 years of age, girls had higher rates of clicking if the occlusion was class II rather than class I. After 13 years, girls with cusp-to-cusp occlusions had greater rates of clicking than other cohorts. The authors concluded that such associations were greater in older children than in younger children.

In Swedish populations, clicking doubled between 7 and 15 years of age.[88] A similar relation was found between 7 to 14 year olds and 15 to 18 year olds in another population.[65] But no significant difference was found between 15 year olds examined again at 20 years.[66,68]

Clicking doubled, from 10% to 20%, between 6 to 8 years and 13 to 15 years in Polish children.[86]

Clicking was significantly higher in 16- to 18-year-old Israeli children than in 10 to 13 year olds.[103] The highest percentage recorded for any population was 44% in adolescents and young adults from Israel.[103] But if the percentages are pooled between 10 to 18 year olds, they do not differ from percentages obtained by pooling data of 15 to 29 year olds from Sweden.[68]

Sounds were about one half as frequent (7% and 4%) in 13- to 15-year-old Finnish adolescents as in 5 to 8 year olds.[104]

Gender

Some differences have been ignored in studies, particularly involving young children (see Table 5-10).

In elderly from Canada, women had more frequent sounds than men.[91] The number of individuals with joint sounds was low. Among Maryland citizens, the percentages were similar in women and men.[133]

In Swedish populations, findings were mixed. Gender was considered important in TMJ function.[42] Fewer women than men had normal TMJ function between 20 and 70 years of age. Differences were observed in joint sounds and deviation on opening. In another population, the frequencies of both clicking (28% versus 21%) and crepitus (40% versus 26%) were greater in women than in men.[53]

No significant difference was found in joint sounds in a comparison of elderly Swedish citizens.[79] Examination showed that at 17 years, the frequency of sounds in girls was not significantly different from that in boys.[87] At 18 and 19 years, women had nearly twice the frequency as men (25% versus 13%).

No difference existed between middle-aged and elderly Australians,[71] and no difference was found in Finnish children between 10 and 16 years[75,104] and younger children.[104]

Significance: The diversity of joint sounds among populations shows the need for improvement in detection. In one study, digital palpation proved superior to stethoscopic examination.[84] Reliability was marginally acceptable (K = 0.62), even with the palpation method.

Numerous recommendations have been made about sounds.[147,148] In sum, sounds should be differentiated from one another (eg, clicking from popping, and crepitus from grating). Little is known of the prognosis of sounds, need for treatment, and long-term results of therapy.

Selected Groups

The findings of most studies suggest that individuals of similar age and gender suffer nearly the same complaints and exhibit similar signs. For most populations, the percentage of complaints was slightly less than reported for populations in nonclinical settings. Muscular tenderness and joint sounds detected by examination were as variable as observed in studies of nonclinical settings. In samples with equal gender ratios, women had more frequent complaints and more frequent signs than men.

Report of Orofacial Pain

Differences reflect the kinds of questions posed to subjects. Investigators asked about generalized orofacial pain, jaw pain, TMJ pain, and ear pain. Whether any of the findings can be considered comparable remains patently unclear (see Table 5-4).

In Virginia, prevalence of jaw pain was 4%, and pain within or surrounding the ear was 8% in Virginia dental students and dental hygienists.[37] Pain localized to the jaw was reported in 22% of nursing students from Minnesota.[112] Orofacial pain was not a major complaint in a small sample of dental students from California.[6] The prevalence of pain of the cervical neck region was less than 1% in these subjects.

Just 15% of dental students from Belgium complained of jaw pain.[123]

Pain in or surrounding the ear was 35% in heavy metal workers from Finland.[97] This latter percentage is inflated because other symptoms (eg, tinnitus, stuffiness, itching, reduced hearing, and pain without infection) were lumped with pain surrounding the ear region.

In Poland, orofacial pain was less than 1% in medical students, 10% in military students, 3% in young soldiers, and 5% in middle-aged soldiers.[13]

Gender

No significant differences were found in pain of the face, jaws, eyes, throat, neck, or ear in college students from California[34] or in dental students and dental hygienists from Virginia.[37] In a small sample of dental students from California, twice as many women reported static jaw pain (8% versus 4%) as men.[149]

The possibility of difference was ignored in a largely male-dominated sample of ship-workers from Sweden[92] and among dental students from Sweden.[150]

Report of Pain on Opening Wide

Information about this pain is limited (see Table 5-4). Just 8% of 25-year-old rural citizens from Norway complained of pain on opening.[85] The pain was twice as common in women as men (11% versus 5%).

Report of Pain on Chewing

The way in which data are expressed produces differences between populations, and the range of reports of pain on chewing is great (see Table 5-4). Chewing pain was present in 2% of rural, 25-year-old Norwegian citizens.[85]

In a sample of 20-year-old Swedish young adults, the prevalence was 51%.[130] This is an inflated percentage because the data were expressed as pain or tiredness and subdivided into frequent and occasional. In a nontreatment group, frequent pain and tiredness occurred in 11% and occasional pain and tiredness in 41%. In a smaller group of these young adults described as needing treatment, pain or tiredness on chewing was frequent in 28% and occasional in 47%.

Gender

No significant differences were found in a heterogenous sample of college students from California.[34] From this same region, significantly more women dental students than men dental students (14% versus 5%) reported chewing pain.[149]

No gender difference was found in 25 year olds from Norway.[85]

Report of Pain on Mandibular Movement

This symptom was of low to moderate frequency among selected groups of individuals (see Table 5-4).[150a] In Sweden, a frequency of 3% was reported by Conscripts and by a sample of 20 year olds.[130] A prevalence of 5% was observed in dental nurses.[120]

Gender

Differences have been found in dental students from California. Significantly more women (14% versus 8%) than men reported jaw pain on movement.[149]

TMJ pain on function was significantly greater (14% versus 3%) in 25-year-old Norwegian women than men of the same age.[85]

Report of Headache

For most populations, the prevalence of headache was low (see Table 5-4). In Swedish soldiers, it was 8%.[107,150a] In a limited sample of 20 year olds from Sweden, no history of headache was reported by 9% of a group needing treatment and by 18% of a group not needing treatment.[130] Extrapolation of percentages yields unusually high prevalences of 91% and 72%, respectively, for subjects with a history of headache. Such differences reflect the importance of asking about recent occurrence of headache.

Gender

Differences have been found in populations from North America and Scandinavia. Significantly more women attending a California university reported headache (15% versus 10%) than men.[34] Subjects suffering headache had more frequent tenderness of the TMJs (15% versus 4%) and muscles of the head and jaw (58% versus 31%) than individuals not suffering headache. Significantly more women dental students and dental hygienists from California reported moderate to severe headache (16% versus 6%) than men dental students.[131]

Within 25-year-old Norwegians, women had significantly more frequent headache (31% versus 24%) than men.[85]

Report of Jaw Fatigue and Stiffness

Conclusions about reports of fatigue and stiffness are limited by the paucity of data (see Table 5-4). Yet populational differences are evident. Thirty-two percent of nursing students from Minnesota suffered this complaint.[112] A prevalence of 2% was reported in a small sample of 20-year-old Swedish young adults.[130]

Gender

Studies showed that significantly more women dental students from California reported jaw fatigue (25% versus 13%) than men dental students.[149]

Report of Difficulty on Opening Wide

Data about difficulty on opening wide are limited (see Table 5-6). No significant difference (9% for both groups) was found between 20-year-old Swedish young perceived as not needing treatment or needing treatment of TMD.[130]

Report of Joint Sounds

Joint sounds were of low to moderate frequency among populations (see Table 5-8). There was remarkable similarity in frequency. In North America, self-reported clicking or popping occurred in 15% and crepitus in 6% of dental students from Virginia.[37] These percentages were similar to the presence of combined clicking and popping in 29% of dental students from California.[149]

In northern Europe, 15% of 20-year-old Swedish young adults[130] had sounds, whereas 22% of male heavy metal workers from Finland had clicking and 6% had crepitus.[97]

In Poland, 10% of medical students, 22% of military students, 17% of young soldiers, and 25% of middle-aged soldiers had both joint sounds and deviation on opening.[13]

Gender

Initial responses showed no significant difference in joint sounds among college students in California; however, direct questioning by examiners indicated that women gave 11% more positive responses than men.[34] This finding is supported by findings from another study of California students. Frequency of clicking was greater (50% versus 39%) in women dental students than in men dental students.[149] Women reported that the clicking disturbed them more (40% versus 30%) than it did the men.

Gender differences have been found in other populations. The occurrence of sounds has been related to other symptoms. Clicking and crepitation were significantly greater in 25-year-old Norwegian women (23% versus 14%) than men of the same age.[85] Among individuals with joint sounds, headache was greater in women (35% versus 20%) than in men. For subjects with sounds, 19% of women and 12% of men reported no headache.

Report of Locking

Joint locking was of minor frequency in these selected groups (see Table 5-8). A history of locking was reported by 8% of nursing students from Minnesota.[112] This frequency corresponded favorably to the 7% frequency found in Finnish heavy metal workers.[97]

The frequency of locking was significantly greater (13% versus 5%) in women dental students than in men dental students from California.[149]

Tenderness on Palpation of Masticatory Muscles

Some variation occurred even for samples from the same locality and for individuals of about the same age (see Table 5-6). Ten percent of a small sample of California dental students had tenderness.[6] Within a larger sample, a prevalence of 48% was found.[131,149] In Minnesota nursing students, the frequency was 24%.[112]

Gender

Significantly more California women dental students and dental hygienists had muscular tenderness (68% versus 33%) than men dental students.[131] Most tenderness was graded as mild. Global tenderness, judged as 4 or more sites, was present in 14 of 16 women. This same relation was observed in college students from California. More women than men (42% versus 26%) had tenderness.[34]

Inconsistencies exist between men of similar ages in different populations from northern Europe. Percentages were less than one half in Finnish workers[97] compared with Swedish soldiers.[107] The latter percentage was not significantly different from the percentage found in nursing students examined from Minnesota.

No gender difference was found in a large sample of Iraqi college students.[151]

As in nonclinical settings, the lateral pterygoids proved the most tender muscle group in all selected groups (see Table 5-10). This finding agrees with the finding in another study. In California college students, tenderness of the lateral pterygoids was nearly twice as frequent in women as in men.[34]

Tenderness on Palpation of TMJs

Tenderness of the TMJs varied within individuals of similar ages and within different populations (see Table 5-6). Generalized joint tenderness occurred in one fourth of Minnesota nursing students.[112] A prevalence of 18% was found by way of the auditory meatus. In contrast, just 3% was found by palpation at the lateral pole of the condyle and 1% by the auditory meatus in Virginia dental students.[37,152]

Generalized tenderness on palpation was found in 1% of Swedish soldiers.[1]

Gender

Most differences between populations probably relate to gender. All Swedish soldiers and nearly all the dental students from Virginia were men, whereas the nursing students from Minnesota were women.

Significantly more California women dental students and dental hygienists had tenderness than men dental students.[131] Of 32 subjects with tenderness, 25 were women. Tenderness of moderate to severe nature was more prevalent in women (12 of 15) than in men. Still, no difference was found among college students from California.[34]

None was found among Iraqi college students,[151] or among Taiwanese university students.[153]

Limitation on Opening Wide

The frequency was low in most populations (see Table 5-8). Only 1% was detected (<40 mm) in dental students and hygienists from California[131] and 4% in college students from California.[34] Limitation among the college students was not gender related but was significantly related to pain on opening wide (17% versus 3%) and to awareness of joint sounds (21% versus 8%).

Asymptomatic university students from Taiwan had significantly greater maximal mouth opening compared with symptomatic students.[153]

Only 3 of 121 Belgian dental students had limited opening.[123] They were women.

In Swedish 20 year olds, limitation has been used as a basis for treatment.[130] The frequency was twice as great (16% versus 8%) in a group needing treatment than in a group not needing treatment.

Mild limitation on lateral movement was found in 71% of college students from California.[34]

Deviation on Opening

Frequencies found for deviation on opening were variable (see Table 5-8). A prevalence of just 3% was found in nursing students from Minnesota,[112] whereas a prevalence of 18% was found in college students from California.[34]

Comparative study of two small groups of 20 year olds from Sweden confirmed this variability. In the group not needing treatment, 15% deviated on opening, whereas in the group needing treatment, 50% deviated 2 mm or more on opening.[130]

Detection of Joint Sounds

Much variation occurred in findings between populations (see Table 5-8). Some differences resulted from the manner in which the noises were detected. Clicking was found in 17% and crepitus in 12% of California college students.[34] Sounds were detected by palpation and stethoscope. In a small sample of dental students from California, the frequency was 72% when sounds were detected by biaural stethoscope.[6]

In male Swedish draftees, clicking or popping was found in 8%.[145] Sounds from the draftees were reported as being "heard."

Joint sounds have been related to other signs. In dental students, clicking correlated with tenderness on palpation in at least one masticatory muscle.[100,152] Various kinds of joint sounds were found, indicating different types of disk disorders in these students. Late opening sounds occurred in 45% of students.

Crepitus was absent in Swedish children and young adults ranging from 9 to 28 years old.[80] It was recorded in less than 1% of Swedish soldiers.[145,107]

Gender

Significantly more women have been found with joint sounds than men. In California college students, the frequency was 35% in women and 22% in men.[34] In dental students and dental hygienists, more women had clicking (36% versus 24%) than men dental students.[131] Five of 7 subjects with crepitus were women.

Gender effects were absent among Iraqi college students[151] and university students in Taiwan.[153]

Private/Clinic Dental Patients

Significance: The occurrence of signs and symptoms in patients presenting to private clinicians or clinics for routine dental care was equal to or slightly less than that found in nonclinical settings. Usually samples from populations at large were obtained from subjects residing in a specific locality and were comprised of individuals of similar races. Most clinic populations, particularly those in large industrialized localities, are comprised of heterogenous cultures. This heterogeneity explains some variation between clinics when comparing the same signs and symptoms.

Report of Orofacial and Related Pain

As in studies in nonclinical settings and selected groups, investigators differed in defining the site of the complaint (see Table 5-4). In North America, orofacial pain was reported by 40% of a small number of dental patients commingled with TMD clinic cases from New York.[154]

Orofacial pain ranged from 15% in a small sample of asymptomatic dental patients from The Netherlands.[140] TMJ pain was reported by 17% of the 20 to 50 year olds.

Jaw pain was reported by 11% of Pennsylvania adults between 19 and 30 years of age.[155] TMJ pain was recorded at 47% in dental patients from New York.[154]

Jaw pain occurred in 66% of Swedish dental patients.[89] Their ages ranged from 20 to 82 years.

Age

No significant difference was observed for pain and soreness around the face, ear, eye, or cervical neck in patients from California younger than 30 years or 60 years and older.[156]

Cervical neck pain during the day was found most commonly in 50 to 59 year olds in a sample from New York.[157] The prevalence reached 45% in an older dental population from New York.[15]

Gender

As in asymptomatic populations, gender differences existed. In a California clinic, the frequency of face and ear pain was more common in women (24% versus 9%)

than in men.[156,158] Significantly more women than men reported orofacial pain in a sample from Virginia.[37] This same relation was found for ear pain during the day (not night) from New York.[157] The frequency was 7% for females and 4% for males.

Jaw ache and tiredness was reported more frequently by women than in men among elderly from British Columbia.[91] The total of 9% agrees exactly with the 9% in jaw fatigue determined by difference between positive and negative responses observed in subjects from Texas.[159]

Pain of the cervical neck region was found in 11% of dental patients from New York.[157] It was significantly greater in females (5% versus 2%) during the night (not day) than in males.

Chronic neckache was significantly greater in women from California (18% versus 7%) than in men from the same locality.[158]

Report of Pain on Opening Wide

Pain on opening wide was found in 6%[37] and 22%[156,158] of large samples of dental clinic patients from Virginia and California, respectively (see Table 5-4). A frequency of 10% to 11% was reported by elderly from California clinics.[158,160]

In a Virginia clinic, significantly more women reported pain on opening wide than men.[37]

Report of Pain on Chewing

Significantly more women than men reported pain on chewing in a sample from Virginia.[37]

Report of Pain on Mandibular Movement

Pain on mandibular movement was reported in 5% of dental patients from California (see Table 5-4).[160]

Report of Headache

The occurrence of headache ranged from 13% to 43% in dental patients from California (see Table 5-4).[156,158] A frequency of 25% was reported by Virginia patients.[37] Complaints of headache or dizzy spells were not significantly different among Texas dental clinic patients giving positive or negative responses to tenderness of the masticatory muscles or to pain on mandibular retrusion.[159]

Headache occurred in 43% of dental patients from The Netherlands.[140]

Age

Differences occurred in some clinic groups. Chronic headache was significantly greater in California subjects younger than 30 than in subjects 60 years and older.[156] Daily headache was significantly greater in 20 to 49 year olds than in other ages from a sample in New York.[157]

Gender

Significantly more women than men reported headache as a frequent symptom in a Virginia clinic.[37] Chronic headache was significantly greater (25% versus 11%) in women than in men from California.[158] Headache was significantly greater in females than males during the day (21% versus 14%) and at night (6% versus 3%) in a sample from New York.[157]

From Sweden, significantly more women (40% versus 29%) than men had headache.[89] Women tended to describe this symptom as more severe than did men.

Report of Jaw Fatigue and Tiredness

In a group of California dental patients, 38% experienced tiredness of the jaws (see Table 5-6).[158] Tiredness was significantly more common (21% versus 8%) in subjects younger than 30 than in individuals 60 years and older.[156] Significantly more women (17% versus 8%) than men complained of this problem.

Tired jaws correlated significantly with tenderness of the masticatory muscles or pain on mandibular retrusion in patients from Texas.[159] In subjects giving positive responses to palpation, 41% reported tiredness, whereas in subjects giving negative responses, 32% mentioned tiredness.

Report of Difficulty on Opening Wide

In the California group (see Table 5-6), significantly more subjects younger than 30 years had difficulty opening wide (22% versus 11%) than patients 60 years and older.[156] More women than men (18% versus 8%) had difficulty.[158]

Report of Joint Sounds

As in nonclinical settings, joint sounds varied widely (see Tables 5-8 and 5-9). Clicking or popping was reported by 6% of dental patients from Virginia[37] and occurred in 45% of patients from California.[156,158,160] The dissimilarity was not attributed to unequal size of samples. Both populations were large.

Crepitus ranged from 6% in a large population from New York[157] to 17% of patients from California.[156,158,160]

Age

Differences were found in heterogenous samples from New York and California. In New York, the greatest prevalence (31%) occurred in 30 to 39 year olds.[157] In California, more individuals younger than 30 years reported clicking or popping (45% versus 23%) than subjects 60 years and older.[156] No age difference was found for crepitus.

Gender

Joint sounds were significantly greater in females than males during the day (23% versus 17%) in a sample from New York.[157] No differences were found for the night.

In California, significantly more women complained of clicking or popping (36% versus 27%) and crepitus (17% versus 10%) than men.[158]

Report of Locking

No report of locking was found in the literature.

Tenderness on Palpation of Masticatory Muscles

In North America (see Tables 5-6 and 5-7), tenderness was 15% in samples from New York[126] and California.[156]

Thirty-three percent of dental patients from Norway had tender muscles.[45]

Age

In the group from California, muscle pain on palpation was significantly greater (24% versus 12%) in individuals younger than 30 years than in subjects 60 years and older.[158] This difference contrasts with findings from studies in New York. Tenderness of the lateral pterygoid muscle increased with advancing age.[126] Pain was found in 8% of subjects between 10 and 19 years and in 32% of those between 80 and 89 years.

Other important disparities were found in a sample from Texas.[159] Comparison of subjects giving positive responses on palpation of the muscles or pain on mandibular retrusion found a 37% prevalence in 50 to 59 year olds and just 20% in 80 to 89 year olds. The same pattern was observed in subjects giving negative responses, which indicated that age was not a significant factor in discriminating between patients with and without these problems. Furthermore, tenderness did not correlate with maximal mouth opening (see Table 5-13), headache (41% positive versus 32% negative) or crepitus (70% positive versus 57% negative).

Gender

No significant difference was found in tenderness of the lateral pterygoids in patients (females 16% versus males 13%) from New York.[126] None was found for several masticatory muscles in a mixed sample of elderly from British Columbia.[91] But tenderness was significantly greater in women than men (19% versus 10%) in a sample from California.[158]

Study of a Norwegian sample showed that tenderness of the masticatory muscles and TMJs was not statistically related to gender or age.[45]

Comparison of specific muscle groups was limited because samples were small (see Table 5-10). Overall, the percentage within each group was the lowest reported among all populations.

Tenderness on Palpation of TMJs

Values (see Table 5-6) ranged from 4% in patients from New York[126] to 45% in patients from California.[156] The tenderness reported for New York patients was derived from palpation at the lateral pole of the condyle. Just 1% were found tender by palpation of the auditory meatus.

Age

No significant differences were found on palpation of the TMJs in a population from New York.[126] On the other hand, Californians younger than 30 years showed greater tenderness (39% versus 23%) than subjects 60 years and older.[156]

Gender

Palpation of the lateral TMJ region did not differ between genders among New York patients.[126] None was found between elderly subjects in British Columbia.[91] But significantly more women than men (36% versus 24%) were tender in a California sample.[156]

No difference was found in a large sample from Norway.[45]

Limitation on Opening Wide

Limitation on opening wide was found in 4% of the patients from California (see Table 5-8)[156,158,160] and in 13% of the Iowa patients.[161]

In Sweden, 35% of 80 dental patients had limitation.[89] Nine percent had severe limitation and 26% had mild limitation.

Age

Limitation was less in young adults than older adults in a population from New York.[126] The frequency was 3% in 20 to 29 year olds and 26% in 80 to 89 year olds. No difference was found between patients younger than 30 years and 60 years and older from California.[156]

Gender

Although the frequency of females with an opening of 37 mm or less was higher than that of males (7% versus 6%), no significant difference was found in patients from New York.[126] None was found in patients from California[158] or in elderly from British Columbia.[91] Limitation was set at 35 mm in the elderly sample.

Deviation on Opening

Deviation on opening was found in 21% of older patients from California (see Table 5-8).[156,158,160]

For the group from Sweden, the frequency was 69%.[89] This finding was considered minor; 3% had severe and 66% had mild signs.

Age

No significant difference was found in subjects younger than 30 years and 60 years and older in a sample from California.[156] None was found in a population from New York.

Gender

No significant difference (females 18% versus males 17%) was found in a population from New York[126] or in a sample of elderly British Columbians.[91] But women showed more significant deviation than men (39% versus 19%) in a sample from California.[156]

Detection of Joint Sounds

Clicking or popping occurred in 52% of dental patients from California (see Table 5-8).[156,158,160]

In Iowa, about 15% of 1000 patients had clinically evident sounds.[161] Clicking was the most prevalent sound. The frequency of crepitus was low. Forty-four percent had reduction of the disk on opening, and 42% had partial subluxation. None of the patients presented with diskal displacement without reduction. One third had present or past discomfort. No significant difference existed between individuals with subluxation, diskal reduction, or crepitus. Patients with crepitus averaged 54 years. Individuals without crepitus averaged 34 and 33 years, respectively.

Clicking or popping was detected in 10% and crepitus in 1% of young German men.[162]

Age

In New York, subjects younger than 9 years and between 10 and 19 years of age differed from other age groups.[126] None had sounds at the youngest age, whereas 26% had sounds by 19 years. Crepitation was absent in both young groups. In California, joint noise was slightly higher (56% versus 41%) in subjects 60 years and older than in individuals younger than 30 years.[156]

Gender

Significantly more females (39% versus 29%) had sounds than males in patients from New York.[126]

This same relation was found among elderly of British Columbia.[91] No percentages were given for each sex, but the overall percentage was significantly lower than that reported for New York patients of the same age.

A greater frequency of females than males was observed in patients from other clinics. Women were found with joint sounds more frequently than men (55% versus 40%) in a sample from California.[158]

TMD Clinic Cases

Significance: The most impressive findings are those comparing TMD patients with asymptomatic subjects from the same populations. Because of the heterogeneity of samples, age-related differences for this group are probably less reliable than those found by comparison of specific age groups selected from nonclinical settings. Studies in which sufficient data exist on gender suffer from the same concerns.

Age

Comparison of symptomatic samples across the world showed that most patients are 30 to 50 years of age (see Table 5-1). In the United States, 69% of patients from Georgia were younger than 40 years,[135] whereas most patients from Illinois fell between 31 and 50 years of age.[163] In New York, 57% were between 21 and 40 years.[164,165] In Tennessee, 62% were between 20 and 50 years of age. Such results are consistent with the finding of a mean of 37 years for Virginia patients.[166]

This age range characterizes other areas from the Americas. A sample from Canada found that the greatest number of symptomatic subjects were between the ages of 36 and 41 years.[167] In Argentina, the frequency was slightly less between 20 and 30 years than at more advanced age.[168]

In England, young women were reportedly the most susceptible individuals.[60] Forty percent were between 18 and 30 years of age.

In Scandinavia, 87% of the Norwegian patients were younger than 49 years.[169] Most patients fell between 20 and 50 years of age.[52] Comparison of samples from Sweden showed that most presented for examination between 19 and 55 years,[96] and specifically between 20 and 39 years.[129]

Interestingly, age was ruled out as significant factor in studies on signs and symptoms of adults in Australia.[46] Several reasons may account for the absence of an age effect. The mean age for patients and for asymptomatic subjects used for comparison was 40 years. The range was narrow in both groups. The total number of patients above and below 40 years was only 136, and the number of comparable subjects was 55. Finally, the heterogeneity in patients presenting for treatment is large in clinics of this kind.

Gender

Differences existed in patients presenting for diagnosis or treatment. Based on ratios for clinic samples, women outnumbered men by 2:1 to 9:1 across the world (see Table 5-1).

In the United States, ratios ranged from 65% women to 35% men in a small group in California[6] to 90% women to 10% men in a group from Virginia.[170] This relation is consistent for other samples from California,[118,149] Virginia,[10,166] Georgia,[135] Illinois,[163] Maryland,[38] Minnesota,[101,127] New York,[154,164,165] Tennessee,[171] and Washington.[84]

Significantly more women than men visited clinics in Canada[99,172] and in Argentina.[168]

In England, women outnumbered men by about 3.5 to 1 in several studies.[60,136,173] An even higher ratio was found in a sample from The Netherlands.[140]

In Scandinavian studies, Norwegian women outnumbered men by about 4 to 1.[52,85,169] Slightly lower ratios have been found in samples from Sweden.[41,89,113,121,129,141,174,175] Exceptions included a selected group of young adults designated as needing treatment[130] and a group of tinnitus patients surveyed for TMD.[176] In these samples, no major gender differences were reported.

Women at all ages were three times as likely as men to visit TMJ clinics in Greece.[177]

Report of Orofacial and Related Pain

The range for pain of the orofacial region was wide across populations (see Table 5-4). As reported for individuals in nonclinical settings, selected groups, and private/clinic dental patients, the location of pain was not always well defined or was expressed differently from one study to the next.

Most studies showed that the frequency of pain was much greater than reported by subjects from nonclinical, selected, or dental clinic settings. In North America, orofacial pain occurred in 98% of a large sample from Illinois.[163] Pain localized to the jaw was reported by 11% and to the TMJs in 83% of patients from Tennessee.[171] Jaw pain reached 94% of cases from Virginia.[166] Facial pain occurred in 66% and pain localized to the TMJs was 11% in a sample from Minnesota.[127]

A history of head, ear, or face pain was significantly more common (90% versus 20% to 27%) in TMD patients than in a group of asymptomatic subjects visiting a health center in Maryland.[38] Pain of the cervical neck was as low as 1% in a sample from New York[154] but was 45% in a large sample from New York.[164] Complaints of neck pain were more common among patients diagnosed with myofascial pain dysfunction (MPD) of the masticatory muscles than in patients with disk interference disorders (DD) primarily.[172] This complaint was more bilateral than unilateral and was found in 66% of MPD patients compared with 36% of DD patients. Face, head, or neck pain was significantly greater (94% versus 85%) in patients from Virginia diagnosed with myogenous pain than in patients with arthrogenous pain.[166]

The same relation was found in Australian patients diagnosed with myogenous facial pain (62% versus 39%) and unilateral static pain (53% versus 7%) compared with patients diagnosed with arthrogenous facial pain.[137]

In The Netherlands, TMJ/jaw pain was significantly greater in patients with myofascial pain (83% versus 17%) than in asymptomatic matched subjects.[140] The frequency of orofacial pain was 11%. No significant differences were found between TMD patients and matched subjects for pain of the forehead (34% versus 33%), temples (14% versus 17%), face (12% each), top of head (24% versus 16%), back of head (9% versus 11%), or neck (34% each).

Comparative studies conducted in Sweden showed that headache, pain of the face or jaws, or pain on moving the mandible were not significantly greater in juvenile arthritic patients than in asymptomatic subjects.[80] No significant differences were found in difficult opening or taking a big bite, in tiredness of the jaws, or in report of joint clicking between groups. None was found for lateral tenderness of the TMJs or for TMJ clicking determined by palpation.

In Norwegians suffering myofascial complaints, dynamic pain of TMJs was concordant with tenderness of the masseter or temporalis muscles.[111]

Age

Facial pain was not significantly related to age in a large heterogenous sample from New York.[165] But pain localized to the TMJ region was more frequently reported between 31 and 50 years than at any other age. Based on a much smaller sample from Australia, age was not considered a significant factor in the endorsement of orofacial pain between TMD cases and asymptomatic individuals.[46]

Gender

Because the literature reveals that women are overly represented in clinic populations, it is often assumed that more women suffer orofacial pain than men. But the reasons for this gender difference in presentation of chronic orofacial pain are not clear. So much ambiguity exists between studies that uncertainty remains (see Table 5-1). The following examples demonstrate the diversity.

In cases from California, static jaw pain was significantly greater (73% versus 53%) in women than in men.[149] TMD pain was reported more frequently by women (84% versus 16%) than by men from Washington.[84]

But no significant gender difference was found in static facial pain in an Australian sample.[137] The ratio of females to males admitted for diagnosis was 4 to 1.

No difference was found for initial symptoms, including facial pain, in a sample from England.[173]

Finally, pains of the jaw/face (44% versus 29%), temple (44% versus 28%), in or near the ear (63% versus 49%), and top of head (21% versus 5%) were significantly greater in Swedish women (44% versus 29%) than in men.[178] The following pains were not significantly different: cheek (40% versus 35%), forehead (23% versus 14%), throat (16% versus 9%), eyes (21% versus 12%), teeth and gums (30% versus 24%), and tongue (7% versus 5%).

To settle the uncertainty about gender, extensive analysis was conducted on chronic orofacial pain in women and men visiting a multidisciplinary orofacial pain center. The findings showed minimal gender difference in symptom presentation or sensitivity to pain.[179] No statistically significant differences were found between women and men in pain intensity, chronic pain unpleasantness, pain-related suffering, meanings of pain to the individual, illness behavior, orofacial pain symptoms, the personality factor of neuroticism, or sensitivity to experimental pain.

Report of Pain on Chewing

In the group from Virginia (see Table 5-4), pain on chewing was a major complaint in 81% of patients with myogenous pain and in 68% with arthrogenous pain.[166]

Biting pain was greater (35% versus 7%) in a Swedish sample of TMD patients than found in the population at large.[41] None was reported in a small sample of Swedish patients with juvenile rheumatoid arthritis.[80]

Gender

Gender differences were observed in a sample from California.[149] More women than men (76% versus 66%) reported this problem.

Report of Pain on Opening Wide

Pain on opening was prevalent in the TMD cases (see Table 5-4). It occurred in 79% of cases from Virginia[166] and in 42% of TMD patients compared with 7% in community-dwelling individuals from Maryland.[38]

Pain on opening wide was significantly greater in Dutch patients with myofascial pain than in matched, asymptomatic subjects.[140]

In Sweden, pain on moving the mandible was greater (10% versus 3%), but not statistically greater, in patients with juvenile rheumatoid arthritis than in matched, asymptomatic individuals.[80] A similar relation was found in other populations. Comparison of a small sample of TMD patients with a large number from the population at large showed that this pain was greater (42% versus 12%), but not statistically greater, in the patients.[41]

Report of Pain on Mandibular Movement

In a Maryland sample (see Table 5-4), functional pain was significantly greater in TMD patients (42% versus 5% to 8%) than in asymptomatic individuals.[38]

This finding is consistent with studies conducted in Sweden. Pain on lateral jaw motions was significantly greater (27% versus 4%) in TMD patients than in the population at large.[41] A similar relation was found for pain on gaping (42% versus 12%). Differences in age may be significant because only 3% of young adults needing treatment experienced this pain.[130]

Studies of a large population from England found that 64% had this pain.[173]

Gender

Findings differ between clinics. Jaw pain on movement was significantly greater in women (86% versus 77%) than in men studied from California.[149]

No significant difference was found in a sample from Australia.[137] Still, the authors found that unilateral pain on movement was significantly greater (59% versus 27%) in patients diagnosed with arthrogenous complaints compared with myogenous complaints.

No significant difference was found (37% versus 34%) in a large clinical study from Sweden.[178]

Report of Headache

Evidence from most clinical studies showed that the occurrence of headache was significantly greater in patients symptomatic for orofacial pain than in populations from nonclinical settings, selected groups, and private/clinic dental patients (see Table 5-4).

In North America, about 20% of cases from New York diagnosed with TMD reported headache.[165] In another clinic, 76% had headache.[164] In a sample from California, the frequency was nearly twice (63% versus 33%) as common among TMD patients as among asymptomatic individuals.[6] Because both specificity and sensitivity were low, the authors concluded that the clinical relevance should be questioned.

A study from Australia showed that headache was significantly higher (21% versus 11%) in patients with myogenous complaints than in patients with arthrogenous complaints.[137] Other studies do not always confirm this relation.

Patients sampled from The Netherlands with different classes of headache (tension, migraine, and combination) were studied for TMD signs and symptoms.[142] Fifty-five percent had concomitant TMD pain; 51% was of myogenous origin and 4% of arthrogenous origin. Tension headache patients had dynamic pain with greater frequency than the migraine and combination groups (33%, 10%, and 15%, respectively).

In Sweden, no significant differences were found in frequency of headache (once or more per week) among patients diagnosed with TMJ crepitus, TMJ tenderness on palpation, or neither crepitus nor tenderness.[113] In another sample of patients seeking treatment of headache, no statistically significant difference was found between subgroups of patients with either arthrogenous or myogenous complaints.[180] The frequencies for headache or joint pain occurring more than once per week were 46% for patients with reversible disk displacement, 70% for patients with permanent disk displacement, and 58% patients with myogenic pain.

Comparison of Swedish TMD patients with the population at large showed that headache was more frequent (68% versus 47%) in the patients.[41] This difference was significant with daily headache (11% versus 3%) and headache once per week (29% versus 15%). No difference was found with headache 1 to 2 times per month and an absence of headache was greater (53% versus 32%) in the population at large.

Another study from Sweden found that TMD patients reported significantly more headaches (women—78% versus 40%; men—59% versus 29%) than regular dental patients.[89] Occurrence of headache was associated with menstruation, as was tenderness of the masticatory muscles.

Recurrent headache was significantly greater (68% versus 36%) in Norwegian patients with myofascial pain than in subjects of similar age and gender not diagnosed with the pain.[181]

But no significant difference was found for headache in Dutch patients (59% versus 43%) diagnosed with myofascial pain matched against individuals not diagnosed with myofascial pain.[140]

Age

A major study relating headache with TMD was conducted on patients from New York.[165] Headache was present in less than 1% of 10 to 20 year olds and 71 to 80 year olds. The highest frequency of about 5% occurred between 31 and 50 years.

This report agrees with findings of more than 86,000 Virginia patients visiting medical centers for various health reasons (Fig. 5-2). Headache peaked between 15 and 35 years of age (25% versus 10%) then decreased significantly after 65 years of age.[182] Migraine peaked between 25 and 45 years and was practically nonexistent (20% versus 1%) after 65 years of age. Tension headache ran a course similar to migraine (20% versus 5%).

Headache decreased slightly (61% versus 54%) between Greek TMJ clinic patients younger than 30 years and 50 years and older.[177]

Gender

Generally, no major gender difference was found for tension headache or generalized headache in over 86,000 patients from Virginia.[182] Migraine peaked in women between 25 and 35 years, but was later in men at 35 to 45 years.

Headache was significantly greater (55% versus 34%) in Swedish women than in men.[178]

No statistically significant difference (63% versus 53%) was found between Greek women and men visiting TMD clinics.[177]

Report of Jaw Fatigue and Tiredness

Variation in age may explain disparities in findings among studies (see Table 5-6). In Swedish studies, fatigue or tiredness was reported in 9% of young adults needing

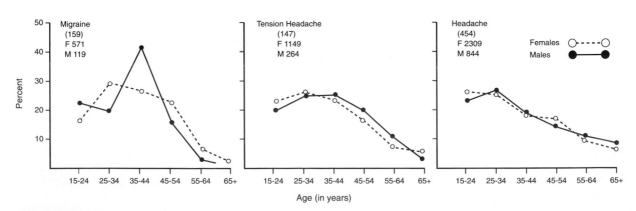

Figure 5-2.
Comparison of different types of headache with age. (Harkins SW, Kwentus J, Price DD. Pain and suffering in the elderly. In Bonica J [ed]. Management of pain. Philadelphia: Lea & Febiger, 1990:552.)

treatment.[130] The symptom occurred in 60% of 10 adult cases of various ages.[175] Jaw fatigue was not a significant complaint of patients diagnosed with TMJ crepitus, with TMJ tenderness on palpation, or with neither crepitus nor tenderness.[113]

Jaw stiffness was significantly greater in Dutch patients diagnosed with myofascial pain than in matched, asymptomatic subjects.[140]

Gender

In a sample from California, more women than men (85% versus 69%) had this complaint.[149] A similar relation was found (46% versus 25%) in a Swedish sample of women and men.[178]

Report of Difficulty on Opening Wide

An inability to open wide results primarily from muscular or joint disorders or from a combination of both disorders. Although limitation is prevalent among TMD patients (see Table 5-4), few studies disclose whether the disorder is primarily myogenous or arthrogenous. Little information is available about the longevity of restriction.

In North America, 63% of patients reporting to an Illinois TMJ Research Center reported limitation of jaw motion.[22]

In Swedish populations, difficult opening was significantly greater (35% versus 6%) in a small sample of TMD patients than in people of the general population.[41] In another study, no significant differences were found among TMD patients diagnosed with crepitus, with tenderness on TMJ palpation, or with neither crepitus nor tenderness.[113]

Based on complex statistical analyses, restricted opening had the highest discriminant power of all symptoms studied in a sample from The Netherlands.[140] Limitation on opening was significantly greater in patients diagnosed with myofascial pain than in matched, asymptomatic subjects.

Age

No significant difference was found between Greek TMD patients younger than 30 years and older than 50 years.[177]

Gender

Swedish women had more difficulty opening wide (36% versus 21%) than men.[178] No difference was found in samples from England[173] and Greece.[177]

Report of Joint Sounds

Some evidence suggests that the presence of joint sounds may be a useful predictor of dysfunction. Discriminant functional analyses conducted in The Netherlands showed that sounds made during mandibular movement could be used to differentiate patients with myofascial pain from asymptomatic dental patients.[140]

The following conclusion tends to support the statistical analyses. Joint sounds were reported significantly more often (79% versus 39%) in a sample of Swedish TMD patients than in a study of the population at large.[41]

However, the range in frequency of sounds is too variable to agree fully (see Table 5-8). Sounds were reported in 79% of young and middle-aged adults from California.[149] But clicking or popping was reported by just 12% of cases from England.[136] This percentage does not differ from the frequency in several populations from non-clinical settings.

In the group from Virginia, bothersome joint noise was more prevalent in patients diagnosed with primarily arthrogenous disorders (85% versus 58%) than in patients with primarily myogenous disorders.[166]

In Australia, no difference was found between patients with myogenous disorders (clicking 23% versus 24%, crepitation 9% each) compared with patients with arthrogenous disorders. This finding reveals the complexity of relying on patient self-reports.

The following statement illustrates the problem with reporting of sounds. Crepitus was reported by 5% of Swedish patients exhibiting TMJ tenderness and by 55% with clinically distinct crepitus.[113] Furthermore, clicking did not prove significantly different among patients diagnosed with TMJ crepitus detected by stethoscope, with TMJ tenderness on palpation, or with neither crepitus nor tenderness.

Age

A minor relation was found between age and joint sounds. In a sample from New York, the highest frequencies of clicking and crepitus (5% and 4%) occurred between 41 and 50 years of age.[165] The lowest (less than 1% each) occurred in 10 to 20 year olds and in 71 to 80 year olds.

Gender

No significant difference was found in a sample from California.[149] The frequency of clicking was about 90%, and the disturbance to the patient was about 86%. None was found between TMD patients and asymptomatic individuals in another California sample.[6]

None was found in a Swedish sample (women 58% versus men 47%),[178] and for clicking or crepitation in an Australian sample.[137]

Contrary to findings of other symptoms, more men than women presented with a complaint of clicking in a sample from England.[173]

Report of Locking

Comparative study of patients with orofacial pain from Virginia showed that 76% with primarily disk disorders complained of locking, whereas 66% with primarily myogenous pain described locking.[166] The results were not statistically significant (see Table 5-8).

In Swedish clinics, report of locking was significantly greater (26% versus 7%) in a limited sample of patients compared with the population at large.[41] Locking was not significantly related to crepitus, to TMJ tenderness on palpation, or to the absence of crepitus or tenderness.[113]

No difference was found in a sample from The Netherlands.[140]

Gender

Differences were reported in a sample from California.[149] The frequency was greater in women (64% versus 50%) than in men.

In patients from Australia, no statistically significant gender difference (0% versus 4%) was found between patients with either myogenous pain or arthrogenous complaints.[137]

No significant difference was found (women 17% versus men 12%) in a Swedish sample.[178]

Tenderness on Palpation of Masticatory Muscles

Evidence is overwhelming that tenderness of the masticatory muscles is significantly greater in patients reporting with TMD complaints than in individuals sampled from nonclinical settings, selected groups, and private/dental clinics (see Table 5-6). A similarity in clinical findings has been found between patients from the same locality reporting to a university TMD clinic and a private clinic practice. In Norway, 90% of patients treated at a university setting and 95% of a group seeking treatment at the clinical practice had tenderness.[183]

Muscle palpation has been studied more often in clinic samples from North America than in samples from clinics around the world. The presence of tenderness ranged from 40% in cases from Washington[84] to 96% in cases from Maryland.[38] Compared with community-dwelling individuals from the Maryland sample, 96% of patients had four or more masticatory muscles tender to palpation, whereas 75% of community-dwelling non-patients had four or more muscles tender to palpation.

Enrollees in a Washington Health Maintenance Organization diagnosed with TMD (CLCA) had significantly greater mean scores for extraoral muscle pain on palpation (5.5%) than community subjects free of TMD (COCO) pain (1.2%), but not so when compared with community cases (COCA) of TMD (3.8%).[84] This same relation was found for intraoral palpation (3.4%, with 2.8% each for TMD cases versus 1.8% for asymptomatic subjects).

In a sample from California, the number of masticatory muscles tender to palpation was significantly greater (2.6% versus 0.2%) in TMD patients than in asymptomatic individuals.[6] The same relation was found with tenderness on palpation of the cervical area (1.3% versus 0.05%). High specificity and sensitivity scores were found for the masticatory muscles but not for palpation of the cervical muscles. The authors concluded that palpation of masticatory muscles was a valuable finding.

The presence of widespread tenderness in so many patients diagnosed with orofacial myogenous pain suggests a possible relation with patients diagnosed as having generalized bodily complaint of fibromyalgia. Among Canadian patients with myofascial pain of the masticatory muscles, 52% had pain on palpation of the neck muscles compared with 15% of patients with other causes of joint pain.[172]

Studies in other localities showed that tenderness of the neck and shoulder muscles was a common occurrence even among asymptomatic subjects. Tenderness was found in about 63% of subjects,[184] which compares favorably with the values of 59% for healthy volunteers but is less than the 75% found in patients with TMD and paraspinal muscular pain.[38]

Associations have been made between tenderness and other complaints, but the findings are inconsistent. In The Netherlands, tenderness proved significantly different between three subgroups of headache patients.[142] Tenderness of the masseter and temporalis muscles was significantly more frequent in combination headache patients than in tension headache or migraine patients.

In Swedish clinics, patients diagnosed with myalgia had 2 or more muscles tender to palpation compared with individuals diagnosed with arthritis-arthrosis or disk disorders (78% versus 33% versus 15% for 3 or more muscles).[129] In a smaller sample, tenderness of the masticatory muscles or TMJ was not significantly different between patients with either TMJ crepitus or TMJ tenderness on palpation, compared with individuals with neither crepitus nor tenderness.[113]

Compared with asymptomatic individuals, no significant relation was found between pain on palpation and joint sounds in patients from Georgia.[135]

Age

Statistically significant differences were found between Greek women younger than 30 years and men 50 years and older (73% versus 50%) and between men younger than 30 years and women 50 years and older (72% versus 61%).[177]

Gender

In adults of the Washington Health Maintenance Organization, no significant gender or age differences were found among the CLCA, COCA, and COCO groups.[84]

In Swedish patients, tenderness was the single significant difference (66% women versus 43% men) between patients with myalgia, arthritis-arthrosis, or disk disorders.[129]

Tenderness of Specific Muscles

The lateral pterygoid proved the most tender muscle in seven of nine studies from North America (see Table 5-10)[22,101,135,149,154,164,170] and in one study from Sweden.[113]

This muscle group was the most frequently involved in TMD patients examined from Canada.[99] Exceptions include the medial pterygoid from a diverse sample of different ages and ethnic groups from New York,[165] the masseter in a smaller number of patients from Minnesota,[127] and the temporalis attachment at the coronoid and trapezius in myofascial pain cases from Norway.[111]

This widespread tenderness has been evidenced in more distant areas, such as the sternocleidomastoid, cervical neck, splenius capitis, and trapezius muscles.[101,135,154,164,170,171]

Tenderness of specific muscles has been found to vary within subgroups of patients. Patients with primarily arthrogenous disorders had significantly less tenderness of the lateral pterygoid than patients diagnosed with myogenous or combined arthrogenous and myogenous disorders.[170] Patients with myogenous disorders had greater tenderness in the superficial masseter than patients diagnosed with either joint or muscle and joint disorders. The frequency for the sternocleidomastoid muscle was lowest in the myogenous group compared with the other groups.

Tenderness on Palpation of TMJs

Wide variability exists because of differences in the regions palpated and between samples of different clinics (see Table 5-6). In a sample from Tennessee, TMJ tenderness was found in 92% of cases.[171] In New York, 25% had tenderness found by posterior palpation.[154] Both the lateral (CLCA—57%; COCA—35%; asymptomatic subjects—9%) and intrameatal aspects of the TMJs were significantly more painful to palpation in TMD clinic cases than in community subjects reporting no TMD pain.[84] No difference was found between clinic and community cases suffering with pain.

Comparison of TMD patients from England with matched, asymptomatic subjects showed that tenderness was significantly greater (59% versus 18%) among patients.[60] Sixty-three patients with tenderness had it at the lateral pole of the condyle.

In Swedish clinics, tenderness of the TMJs was recorded as 4% in patients with diskal disorders but was 78% in patients with myogenous disorders.[129] Tenderness was 21% at the lateral pole of the condyle and 15% by posterior palpation in cases with crepitus.[113]

Division of patients into subgroups having crepitation (E-1 TM), tenderness on palpation (E-2 TM), and neither of the two (R) showed that crepitus was significantly greater in E-1 versus R, with R having the least crepitus.[113] Reproducibility for TMJ tenderness was considered less than acceptable based on low specificity and low Scott's Pi (a measure of sensitivity) for tenderness of the TMJ.

Palpation of the TMJs by the auditory meatus proved significantly more tender in patients with juvenile rheumatoid arthritis (15% versus 0%) than in matched, asymptomatic subjects.[80]

Age and Gender

In Washington, no age or gender differences were found between either CLCA or COCA cases, or asymptomatic community subjects.[84]

No significant gender difference was found in an Australian sample.[137]

Although TMD was reported as being most common in English women between 18 and 30 years of age, tenderness of the TMJs did not differ significantly between women suffering from TMD (48% versus 41%) and asymptomatic subjects of the same age.[60]

In Sweden, an age relation was found between crepitation and TMJ tenderness. Crepitation increased significantly with age. No crepitation was found at 16 to 24 years, 20% was found at 25 to 49 years, and 80% was found at 50 to 88 years.[113] Palpable tenderness increased from 19% in young adults to 27% in the middle aged and 45% in older adults. No gender difference was found in this population.

Limitation on Opening Wide

Comparison of symptomatic and asymptomatic subjects shows that patients had restricted opening (see Table 5-8). In a heterogenous sample from California, limitation on opening was uneven with respect to other symptoms, and restricted opening alone was judged unreliable for assessing TMJ problems.[118] The author concluded that it can be useful when other signs and symptoms are known.

In Washington (see Table 5-12), the mean and range for jaw opening without pain (37 mm versus 42 mm versus 47 mm) and maximal unassisted opening (45 mm versus 49 mm versus 51 mm) proved significantly less in CLCA clinic cases than for either COCA cases or COCO subjects without TMD pain.[84] For maximal assisted opening, TMD clinic cases proved significantly less than found for the community group (47 mm versus 52 mm).

In Norway, about one half of TMD patients had limited opening.[111] No significant difference (50% each) was found between TMD patients examined in a university setting and individuals seeking treatment of TMD in a clinical practice.[183]

Studies from Sweden showed that when age and gender were excluded, restricted opening ranged from 8% to 50% (mean = 16%).[129] When the patients were diagnosed into subgroups, the percentages were myalgia—8%, disk disorder—27%, and arthrosis-arthritis—50%. In another study, juvenile rheumatoid arthritics had significantly less opening (28% versus 3%) than matched, asymptomatic subjects.[80]

In The Netherlands, limitation was found in headache patients with TMD pain.[142] Compared with headache patients without TMD pain, maximal mouth opening was significantly less (48 mm versus 53 mm) in the pain group. The mean distance between maximal active opening and passive opening was greatest in the pain group.

Age

In a Maryland sample, an opening of less than 40 mm was found in 33% of TMD patients. This restriction differed from the 5% of community-based adults younger than 56 years and 13% of adults 56 years and older.[38]

Among Greek TMD patients, significant differences (46% versus 25%) were found between women younger than 30 years and older than 50 years.[177] None was found between men patients.

Gender

In Washington, vertical and protrusive jaw motions were significantly greater in males than in females.[84] Males had consistently larger openings (3 to 5 mm) and protrusive movements (0.5 to 1.0 mm) than females. These differences were attributed to greater physical stature in males than females.

No significant difference was found in an Australian sample.[137]

The highest prevalence of restricted opening was 53% among Swedish women.[185] Seven years after treatment, it averaged 22%.

Deviation on Opening

Results from different cultures are incongruent (see Table 5-8). No statistically significant difference was found between TMD cases and community-based individuals from Maryland.[38] The author argued that this finding indicates that the clinical observation of deviation is unrelated to the clinical presentation of orofacial pain or joint noises.

Comparison of subjects from Washington showed deviated opening patterns were more frequent in CLCA cases (29% versus 13%) than in COCO subjects without TMD pain, but not different (26%) from COCA cases.[84] The deviation (more than 4 mm) was striking for CLCA cases (25% versus 15%) compared with COCO subjects.

TMD patients from England had significantly greater deviation (79% versus 54%) than matched, asymptomatic individuals.[60]

Association with other symptoms has been variable. In Sweden, deviation was 14% in cases with headache,[142] but was 83% in another study of headache patients.[89]

No significant difference was found (60% versus 53%) between Norwegian TMD patients treated at a university setting and individuals seeking TMD treatment at a clinical practice.[183]

Gender

No significant difference was found in an Australian sample.[137]

Detection of Joint Sounds

Great variation was found in detection of joint sounds, probably due to different methods. On an average, joint sounds were more prevalent in patients suffering from TMD than in subjects from nonclinical settings, selected groups, and private/dental clinics (see Table 5-8).

Assessment of joint sounds by palpation showed that clicking was significantly higher (43% versus 25%) in CLCA patients from Washington than in COCO community subjects (43% versus 25%) and in COCA cases (33%).[84] No significant difference was found in crepitus or grating between these groups. The authors concluded that sounds detected by palpation had marginal levels of reliability (K = 0.62) and those detected by stethoscope were unreliable (K = 0.26).

Sounds were twice as prevalent (65% versus 33%) in TMD patients as in community-based individuals from a large Maryland population.[38]

Differences in specific sounds have been observed. In large samples, clicking or popping ranged from 8% in patients examined from Tennessee[171] to 92% in a sample from Illinois.[163]

Crepitus was present in 8% of CLCA cases from Washington[84] but was 34% in patients from Minnesota.[127]

In Sweden, crepitation (33% versus 9% versus none) and TMJ tenderness on palpation (63% versus 23% versus 4%) were significantly greater in patients with arthritis-arthrosis compared with subjects suffering from myalgia or disk disorders.[129] Clicking was significantly more frequent in patients with disk disorder (69% versus 31% versus 13%) than in myalgia and arthritis-arthrosis patients. In another study, crepitus was significantly greater (15% versus 0%) in juvenile rheumatoid arthritics than in asymptomatic subjects.[80]

Age

In a Greek population aged 30 and younger, clicking was more prevalent (86% versus 50%) in women than in men.[177] No age or gender difference existed beyond the age of 50 years.

Need or Demand for Treatment

Estimated Need by Clinician

Because need for treatment of the occlusion has been emphasized by some clinicians, much disparity exists among populations across the world (Table 5-14). Most practitioners grouped estimates for occlusal problems with need for treatment of pain, limited opening, muscle tenderness, and joint sounds.

Few estimates of need have been made for populations in North America. Five percent of California university students were judged in need of treatment.[34]

Table 5-14
Percentages for Populations Estimated to Need or
Seeking Treatment for at Least One Symptom and Sign

Country	%	Characteristic	Reference
Estimated Need by Clinician			
Denmark	10	Children for treatment	D1
	20	Children for observation	
Hungary	20	Citizens for treatment	Hu
Poland	33	Children for treatment	P2
	7	Children for specialist care	
Sweden	21	Dental nurses for treatment	S1
	25–30	Shipworkers for treatment	S14
	27	Young adults for treatment	S50
California	5	Students for treatment	C3
Subject Demand for Treatment			
Finland	27	Citizens	F8
Sweden	13	Dental students	S28
	90	TMD patients	S42
	2	Adolescents for embarassing joint sounds	S49
	13–19	Citizens	S47
	3	Young adults	S50
Virginia	15	Citizens	Vo
	21	Dental students	Vs
	14	Dental patients	V
Sought Advice or Treatment			
Finland	5	Workers	F5
Sweden	7	Citizens	S5
Minnesota	7	Nurses	Mn3
Pennsylvania	6	Citizens	Pa

Need for treatment was estimated at 20% to 30% for urbanized adults in Hungary,[106] shipworkers,[92] and young adults sampled from Sweden.[130]

Among Danish children, 10% were estimated in need of treatment and another 20% in need of observation.[98] Of Polish children, 33% were judged as needing treatment and another 7% as requiring specialist care.[81]

Subject Demand for Treatment

The percentages differed depending on the kind of subject interviewed and the types of questions asked (see Table 5-14). Some screening involved questions about need for occlusal treatment. Usually, subjects were given little opportunity to discern major symptoms from occlusal problems.

Demands for treatment by subjects from Virginia ranged from 15% for citizens interviewed from the general population to 14% for dental patients visiting a clinic and 21% for dental students.[37] Clearly, the greater response by dental students reflected more awareness about TMD than in the other groups.

The greatest variation occurred among Swedish populations. About 13% of a small sample of dental students felt the need for treatment.[150] This percentage differed little from requests for treatment by Swedish citizens at 13% to 19%.[53] Yet just 2% to 3% of adolescents and young adults demanded treatment.[94,130] On the other hand, 90% of TMD patients requested treatment.[178]

Sought Advice or Treatment

Generally, the percentages (5% to 7%) of individuals seeking advice or treatment are about one fourth of the clinician estimates of subjects in need of treatment (see Table 5-14).

Percentages reported for populations from Pennsylvania[155] and Minnesota[112] closely correspond with percentages for populations from Finland[44] and Sweden.[40]

References

1. Mausner JS, Kramer S. Mausner & Bahn epidemiology: an introductory text. Philadelphia: WB Saunders, 1985.

1a. Solberg WK. Epidemiology, incidence, and prevalence of temporomandibular disorders: a review. In Laskin DM et al (eds). The president's conference on the examination, diagnosis, and management of temporomandibular disorders. Chicago: American Dental Association 1983:30.

2. Baume LJ. Standardization in reporting epidemiologic findings. Second Conference on Oral Biology. J Dent Res 1963;42:245.

3. Agerberg G. Mandibular function and dysfunction in complete denture wearers—a literature review. J Oral Rehabil 1988;15:237.

4. Greene CS, Marbach JJ. Epidemiologic studies of mandibular dysfunction: a critical review. J Prosthet Dent 1982;48:184.

5. Riolo ML, TenHave TR, Brandt D. Clinical validity of the relationship between TMJ signs and symptoms in children and youth. ASDC J Dent Child 1988; 55:110.

6. Cacchiotti DA, Plesh O, Bianchi P, McNeill C. Signs and symptoms in samples with and without temporomandibular disorders. J Craniomandib Disord Facial Oral Pain 1991;5:167.

7. Helkimo M. Studies on function and dysfunction of the masticatory system. II. Index for anamnestic and clinnical dysfunction and occlusal state. Swed Dent J 1974;67:101.

7a. Helkimo M. Studies on function and dysfunction of the masticatory system. Proc Fin Dent Soc 1974;70:37.

7b. Helkimo M. Studies on function and dysfunction of the masticatory system. IV. Age and sex distribution of dysfunction in the masticatory system in Lapps in the north of Finland. Acta Odontol Scand 1974;32:255.

8. Helkimo M. Epidemiological surveys of dysfunction of the masticatory system. In Zarb GA, Carlsson GE (eds). Temporomandibular joint: function and dysfunction. St. Louis: CV Mosby 1979:175.

9. Van der Weele L Th, Dibbets JMH. Helkimo index: a scale or just a set of symptoms? J Oral Rehabil 1987;14:229.

10. Nielsen L, Melsen B, Terp S. Clinical classification of 14–16-year-old Danish children according to function status of the masticatory system. Community Dent Oral Epidemiol 1988;16:47.

11. Harkins SW, Bush FM, Price DD, Hamer RM. Symptom report in orofacial pain patients: relation to chronic pain, experimental pain, illness behavior, and personality. Clin J Pain 1991;7:102.

12. Mohl ND, McCall WD, Lund JP, Plesh O. Devices for the diagnosis and treatment of temporomandibular disorders: introduction, scientific evidence, and jaw tracking. J Prosthet Dent 1990;63(pt 1):198.

13. Wigdorowicz-Makowerova N, Grodzki C, Panek H, Maslanka T. Plonka A. Epidemiologic studies on prevalence and etiology of functional disturbances of the masticatory system. J Prosthet Dent 1979;41:76.

14. Lignell L, Ransjo K. Maximal gapformaga. Sver Tandlarkarf Tidn 1967;21:859–862.

15. Agerberg G. Maximum mandibular movements in young men and women. Svensk Tandlak Tidskr 1974;67:81.

16. Allen JD, Rivera-Morales WC, Zwemer JD. The occurrence of temporomandibular disorder symptoms in healthy young adults with and without evidence of bruxism. J Craniomandib Pract 1990;8:312.

17. Brussel IJ. Temporomandibular joint diseases: differential diagnosis and treatment. J Am Dent Assoc 1949;39:532.

18. Crooks MC, Ferguson JW, Edwards JL. Clinical presentation and final diagnosis of patients referred to a temporomandibular joint clinic. N Z Dent J 1991;87:113.

19. Dibbets JMH. Juvenile temporomandibular joint dysfunction and craniofacial growth. Groningen, The Netherlands: Rijksuniversiteit te Groningen, 1977. Doctoral thesis.

20. Geering-Gaerny M, Rakosi T. Initial-symptome von Kiefergelenkstornungen bei Kindern im Alter von 8–14 Jahren. Schweiz Monatsschr Zahnheilkd 1971;81:691.

21. Glass EG, McGlynn FD, Glaros AG, Melton K, Romans K. Prevalence of temporomandibular disorder symptoms in a major metropolitan area. J Craniomandib Pract 1993;11:217.

22. Greene CS, Lerman MD, Sutcher HD, Laskin DM. The TMJ-pain dysfunction syndrome: heterogeneity of the patient population. J Am Dent Assoc 1969;79:1168.

23. Ingervall B. Range of movement of mandible in children. Scand J Dent Res 1970;78:311.

24. Kampe T, Carlsson GE, Hennerz H, Haroldson T. Three-year longitudinal study of mandibular dysfunction in young adults with intact and restored dentitions. Acta Odontol Scand 1987;45:25.

25. Kopp S. Subjective symptoms in temporomandibular joint osteoarthritics. Acta Odontol Scand 1977;35:207.

26. Lindquist B. Bruxism in twins. Acta Odontol Scand 1974;32:177.

27. Marciani RD, Haley JV, Roth GT. Facial pain complaints in the elderly. J Dent Res 1984;63(special issue):345. Abstract 1567.

28. Ohno H, Morisushi T, Ohno K, Ogura T. Comparative subjective evaluation and prevalence study of TMJ dysfunction syndrome in Japanese adolescents based on clinical examination. Community Dent Oral Epidemiol 1988;16:122.

29. Ozaki Y, Schigfmatsu T, Takahashi S. Clinical findings in temporomandibular disorders. Bull Tokyo Dent Coll 1990;31:229.

30. Petersen PE, Moller E. Self-reported TMJ-problems, health status and oral functioning among 67 Danes. J Dent Res 1991;70:828. Abstract 35.

31. Rao MB, Rao CB. Incidence of temporo-mandibular joint pain dysfunction syndrome in rural population. Int J Oral Maxillofac Surg 1981;10:261.

32. Seyffart H, Steen-Johnsen S. Belastningsskdommer i tuggeapparatet hos barn. Norske Tannlaegeforen Tid 1956;66:295.

33. Siebert G. Zur Frage okklusaler Interferenzen bei Jugendlichen (Ergebnis einer Untersuchung bei 12- bis 16-jahrigen). Dtsch Zahnarztl Z 1975;30:539.

34. Solberg WK, Woo MW, Houston JB. Prevalence of mandibular dysfunction in young adults. J Am Dent Assoc 1979;98:25.

35. Wänman G, Agerberg G. Relationship between signs and symptoms of mandibular dysfunction in adolescents. Community Dent Oral Epidemiol 1986;14:225.

36. Wilding RJC, Owen CP. The prevalence of temporomandibular joint dysfunction in edentulous non-denture wearing individuals. J Oral Rehabil 1987;14:175.

37. Bush FM, Butler JH, Abbott DM, Carter WH. Prevalence of mandibular dysfunction: subjective signs and symptoms. In Lundeen HC, Gibbs CH (eds). Postgraduate dental handbook. Boston: John Wright, 1982:106.

38. Heft MW. Prevalence of TMJ signs and symptoms in the elderly. Gerodontology 1984;3:125.

39. Locker D, Slade G. Association of symptoms and signs of TM disorders in an adult population. Community Dent Oral Epidemiol 1989;17:150.

40. Agerberg G, Carlsson GE. Functional disorders of the masticatory system: distribution of symptoms according to age and sex as judged from investigation by questionnaire. Acta Odontol Scand 1972;30(pt 1):597.

41. Agerberg G, Carlsson GE. Symptoms of functional disturbances of the masticatory system: a comparison of frequencies in a population sample and in a group of patients. Acta Odontol Scand 1975;33:183.

42. Salonen L, Hellden L, Carlsson GT. Prevalence of signs and symptoms of dysfunction in the masticatory system: an epidemiologic study in an adult Swedish population. J Craniomandib Disord Facial Oral Pain 1990;4:241.

43. Helkimo M. Epidemiological surveys of dysfunction of the masticatory system. Oral Science Review 1976;7:54.

44. Swanljung O, Rantanen T. Functional disorders of the masticatory system in Southwest Finland. Community Dent Oral Epidemiol 1979;7:177.

45. Gustavsen F, Katz RV, Tangerud T, Newitter DA. The prevalence of idiopathic chronic TMJ disorders in adults. J Dent Res 1991;70:828. Abstract 36.

46. Gerke DE, Gross AN, Pilowsky I. The relation of age to temporomandibular joint dysfunction. Clin J Pain 1988;4:17.

47. Serfaty V, Memcovsky CE, Friedlander D, Gazit E. Functional disturbances of the masticatory system in an elderly population group. J Craniomandib Pract 1989;7:46.

48. Harriman LP, Snowdon DA, Messer LB, Rysavy DM, Ostwald SK, Lai CH, Soberay AH. Temporomandibular joint dysfunction and selected health parameters in the elderly. Oral Surg Oral Med Oral Pathol 1990;70:406.

49. Hansson T, Oberg T. En kliniskt-bettfysiologisk undersokning av 67-aringer i Dalby. Tandlakartidning 1971;18:650.

50. Agerberg G, Osterberg T. Maximum mandibular movements and symptoms of mandibular dysfunction in 70-year old men and women. Swed Dent J 1974; 67:147.

51. Duckro PN, Tait RC, Margolis RB, Deshields TL. Prevalence of temporomandibular symptoms in a large United States metropolitan area. J Craniomandib Pract 1990;8:131.

52. Helöe B, Helöe LA. Signs and symptoms of temporomandibular joint disorders in an elderly population. J Dent Res 1977;56:91. Abstract 195.

53. Agerberg G, Inkapööl I. Craniomandibular disorders in an urban Swedish population. J Craniomandib Disord Facial Oral Pain 1990;4:154.

54. TM disorders, guide To dental health. J Am Dent Assoc 1984;108(special issue):64.

55. U. S. Department of Health and Human Service. Broadening the scope: long-range research plan for the nineties. Public Health Service/National Institutes of Health. Bethesda: National Institutes Dental Research, 1990:108. NIH publication 90–1188.

56. Ogura T, Morisushi T, Ohno Sumi K, Hataka K. An epidemiological study of TMJ dysfunction syndrome in adolescents. J Pedodont 1985;10:22.

57. Lipton JA. Orofacial pain in the U. S. adult population. J Dent Res 1991; 70(special issue):429. Abstract 1309.

58. Lipton J, Ship J, Larach-Robinson D. Estimated prevalence and distribution of reported orofacial pain in the United States. J Am Dent Assoc 1993; 124(10):115.

59. Goulet JP, Lund JP, Lavigne G. Jaw pain: an epidemiologic survey among French Canadians in Quebec. J Dent Res 1992;71(special issue):150. Abstract 353.

60. Thomson H. Mandibular joint pain: a survey of 100 treated cases. Br Dent J 1959;107:243.

61. Tervonen T, Knuuttila M. Prevalence of signs and symptoms of mandibular dysfunction among adults aged 25, 35, 50 and 65 years in Ostrobothnia, Finland. J Oral Rehabil 1988;15:455.

62. Khan AA. The prevalence of myofacial pain dysfunction syndrome in a lower socio-economic group in Zimbabwe. Community Dent Health 1990;7:189.

63. Von Korff M, Dworkin S, LeResche L, Kruger A. Epidemiology of temporomandibular disorders. II. TMD pain compared to other common pain sites. In Dubner R, Gebhart GF, Bond MR (eds). Pain research and clinical management 3. New York: Elsevier, 1988:506.

64. Agerberg G, Bergenholtz A. Craniomandibular disorders in adult populations of West Bothnia, Sweden. Acta Odontol Scand 1989;47:129.

65. Nilner M. Functional disturbances and diseases in the stomatognathic system among 7 to 18 year olds. J Craniomandib Pract 1985;3:358.

66. Magnusson T. Five-year longitudinal study of signs and symptoms of mandibular dysfunction in adolescents. J Craniomandib Pract 1986;4:338.

67. Kampe T, Hennerz H, Strom P. Mandibular dysfunction related to dental filling therapy: a comparative anamnestic and clinical study. Acta Odontol Scand 1986;44:113.

68. Magnusson T, Egermark-Eriksson I, Carlsson GE. Five-year longitudinal study of signs and symptoms of mandibular dysfunction in adolescents. J Craniomandib Pract 1986;4:338.

69. Kampe T, Hennerz H, Strom P. Five-year follow-up of mandibular dysfunction in adolescents with intact and restored dentitions: a comparative anamnestic and clinical study. J Craniomandib Disord Facial Oral Pain 1991;5:121.

70. Riolo ML, Brandt D, TenHave TR. Associations between occlusal characteristics and signs and symptoms of TMJ dysfunction in children and young adults. Am J Orthod Dentofacial Orthop 1987;92:467.

71. Mercado MDF, Faulkner KDB. The prevalence of craniomandibular disorders in completely edentulous denture-wearing subjects. J Oral Rehabil 1991; 18:231.

72. Agerberg G, Carlsson GE. Functional disorders of the masticatory system: symptoms in relation to impaired mobility as judged from investigation by questionnaire. Acta Odontol Scand 1973;31(pt 2):335.

73. Wänman A, Agerberg G. Mandibular dysfunction in adolescents: prevalence of symptoms. Acta Odontol Scand 1986;44(pt 1):47.

74. Wänman A, Agerberg G. Two-year longitudinal study of symptoms of mandibular dysfunction in adolescents. Acta Odontol Scand 1986;44:321.

75. Könönen M, Nystrom M, Kleemola-Kujala E, Kataja M, Evälahti M, Laine P, Peck L. Signs and symptoms of craniomandibular disorders in a series of Finnish children. Acta Odontol Scand 1987;45:109.

76. Heikinheimo K, Salmi K, Myllärniemi S, Kirveskari P. Symptoms of craniomandibular disorder in a sample of Finnish adolescents at the ages of 12 and 15 years. Eur J Orthod 1989;11:325.

77. Vanderas AP. Prevalence of craniomandibular dysfunction in white children with different emotional states: calm group. ASDC J Dent Child 1988;55 (pt 1):441.

78. Vanderas AP. Prevalence of craniomandibular dysfunction in white children with different emotional states: non-calm group. ASDC J Dent Child 1989;56(pt 2):348.

79. Osterberg T, Carlsson GE. Symptoms and signs of mandibular dysfunction in 70-year-old men and women in Gothenberg, Sweden. Community Dent Oral Epidemiol 1979;7:315.

80. Forsberg M, Agerberg G, Persson M. Mandibular dysfunction in patients with juvenile rheumatoid arthritis. J Craniomandib Disord Facial Oral Pain 1988; 2:201.

81. Grosfeld O, Jackowska M, Czarnecka B. Results of epidemiological examinations of the temporomandibular joint in adolescents and young adults. J Oral Rehabil 1985;12:95.

82. Norheim RW, Dahl BC. Some self-reported symptoms of temporomandibular dysfunction in a population in northern Norway. J Oral Rehabil 1978;5:63.

83. Dworkin SF, Von Korff M, LeResche L, Truelove E. Epidemiology of tempo-

romandibular disorders. I. Initial clinical and self-report findings. In Dubner R, Gebhart GF, Bond MR (eds). Pain research and clinical management 3. New York: Elsevier, 1988:499.

84. Dworkin SF, Huggins KH, LeResche L, Von Korff M, Howard J, Truelove E, Sommers E. Epidemiology of signs and symptoms in temporomandibular disorders; clinical signs in cases and controls. J Am Dent Assoc 1990;120:273.

85. Helöe B, Helöe LA. Frequency and distribution of myofascial pain dysfunction syndrome in a population of 25 year olds. Community Dent Oral Epidemiol 1979;7:357.

86. Grosfeld O, Czarnecka B. Musculo-articular disorders of the stomatognathic system in school children examined according to clinical criteria. J Oral Rehabil 1977;4:193.

87. Wänman A, Agerberg G. Two-year longitudinal study of signs of mandibular dysfunction in adolescents. Acta Odontol Scand 1986;44:333.

88. Egermark-Eriksson I, Carlsson GE, Ingervall B. Prevalence of mandibular dysfunction and orofacial parafunctions in 7-, 11-, and 15-year-old Swedish children. Eur J Orthod 1981;3:163.

89. Magnusson T, Carlsson GE. Comparison between two groups of patients in respect to headache and mandibular dysfunction. Swed Dent J 1978;2:85.

90. Wänman A, Agerberg G. Subjective report of fatigue in the jaws: an indication of dysfunction. J Oral Rehabil 1988;15:212.

91. MacEntee MI, Weiss R, Morrison BJ, Waxler-Morrison NE. Mandibular dysfunction in an institutionalized and predominantly elderly population. J Oral Rehabil 1987;14:523.

92. Hansson T, Nilner M. A study of the occurrence of symptoms of diseases of the temporomandibular joint masticatory musculature and related structures. J Oral Rehabil 1975;2:313.

93. Gunn SM, Woolfolk MW, Faja BW. Malocclusion and TMJ symptoms in migrant children. J Craniomandib Disord Facial Oral Pain 1988;2:196.

94. Wänman A, Agerberg A. Temporomandibular joint sounds in adolescents: a longitudinal study. Oral Surg Oral Med Oral Pathol 1990;69:2.

95. Budtz-Jörgensen E, Luau WM, Holm-Pedersen P, Fejerskov, O. Mandibular dysfunction related to dental, occlusal and prosthetic conditions in a selected elderly population. Gerodontics 1985;1:28.

96. Martinez C, Barghi N. Prevalence of various types of TMJ clicking. J Dent Res 1981;60:877. Abstract 880.

97. Alanen P, Kirveskari P. Stomatognathic dysfunction in a male Finnish working population. Proc Finn Dent Soc 1982;78:184.

98. Nielsen L, Melsen B, Terp S. Prevalence, interrelation, and severity of signs of dysfunction from masticatory system in 14–16-year-old Danish children. Community Dent Oral Epidemiol 1989;17:91.

99. Zarb GA, Thompson GW. The treatment of patients with temporomandibular joint pain dysfunction syndrome. J Can Dent Assoc 1975;7:410.

100. Bush FM. Malocclusion, masticatory muscle and temporomandibular joint tenderness. J Dent Res 1985;64:129.

101. Fricton JR, Kroening R, Haley D, Siegert R. Myofascial pain syndrome of the head and neck: a review of clinical characteristics of 164 patients. Oral Surg Oral Med Oral Pathol 1985;60:615.

102. Mazengo MC, Kirveskar P. Prevalence of craniomandibular disorders in adults of Ilala district, Dar-Es-Salaam, Tanzania. J Oral Rehabil 1991;18:569.

103. Gazit E, Lieberman M, Eini R, Hirsch N, Serfaty V, Fuch C, Lilos P. Prevalence of mandibular dysfunction in 10–18-year-old Israeli schoolchildren. J Oral Rehabil 1984;11:307.

104. Pahkala R, Laine T. Variation in function of the masticatory system in 1008 rural children. J Clin Pediatr Dent 1991;16:25.

105. Abdel-Hakim AM. Stomatognathic dysfunction in the western desert of Egypt: an epidemiological survey. J Oral Rehabil 1983;10:461.

106. Szentpetery A, Huhn E, Fazekas A. Prevalence of mandibular dysfunction in an urban population in Hungary. Community Dent Oral Epidemiol 1986; 14:177.

107. Ingervall B, Mohlin B, Thilander B. Prevalence of symptoms of functional disturbances of the masticatory system in Swedish men. J Oral Rehabil 1980; 7:185.

108. Williamson EH. Temporomandibular dysfunction in pretreatment adolescent patients. Am J Orthod 1977;72:429.

109. Nilner M, Lassing SA. Prevalence of functional disturbances and diseases of the stomatognathic system in 7–14-year-olds. Swed Dent J 1981;5:173.

110. Wänman A, Agerberg G. Mandibular dysfunction in adolescents. prevalence of signs. Acta Odontol Scand 1986;44(pt 2):55.

111. Helöe B, Helöe LA, Heiberg A. Relationship between sociomedical factors and TMJ-symptoms in Norwegians with myofascial pain-dysfunction syndrome. Community Dent Oral Epidemiol 1977;5:207.

112. Schiffman EL, Fricton JR, Haley DP, Shapiro BL. The prevalence and treatment of subjects with temporomandibular disorders. J Am Dent Assoc 1990; 120:295.

113. Kopp S. Constancy of clinical signs in patients with mandibular dysfunction. Community Dent Oral Epidemiol 1977;5:94.

114. Nilner M. Prevalence of functional disturbances and diseases of the stomatognathic system in 15–18 year olds. Swed Dent J 1981;5:189.

115. Lysell L. How wide is normal? Letters to the editor. J Oral Maxillofac Surg 1984;42:763.

116. Travell J. Temporomandibular joint pain referred from muscles of the head and neck. J Prosthet Dent 1960;10:547.

117. Sheppard JM, Sheppard SM. Maximal incisal opening: a diagnostic index. J Dent Med 1965;20:13.

118. Rieder CE. Maximum mandibular opening in patients with and without a history of TMJ dysfunction. J Prosthet Dent 1978;39:441.

119. Fonseca DM, Paiva MJ, Bonfante G. Temporomandibular joint clicking: a clinical study. J Dent Res 1991;70:643. Abstract 62.

120. Posselt U. The temporomandibular joint syndrome and occlusion. J Prosthet Dent 1971;25:432.

121. Carlsson GE, Svardstrom G. A survey of the symptomatology of a series of 299 patients with stomatognathic dysfunction. Swed Dent J 1971;64:889.

122. Wood GD, Branco JA. A comparison of three methods of measuring maximal opening of the mouth. J Oral Surg 1979;37:175.

123. De Laat A, van Steenberghe D. Occlusal relationships and temporomandibular joint dysfunction: epidemiological findings. J Prosthet Dent 1985;54(pt 1):835.

124. Mezitis M, Rallis G, Zachariades N. The normal range of mouth opening. J Oral Maxillofac Surg 1989;47:1028.

125. Agerberg G. Longitudinal variation of maximal mandibular mobility: an intraindividual study. J Prosthet Dent 1987;58:370.

126. Gross A, Gale EN. A prevalence study of the clinical signs associated with mandibular dysfunction. J Am Dent Assoc 1983;107:932.

127. Butler JH, Folke LEA, Bandt CL. A descriptive survey of signs and symptoms associated with the myofascial pain–dysfunction syndrome. J Am Dent Assoc 1975;90:635.

128. Graham MM, Buxbaum J, Staling LM. A study of occlusal relationships and the incidence of myofascial pain. J Prosthet Dent 1982;47:549.

129. Magnusson T. Patients referred for stomatognathic treatment: a survey of 282 patients. Swed Dent J 1984;8:193.

130. Magnusson T, Carlsson GE, Egermark-Eriksson I. An evaluation of the need and demand for treatment of craniomandibular disorders in a young Swedish population. J Craniomandib Disord Facial Oral Pain 1991;5:57.

131. Pullinger AG, Seligman DA, Solberg WK. Temporomandibular disorders: functional status, dentomorphologic features, and sex differences in a nonpatient population. J Prosthet Dent 1988;59(pt 1):228.

132. Freedman GL, Gordon RL. Unilateral bony ankylosis of the temporomandibular joint: report of a case. J Oral Surg 1968;26:807.

133. Huber MA, Hall EH. A comparison of the signs of temporomandibular joint dysfunction and occlusal discrepancies in a symptom-free population of men and women. Oral Surg Oral Med Oral Pathol 1990;70:180.

134. Dingman R. Menisectomy in treatment of the temporomandibular joint. J Oral Surg 1951;9:2.

135. Kaye LB, Moran JH, Fritz ME. Statistical analysis of an urban population of 236 patients with head and neck pain. patient symptomatology. J Periodontol 1979;50(pt 2):59.

136. Copeland J. Diagnosis of mandibular joint dysfunction. Oral Surg Oral Med Oral Pathol 1960;13:1106.

137. Bezuur JN, Hansson T, Wilkinson TM. The recognition of craniomandibular disorders: an evaluation of the most reliable signs and symptoms when screening for CMD. J Oral Rehabil 1989;16:367.

138. Agerberg G. Maximum mandibular movements in children. Acta Odontol Scand 1974;32:147.

139. Landtwing K. Evaluation of the normal range of vertical mandibular opening in children and adolescents with special reference to age and stature. J Maxillofac Surg 1978;6:157.

140. Hijzen TH, Slangen JL. Myofascial pain-dysfunction: subjective signs and symptoms. J Prosthet Dent 1985;54:705.

141. Carlsson GE, Kopp S, Wedel A. Analysis of background variables in 350 patients with TMJ disorders as reported in self-administered questionnaire. Community Dent Oral Epidemiol 1982;10:47.

142. Schokker RP, Hansson TL, Ansink BJJ. Craniomandibular disorders in patients with different types of headache. J Craniomandib Disord Facial Oral Pain 1990;4:47.

143. Nevakari K. "Elapsio praearticularis" of temporomandibular joint: a pantomographic study of the so-called physiological subluxation. Acta Odontol Scand 1960;18:123.

144. Egermark-Eriksson I, Ingervall B, Carlsson GE. The dependence of mandib-

ular dysfunction in children on functional and morphologic malocclusion. Am J Orthod 1983;83:187.

145. Molin C, Carlsson GE, Friling B, Hedergard B. Frequency of symptoms of mandibular dysfunction in young Swedish men. J Oral Rehabil 1976;3:9.

146. Nilner M. Epidemiology of functional disturbances and diseases in the stomatognathic system. Swed Dent J 1983;17(suppl):1.

147. Gale EN, Gross A. An evaluation of temporomandibular joint sounds. J Am Dent Assoc 1985;111:62.

148. Wabeke KB, Hansson TL, Hoogstraten J, Van der Kuy P. Temporomandibular joint clicking: a literature overview. J Craniomandib Disord Facial Oral Pain 1989;3:163.

149. Pullinger AG, Monteiro AA. Functional impairment in TMJ patients and non-patient groups according to a disability index and symptom profile. J Craniomandib Pract 1988;6:156.

150. Droukas B, Lindee C, Carlsson GE. Relationship between occlusal factors and signs and symptoms of mandibular dysfunction: a clinical study of 48 dental students. Acta Odontol Scand 1984;42:277.

150a. Ingervall B, Hedegard B. Subjective evaluation of functional disturbances of the masticatory system in young Swedish men. Community Dent Oral Epidemiol 1974;2:149–152.

151. Al-Hadi LA. Prevalence of temporomandibular disorders in relation to some occlusal parameters. J Prosthet Dent 1993;70:345.

152. Bush FM, Butler JH, Abbott DM. The relationship of TMJ clicking to palpable facial pain. J Craniomandib Pract 1983;1:43.

153. Shiau YY, Chang C. An epidemiological study of temporomandibular disorders in university students of Taiwan. Community Dent Oral Epidemiol 1992;20:43.

154. Weinberg LA, Lager LA. Clinical report on the etiology and diagnosis of TMJ dysfunction-pain-syndrome. J Prosthet Dent 1980;44:642.

155. Markowitz HG, Gerry RG. Statistical evaluation of temporomandibular disease. Oral Surg Oral Med Oral Pathol 1949;2:1307.

156. Rieder CE, Martinoff JT, Wilcox SA. The prevalence of mandibular dysfunction: sex and age distribution of related signs and symptoms. J Prosthet Dent 1983;50(pt 1):81.

157. Gross AJ, Rivera-Morales WC, Gale EN. A prevalence study of symptoms associated with TM disorders. J Craniomandib Disord Facial Oral Pain 1988; 2:191.

158. Rieder CE. The incidence of some occlusal habits and headaches/neckaches in an initial survey population. J Prosthet Dent 1976;35:445.

159. Rosenbaum M. The feasibility of a screening procedure regarding temporomandibular joint dysfunction. Oral Surg Oral Med Oral Pathol 1975;39:382.

160. Rieder CE, Martinoff JT. The prevalence of mandibular dysfunction: a multiphasic dysfunction profile. J Prosthet Dent 1983;50(pt 2):237.

161. Vincent SD, Lilly GE. Incidence and characterization of temporomandibular joint sounds in adults. J Am Dent Assoc 1988;116:203.

162. Pöllmann L. Sounds produced by the mandibular joint in young men. J Maxillofac Surg 1980;8:155.

163. Perry HT. The symptomatology of temporomandibular joint disturbance. J Prosthet Dent 1968;19:288.

164. Cooper BC, Alleva M, Cooper DL, Lucente FE. Myofascial pain dysfunction: an analysis of 476 patients. Laryngoscope 1986;96:1099.

165. Gelb H, Calderone JP, Gross SM, Kantor ME. The role of the the dentist and the otolaryngologist in evaluating temporomandibular joint syndromes. J Prosthet Dent 1967;18:497.

166. Bush FM, Whitehill JM, Martelli MF. Pain assessment in temporomandibular disorders. J Craniomandib Pract 1989;7:137.

167. Zarb GA, Thompson GW. Assessment of clinical treatment of patients with temporomandibular joint dysfunction. J Prosthet Dent 1970;24:542.

168. Carraro J, Caffesse R, Albano E. Temporomandibular joint syndrome. Oral Surg Oral Med Oral Pathol 1969;28:54.

169. Helöe B, Helöe LA. Characteristics of a group of patients with temporomandibular joint disorders. Community Dent Oral Epidemiol 1975;3:72.

170. Abbott DM, Bush FM, Butler JH, Gunsolley JC. Clinical signs as differentiating predictors of temporomandibular disorders (TMD). J Dent Res 1991; 70(special issue):329. Abstract 509.

171. Hodges JM. Managing temporomandibular joint syndrome. Laryngoscope 1990;100:60.

172. Blasberg B, Chambers A. Temporomandibular pain and dysfunction syndrome associated with generalized musculoskeletal pain: a retrospective study. J Rheumatol 1989;19(suppl 16):87.

173. Rothwell PS. Symptoms of temporomandibular pain dysfunction in 400 patients: time to revise the classic profile? J Dent 1987;15:6.

174. Werndahl L, Seeman L, Carlsson GE. Treatment of patients with TMJ pain and dysfunction. Tandlakartidn 1971;63:560.

175. Helkimo M, Ingervall B. Recording of the retruded position of the mandible in patients with mandibular dysfunction. Acta Odontol Scand 1977;36:167.

176. Rubinstein R, Axelsson A, Carlsson GE. Prevalence of signs and symptoms of craniomandibular disorders in tinnitus patients. J Craniomandib Disord Facial Oral Pain 1990;4:186.

177. Koidis PT, Zarifi A, Grigoriadou E, Garefis P. Effect of age and sex on craniomandibular disorders. J Prosthet Dent 1993;69:93.

178. Agerberg G, Helkimo M. Stomatology of patients referred for mandibular dysfunction: evaluation of a questionnaire. J Craniomandib Pract 1987;5:157.

179. Bush FM, Harkins SW, Harrington WH. Does gender influence symptom presentation in a heterogeneous population of orofacial pain patients? J Dent Res 1991;70(special issue):371. Abstract 845.

180. Isacsson G, Linde C, Isberg A. Subjective symptoms in patients with temporomandibular joint disk displacement versus patients with myogenic craniomandibular disorders. J Prosthet Dent 1989;61:70.

181. Helöe B, Heiberg AN, Krogstad BS. A multiprofessional study of patients with myofascial pain-dysfunction syndrome. Acta Odontol Scand 1980;38(pt 1):109.

182. Harkins SW, Kwentus J, Price DD. Pain and suffering in the elderly. In Bonica J (ed). Management of pain. Philadelphia: Lea & Febiger, 1990:552.

183. Helöe B. Comparison between two groups of patients with TMJ disorder. Community Dent Oral Epidemiol 1979;7:117.

184. Sola AE, Rodenberger ML, Getty BB. Incidence of hypersensitive areas in posterior shoulder muscles. Am J Phys Med Rehabil 1955;34:585.

185. Mejersjö C, Carlsson GE. Long-term results of treatment for temporomandibular joint-pain dysfunction. J Prosthet Dent 1983;49:809.

186. De Kanter RJ, Truin GJ, Burgerdijk RC, Van't Hof MA, Battistuzzi PG, Kalesbeek H, Kayser AF. Prevalence in the Dutch population and a meta-analysis of signs and symptoms of the temporomandibular disorder. J Dent Res 1993;72:1509.

187. Rieder CE. Comparison of the efficacy of a questionnaire, oral history, and clinical examination in detecting signs and symptoms of occlusal and temporomandibular joint dysfunction. J Prosthet Dent 1977;38:433.

The Temporomandibular Joint and Related Orofacial Disorders,
by Francis M. Bush and M. Franklin Dolwick.
J.B. Lippincott Company, Philadelphia, © 1995.

6

Screening

Auniversally accepted diagnostic scheme is needed to manage patients with TM disorders appropriately. Although no scheme has acquired universal acceptance, a general sequence has been proposed that appears useful (Table 6-1). Its goals are lofty—improved decision making and reduced diagnostic failures.[1]

The sequence includes a screening of the patient's general health history. The history gives the clinician an overview of the patient's health and experience in the health care delivery system. The clinician also gains insight into the patient's attitudes about health service and other medical personnel involved in the treatment.[2] This history can be initiated with a self-administered checklist followed by a clinical interview.

After a review of the patient's general health, the clinician should screen for signs and symptoms of TMD. This screening can be initiated with the special questionnaires shown in Figures 6-1 through 6-5. Unfortunately, few assessment instruments involving TMD have been validated. One that has been validated is the Orofacial Pain Symptom Checklist,[3] which was modified from a commonly employed instrument used to evaluate TMD.[4] Many questions from this instrument are included in the questionnaires in this chapter. This self-report instrument assesses specific symptoms that are not biased by psychological disturbance. It has good test-retest reliability for measuring several symptoms and ought to be useful for evaluating treatment outcome. Questionnaire items are divided into four indices: joint movement (JM), parafunction (PI), circumoral complaints surrounding the cheeks and temples (CO), and painful symptoms (PSI). The pain symptom index proved most informative about the disability of the patient.

Additional questionnaires here have been modified from the Registration Questionnaire used in the Temporomandibular Joint and Orofacial Pain Research Center of the Medical College of Virginia Commonwealth University, which opened around 1973.[3,5,6] Questions about pain and emotional suffering as assessed by Visual Analogue Scales (VAS) were drawn from selected publications.[7] The VAS is a 100-mm horizontal line representing a pain or suffering continuum. At one end of the line are the words "No sensation" and at the other end "Worst sensation imaginable."

Table 6-1
Proposed Diagnostic Sequence
for Management of Patients

Identification of perceived abnormality
Initial triage
Gathering of data
Specific tests
Radiography
Comparison of discovery data versus classic signs and symptoms
 of disease
Tentative estimates of probable diagnosis
Acquisition of other data as needed
Refinement of working diagnosis
Tailoring plan of treatment to diagnosis

Modified from Krutchkoff DJ. The clinical diagnostic process: a prerequisite
to excellence in practice. J Am Dent Assoc 1993;124:122.

Patients are instructed to mark the line at the point that corresponds to their perceived amount of sensation. The mark is translated to a numerical value from 0 to 100. The level of sensation or emotion can be judged before and after treatment to measure treatment outcome.

Caveat: Although other instruments can be chosen to assess pain, the high rate of variability over time in reporting of pain among TMD cases may rule against implications for clinical practice.[8] Only pain of the masticatory muscles on palpation has been correlated with report of pain intensity among TMD patients.[9] No significant relation was found between pain intensity and clicking, between pain intensity and range of mandibular motion or between pain intensity and tooth grinding.

Another instrument for assessment is the TMJ Scale, which is available on a fee-for-service basis from Pain Resource Center Inc. (Durham, NC). This inventory recognizes the multidimensional etiology of TMD. Its 10 subscales are organized into a global domain that represents the single best predictor for the presence of TMD. A physical domain assesses joint dysfunction, self-report, and palpation of pain, and a psychosocial domain judges psychological disturbance. Preliminary studies show content validity, test-retest reliability, and some measure of specificity-sensitivity.[10]

Most clinicians agree that screening should be done for psychological disorders because emotional factors impact greatly on the course of TMD. Some may wonder if one self-reported psychological questionnaire is better than another. This issue has been settled to some degree. A comparison of questionnaires responded to by TMD patients revealed important correlations between seven depression scales and between four anxiety tests.[11] Because little difference in reliability was found, the single-question depression and anxiety instrument has been selected (see Fig. 6-4). If more information is needed about the "distress" status of the patient, the clinician can choose from many other questionnaires.

(text continues on p. 229)

LOCATION AND KIND OF PAIN
Do you have pain in, around, or for any of the following?

Yes No

—— —— Ears
—— —— Cheeks
—— —— Temples
—— —— Forehead
—— —— Nose
—— —— Teeth
—— —— Gums
—— —— Neck
—— —— Causing frequent headache
—— —— Causing frequent eyeache
—— —— During yawning or talking
—— —— During sleeping
—— —— Interfering with daily activities
—— —— Interfering with appetite
—— —— Other areas not listed

Date your pain began: Year _____ Month _____

Mark the areas on the diagrams below where you feel painful sensations. Use the following symbols:

Pricking/Burning	Dull Aching	Sharp/Stabbing
xxxx	0000	////
Throbbing	Pressure	Other (specify)
****	====	++++

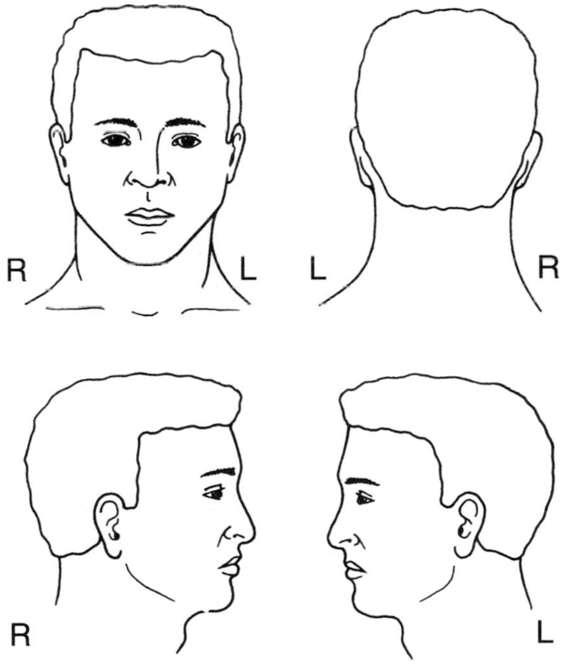

Figure 6-1.
Questionnaire regarding location and kind of pain involved with the current problem, including a diagram of areas of painful sensation to be marked by the patient.

(continued)

Where does your pain occur? Circle the number which best fits your problem.
1. Right side only
2. Mostly on the right side
3. Both sides equally
4. Mostly on the left side
5. Left side only

What is the degree of your suffering?
Check along the line below (with an X) the *intensity* of sensation at your usual level of pain.

	Most Sensation
No Sensation _____	Imaginable

Check along the line below (with an X) the *discomfort* (bothersome, unpleasantness) at your *usual* level of pain.

	Most Discomfort
Not Unpleasant _____	Imaginable

Figure 6-1. *(Continued)*

POSSIBLE CAUSES OF PAIN
Check any of the following circumstances that may be related to onset of your pain: 1 = most likely, 2 = second most likely, and 3 = third most likely.
__ Pain just began
__ Accident (eg, whiplash)
__ Psychological stress
__ Dental treatment
__ Oral habits
__ Following surgery
__ Following illness
__ Other not listed

Circle any of the following factors that may affect your pain: 1 = decreases pain, 2 = little change, 3 = increases pain.

1	2	3	Caffeinated drinks (cola, tea, chocolate)
1	2	3	Alcohol-containing drinks
1	2	3	Monosodium glutamate (MSG)
1	2	3	Onions, garlic
1	2	3	Spicy food
1	2	3	Nitrites (bacon, hot dogs, ham)
1	2	3	Bright lights
1	2	3	Loud noise
1	2	3	Weather changes (dampness)
1	2	3	Massage
1	2	3	Pressure
1	2	3	Mild exercise
1	2	3	Staying still
1	2	3	Fatigue
1	2	3	Menstruation
1	2	3	Sexual intercourse
1	2	3	Urination, defecation
1	2	3	Tension on the job or home
1	2	3	Others not listed (specify: _____)

Figure 6-2.
Questionnaire about possible causes of pain and stimuli affecting the problem.

PHYSICAL SYMPTOMS
Do you have jaw problems with any of the following?

Yes   No

—   —   Opening your mouth wide
—   —   Moving your jaw from side to side
—   —   Your jaw deviating to the side on opening
—   —   Clicking in the joint during movement
—   —   Popping in the joint during movement
—   —   Grating (grinding) in the joint during movement
—   —   Fatigue, tightness, or stiffness
—   —   Numbness
—   —   Arthritis in the joint
—   —   Trauma to your joint

Do you have neck problems with any of the following?

Yes   No

—   —   Injury
—   —   Pain
—   —   Hurt when turning or bending head
—   —   Noises on movement
—   —   Neck gets stuck in one position
—   —   Numbness
—   —   Disturbs your sleep

Do any of these occlusal activities cause you difficulty?

Yes   No

—   —   Chewing hard foods hurts your teeth
—   —   Bite feels uncomfortable
—   —   Teeth "don't fit together"
—   —   Teeth feel loose
—   —   Teeth are wearing down
—   —   Clamping (clenching) your teeth
—   —   Shifting of your teeth
—   —   Teeth are sensitive to cold
—   —   Teeth are sensitive to hot

Figure 6-3.
Questionnaire about problems associated with the jaws, neck, and occlusion.

EMOTIONAL STATUS
Check along each of the lines below (with an X) the intensity of FEELING as it relates to your usual level of pain.

None   Most Severe
                                         Immaginable

Depression   ————————————
Anxiety   ————————————
Frustration ————————————
Anger   ————————————
Fear   ————————————

Circle any of the numbers that best fits your current problem.
How depressed are you?
Never   Often
        0   1   2   3   4
Do you consider yourself more calm than tense?
Calm   Tense
        0   1   2   3   4

Figure 6-4.
Questionnaire regarding the emotional status of the problem. Price DD, McGrath PA, Rafii A, Buckingham B, The validation of visual analog scales as ratio measures for chronic and experimental pain, Pain 1983;17:45, and Gale EN, Dixon DC, A simplified psychologic questionnaire as a treatment planning aid for patients with temporomandibular joint disorders, J Prosthet Dent 1989;61:235).

HEALTH CARE PROVIDERS AND TREATMENT

Have you seen any of the following health care providers for your problem?

Yes	No	
—	—	General dentist
—	—	Oral Surgeon
—	—	Orthodontist
—	—	Periodontist
—	—	Endodontist
—	—	Prosthodontist (dentures, bridges)
—	—	General physician
—	—	Otolaryngologist (ear, nose, throat)
—	—	Neurologist
—	—	Internist
—	—	Psychiatrist
—	—	Clinical psychologist
—	—	Chiropractor
—	—	Physical therapist
—	—	Occupational therapist
—	—	Radiologist
—	—	Others not listed (specify: _____)

Circle one of the following numbers for any treatment that you actually received for your current problem: 1 = complete improvement, 2 = little change, 3 = worse.

1	2	3	Dental restorations (removal)
1	2	3	Dental restorations (fixed)
1	2	3	Dental extraction
1	2	3	Endodontic (root canal) therapy
1	2	3	Dental occlusal adjustment
1	2	3	Dental oral appliance (splints, guards)
1	2	3	Orthodontics
1	2	3	Orthognathic surgery
1	2	3	Periodontal surgery
1	2	3	TMJ surgery
1	2	3	Ultrasound
1	2	3	Transelectric nerve stimulation (TENS)
1	2	3	Muscle stimulation
1	2	3	Massage therapy (myofascial release)
1	2	3	Heat
1	2	3	Cold
1	2	3	Vapocoolant spray
1	2	3	Nerve/muscle injection
1	2	3	Joint injection
1	2	3	Psychotherapy (counseling)
1	2	3	Hypnotherapy
1	2	3	Relaxation therapy
1	2	3	Biofeedback
1	2	3	Acupuncture, acupressure
1	2	3	Radiation therapy
1	2	3	Hospitalization
1	2	3	Others not listed (specify: _____)

Figure 6-5.

Questionnaire about health care providers and kinds of treatment related to problem.

(continued)

Circle one of the following numbers for any medications that you have taken for your current problem: 1 = decreased problem, 2 = little change, 3 = increased problem.

1	2	3	Analgesics (eg, aspirin, ibuprofen)
1	2	3	Narcotics (eg, codeine)
1	2	3	Minor Tranquilizers (eg, Valium)
1	2	3	Major Tranquilizers (eg, Thorazine)
1	2	3	Antidepressants (eg, amitriptyline)
1	2	3	Barbiturate/hypnotics (eg, Nembutal)
1	2	3	Stimulants/antihistamines (eg, Antivert)
1	2	3	Antiseizure (eg, Tegretol)
1	2	3	Antimigraine (eg, Cafergot)
1	2	3	Antiarthritics (eg, cortisone)
1	2	3	Antibiotics (eg, penicillin)
1	2	3	Others not listed (specify: _____)

Figure 6-5. *(Continued)*

Initial Contact

The initial contact should help the patient feel cared about and inspire a sense of trust in high-quality practice.[12] Whether the appointment administrator greets the patient in person or by phone, the meeting should be cordial and concerned with the details of the appointment. Specific questions should include the following:

1. How may I help you?
2. May I ask you some questions about your appointment or your visit?
3. Whom may we thank for referring you?

Additional information about the patient's problem can be obtained from a self-administered questionnaire. The necessary form can be mailed to the patient and completed before examination. The questionnaire should be accompanied by an appointment card, a map, and a letter discussing the details of patient registration.

The appointment administrator should greet new patients by name and introduce him or herself. The introduction should be done while standing. The administrator asks for completed forms and requests that the patient complete any other forms. The staff should assist with completion of these forms, particularly if insurance is involved. The appointment administrator should review the forms for completeness and notify the assistant that the patient has arrived.

Symptom History

A questionnaire allows patients to organize their thoughts and to gather data about prior diagnosis and treatment. Its completion saves time that the clinician can devote to interviewing and examining the patient. The clinician should pay particular attention to the regions the patient marks as painful on the anatomic diagrams (see Fig. 6-1).

The Interview

After the clinician reviews the questionnaire, he or she should discuss the data with the patient. This discourse is crucial because reliance on data obtained from health questionnaires has proved inadequate for assessing the problems of some patients. In a study of 415 dental patients, 15% of the vital information about health status obtained in the interview was not documented in the questionnaire.[13]

Nature of the Complaint

Notes from an interview should be recorded on a separate sheet of paper. The interview should focus on the patient's complaint and on correcting myths or misinformation about the problem. The interviewer should explain reasons for asking questions. Patients speak more freely if they understand a question's purpose. Most appreciate the opportunity to talk about their problem.

The interviewer should provide good eye contact and perhaps physical contact if the patient is tense. Although patients may have visited other doctors in search of a solution to their problems, they may not have received a diagnosis or may not have understood what the doctor told them; therefore, the interviewer should talk in terms the patient can understand and should listen carefully to the patient. If the clinician has any doubts about the patient's comprehension of a statement, he or she should ask the patient to repeat what was said.

The clinician should direct the course of the interview, which should flow without interruption. Along with the symptom checklist, communication should be guided towards a history of the patient's problem. Care should be made not to judge the patient as the problem. Clinicians should avoid forming early opinions or having a critical attitude about their own assumptions.[2] They should listen attentively, particularly for "hidden questions." The clinician must not allow the patient to dominate the conversation for longer than five minutes without interruption. Although the patient in pain may exhibit anger or hostility, the clinician should exhibit neither. The patients' true concerns should be answered.

Remember that the goals are to identify the chief complaint, reconstruct the circumstances that led to its onset, and determine any factors that may have modified the problem (see Fig. 6-3). Achieving these goals is not easy. Patients often have diffuse symptoms and may have difficulty locating the site of the complaint.

Leading questions should include the following:

1. What is your chief complaint?
2. Has your condition changed within the past 24 hours?
3. Can you tell me the time of onset?
4. Can you place a finger on a specific location that bothers you?
5. Where else does it hurt?
6. How has the complaint affected your daily activities?
7. Have any of your doctors diagnosed your condition?

Dialogue about associated pains and miscellaneous symptoms should occur. Some complaints may represent disorders other than TMD and may compromise success in treatment. These include aching in the teeth, sinuses, ears, head, or neck.

Significance: The chief subjective features of TMD should be kept in mind: dull aching pain in or around the jaw and ear that may become sharp or throbbing during function.[14] Pain with the jaw at rest should signal the clinician that the problem probably originates from another source. *Caveat:* Complaints of numbness or swelling should be heeded because of potential involvement with neoplasia.

Patients may complain of nuisances such as ill-fitting eyeglasses, shape or color of teeth, or facial changes associated with aging. These complaints usually have little effect on the outcome of the current problem and should be referred appropriately.

Etiology

The interview offers an opportunity to discuss possible etiologies of the complaint. Events in the history such as oral habits, physical trauma, or whiplash should be discussed, and details of their occurrence should be documented (see Fig. 6-2).

Significance: As a general rule, subtle events play little role in current complaints.

Social Interactions and Psychological Needs

Some clinicians feel uncomfortable discussing the patient's social history or psychological needs. The social history encompasses work, relationships, and play.[14] If the solo practitioner believes that the patient's complaints arise from social or psychological imbalance and does not want to deal with them, the patient should be referred appropriately. In a multidisciplinary setting, these matters can be managed by a clinical psychologist.

Key features of social interaction may be determined from the questionnaire. A "yes" response for the interference of pain with daily activities[3] or for the depression and anxiety subscales[11] probably signals pending problems. Avoidance of social activities, work, and parenting and interruptions in healthful sleep patterns are powerful indicators of problems that require decisions.

Significance: Unless a major event has occurred recently, most social or psychological factors can be ruled out as affecting the current problem.

Medications

Discussion about the use of medication is necessary. Specific questions provide the clinician with some understanding of the severity of problem, drug interactions, and potential abuse. The clinician who discovers a patient with a history of many different kinds of medications or with long-standing use of pain relief medication should obtain a satisfactory reason from the patient and documentation from their doctors about past and present needs.

Significance: Successful management may require medication. Some patients may be overmedicated, whereas others who refuse may be helped by it.

Other Treatments, Insurance, and Costs

To assess outcome, details of previous treatments should be reviewed. Treatments such as physical therapy, oral appliances, or joint surgery may be viewed by the patient as worthless for various reasons. Many patients will not wear an ill-fitting oral appliance. Massage therapy to the jaw for a disorder arising in the neck is another example. The patient may have negative feelings about the results of surgery of the TMJ, even though it may be judged successful by surgical standards.

Often, health care providers are confronted by unwanted dialogue about insurance coverage or excessive costs of previous treatment. Such matters must be resolved expeditiously. Questions about insurance should be directed to the administrator in charge of coverage. Consideration about prior fees or treatment from another clinician should be approached cautiously. A financial agreement between the patient and another clinician should be resolved between those parties. Patients must be informed of the current status of their oral health, but disparaging remarks by a clinician about a patient's prior services is unethical (see the 1992 American Dental Association's *Ethics and Code of Professional Conduct*).[15]

Significance: The review of questionnaire data and interview about prior health care are time-consuming activities. Clinicians should educate themselves to accept payment for time spent in this manner, and patients should pay accordingly.[2]

References

1. Krutchkoff DJ. The clinical diagnostic process: a prerequisite to excellence in practice. J Am Dent Assoc 1993;124:122.
2. Helöe B. Clinical examination of patients with orofacial pain. Endodontics and Dental Traumatology (Copenhagen) 1988;4:139.
3. Harkins SW, Bush FM, Price DD, Hamer RM. Symptom report in orofacial pain patients: relation to chronic pain, experimental pain, illness behavior, and personality. Clin J Pain 1991;7:102.
4. Solberg WK. Occlusion-related pathosis and its clinical evaluation. In Clark JW (ed). Clinical dentistry, vol 2. Philadelphia: Harper & Row 1985;35:1.
5. Bush FM, Whitehill JM, Martelli M. Pain assessment in temporomandibular disorders. J Craniomandib Pract 1989;7:137.
6. Harkins SW, Price DD, Bush FM, Small R. Geriatric pain. In Wall PD, Melzack R. Textbook of pain. Edinburgh: Churchill-Livingstone 1984;42:769.
7. Price DD, McGrath PA, Rafii A, Buckingham B. The validation of visual analog scales as ratio measures for chronic and experimental pain. Pain 1983;17:45.
8. Raphael KG, Marbach JJ. A year of chronic TMPDS: evaluating patients' pain patterns. J Am Dent Assoc 1992;123:53.

9. Raphael KG, Marbach JJ. A year of chronic TMPDS: relating patient symptoms and pain intensity. J Am Dent Assoc 1992;123:49.

10. Levitt SR, McKinney MW, Lundeen TF. The TMJ scale: cross-validation and reliability studies. J Craniomandib Pract 1988;6:17.

11. Gale EN, Dixon DC. A simplified psychologic questionnaire as a treatment planning aid for patients with temporomandibular joint disorders. J Prosthet Dent 1989;61:235.

12. Pride J. New patient examination and consultation: providing the initial contact. J Am Dent Assoc 1992;123:80.

13. Fenlon MR, McCartan BE. Validity of a patient self-completed health questionnaire in a primary care dental practice. Community Dent Oral Epidemiol 1992;20:130.

14. Solberg WK. Temporomandibular disorders: physical tests in diagnosis. Br Dent J 1986;160:273.

15. American Dental Association. ADA principles of ethics and professional conduct. Chicago: American Dental Association, 1992.

The Temporomandibular Joint and Related Orofacial Disorders,
by Francis M. Bush and M. Franklin Dolwick.
J.B. Lippincott Company, Philadelphia, © 1995.

7

Basic Examination

The goal of the basic examination is to provide the clinician with valid indices to avoid erroneous conclusions. The validity of present measures for diagnosing or evaluating treatment outcome in TMD patients is open to question. Arguments for and against the validity of some items are reviewed in the publications listed in this chapter's References and in Chapter 5. Issues surrounding the validity of specific signs and symptoms of TMD may never be resolved.

Content validity has been shown in some studies because the measures used to assess signs and symptoms have proven to be reliable indicators of the disorder. Construct validity has been proved by comparing certain measures of patients with different diagnoses against healthy individuals matched for age and gender. Criterion validity has been supported by findings of significant correlations between disparate samples of patients examined with different indices. Because of uncertainty about the validity of some measures, the measures adopted here are those currently used by practitioners around the world.

Several objective tests aid in the differential diagnosis of TMD from mimicking disorders. The examination measures described here have been obtained from many sources, including the Virginia Commonwealth University Pain Questionnaire and Examination Form developed in 1974, the Helkimo Index,[1] modified forms of W.K. Solberg,[2–4] the guidelines for examination and diagnosis of TMD,[5] the Craniomandibular Index,[6,7] the Clinical Diagnostic Criteria for TMD,[8] and Cranio-Cervical Dysfunction Criteria.[9,10] The suggested guidelines for clinical normality versus TMJ abnormality[11] have been incorporated into the examination measures. Other measures have evolved from general observations drawn from clinical experience.

These measures are divided into seven parts (Table 7-1). The first four measures usually supply the most reliable information about the status of the TMJs. To rule out mimicking disorders, collateral measures are described for other head and neck disorders (Table 7-2).

Table 7-1
Physical Tests for Examination of Masticatory Muscles, TMJs, and Occlusion

Range of Motion

Pain free opening
Active range of motion (AROM)
Passive range of motion (PROM) or passive stretch opening
Restriction on opening
Deviation on opening

TMJ Function

Anterior–posterior movement
Lateral movement
Joint sounds
Diagnostic manipulation

Muscle Palpation for Tenderness

Masticatory muscles

TMJ Palpation for Tenderness

Lateral surface
Superior surface
Dorsal surface—external auditory meatus

Loading Tests

Resistance tests
Unilateral bitestick
Intercuspal clenching and bilateral bitestick

Elevator Muscle Function

Closure—clench
Masseter function

Occlusal Analysis

Intercuspal contacts
Retruded contact position (RCP) to intercuspal position (IP)
Gross occlusal interferences
Dental wear

*Modified from Solberg WK. Temporomandibular disorders: data collection and examination. Br Dent J 1986;160:317–322.

Facial Appearance

Initially, the examiner should observe the patient's overall facial form. The condition of the eyes, ears, skin, and lips should be noted. Although most asymmetry of the face and head is of developmental origin, recent evidence of swelling, hypertrophy, or lesions may be related to systemic or neoplastic conditions that mimic TMD symptoms.

Range of Jaw Motion

The patient is asked to **"open as wide as you can."** The following measures are determined.

Table 7-2
Evaluation of Dental Condition, Swallowing, Sinuses,
Salivary Glands, and Lymph Nodes

Dental Condition

Visual inspection
Exploration
Percussion
Mobility
Thermal sensitivity
Vitality testing
Transillumination
Bitesticks
Probing
Palpation

Swallowing

Sinuses

Palpation
Transillumination

Salivary Glands

Palpation

Lymph Nodes

Palpation

Cranial Nerves

Sensory testing
Motor testing

Active range of motion (AROM) is the opening under voluntary effort. AROM is tested by measuring the opening between the upper central incisors and lower central incisors with a millimeter ruler or Boley gauge as the patient opens fully (Fig. 7-1). Data are recorded (Table 7–3).

Restricted opening is judged at 35 mm or less for men and 30 mm or less for women. These values allow for differences in physical stature and vertical overlap of the anterior teeth. For further reliability, the examiner may measure the difference between the alveolar crests. From extrapolation of interincisal distance, measurement at the alveolar crests would establish limits at 39 mm or less for men and 34 mm or less for women.

Pain-free opening involves stretching of the mandible in an inferior direction to the greatest extent possible without report of pain. A sensation of facial pressure or tightness by the patient can be excluded from the record. The presence of pain should be considered abnormal.[11]

  Significance: Monitoring the range of motion provides insight about the status of pain and mandibular mobility caused by joint or muscular problems. The patient's progress can be judged by comparing initial measurements with measurements made during the course of treatment.

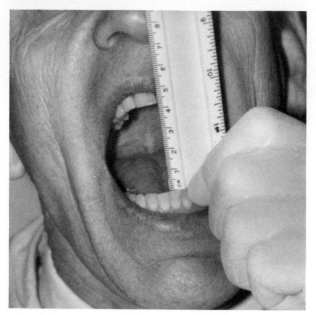

Figure 7-1.
Measurement of voluntary opening is made between the maxillary and mandibular central incisors as the patient opens fully.

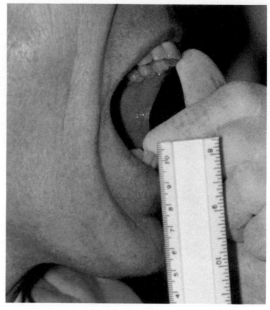

Figure 7-2.
Measurement of passive range of opening is made between the maxillary and mandibular central incisors as the examiner pushes downward on the patient's mandible.

Restriction, or hypomobility, may represent either joint or muscle disorder. Excessive movement, or hypermobility, usually represents joint laxity related to instability of the capsular attachment and disk–condyle relation. Hypermobility should be considered normal, unless there is a history of joint locking in the open position or there is pain or discomfort that prevents normal function during wide opening.[11]

Passive range of motion (PROM) or passive stretch opening is determined as the examiner pushes gently downward on the patient's mandible (Fig. 7-2). Usually the opening is increased by an average of 2 mm. The PROM is positive if the opening is 37 mm or less for men and 32 mm or less for women (see Table 7-3). Measurements made between the alveolar crests are positive at 41 mm or less for men and 36 mm or less for women.

    Significance: If AROM is painful and PROM is not, the problem is probably muscle related. An increased opening or "springy" feeling detected by the examiner suggests muscular restriction. A "hard" feeling suggests adhesion, arthrosis, or possible contracture.

Lateral deviation is measured at the midline as the patient opens the mouth fully and then closes the teeth together. If the deviation is more than 2 mm, it should be considered positive (see Table 7-3).

Table 7-3
Measurements for Range of Mandibular Motion

Maximum opening (maxillary central incisor to mandibular central
 incisor): _____ mm (mean range for most individuals = 40–60)
Passive stretch opening: _____ mm (mean range = 42–62)
Lateral deviation on opening or closing: right _____ mm;
 left _____ mm (>2)
Pain on opening: _____ positive; _____ negative

Significance: The absence of deviation should be considered normal. Unilateral deviation indicates an inability to translate the condyle properly from the restricted side. Reduced tenderness on palpation suggests a disk disorder or adhesion. A repeatable deviation from straight opening that has been present for many years and is unrelated to other symptoms should be regarded as compensatory and, therefore, clinically normal.[11]

TMJ Function

The patient is asked to **"move the lower jaw as far as possible in a forward direction."**

Anterior–posterior movement is measured as the patient moves the mandible from the intercuspal position to full protrusion. The measurement is made at the diastema between the labial surfaces of the maxillary incisors and the diastema between the labial surfaces of the mandibular incisors. Unless the incisors are end-to-end at the intercuspal position, the measurement is considered positive if less than 7 mm (Table 7-4). The presence of pain should be noted.

The patient is asked to **"move the lower jaw as far as possible to the left and then to the right".**

Laterotrusion involves movement to each side. This measurement is made at the diastema between the maxillary central incisors to the diastema between the mandibular central incisors as the patient extends the mandible fully to the right and then to the left (Fig. 7-3). If the diastemata differ at the intercuspal position, a correction is made in the final measurement. The measurement should be considered positive if less than 7 mm to each side. This horizontal movement should be symmetrical to be considered normal. The presence of pain should be noted.

Joint sounds are assessed by palpation, listening, and asking the patient. The patient is asked to **"open as wide as possible"** and then to **"move the lower jaw from side to side as far as possible."** To be judged positive, sounds should be audible to the patient and the examiner, and the uncoordinated disk movement should be palpable by the examiner. Uncoordinated disk movement is determined by palpating across the joint capsule during unrestricted opening and closing movements. If doubt exists, further palpation is done by inserting the little finger into the patient's auditory

Table 7-4

Tests for TMJ Function

Anterior–posterior movement _____ (<7 mm)

	Right		Left	
	Pos.	*Neg.*	*Pos.*	*Neg.*
Laterotrusion (<7mm)	___	___	___	___
Reciprocal click (eliminated with repositioning)	___	___	___	___
Reproducible opening click	___	___	___	___
Reproducible laterotrusive click	___	___	___	___
Reproducible closing click	___	___	___	___
Nonreproducible opening click	___	___	___	___
Crepitus (fine)	___	___	___	___
Crepitus (coarse)	___	___	___	___
Popping (audible without stethoscope)	___	___	___	___
Locked open	___	___	___	___
Locked closed	___	___	___	___
Diagnostic reduction	___	___	___	___

meatus. Additional testing can be done by asking the patient to **"chew gum or wax."** The location of sounds is related to the position of the jaw during the respective movements.

For clicking to be judged as *reciprocal*, the noise must be reproducible on opening and closing, starting from full intercuspation and extending to full opening. *Reproducible* clicks may exist exclusively during opening, laterotrusion, or closing. Some are nonrepeatable; they are considered *nonreproducible* clicks. *Fine crepitus* is a weakly perceived grating sound suggestive of mild bone-on-bone contact. *Coarse crepitus* is a strongly perceived grating sound suggestive of gross bone-on-bone contact. *Popping* is a loud sound detected on opening that is audible to the examiner without the aid of a stethoscope.

Significance: Joint sounds indicate disk disorders. Crepitus implies degeneration of the disk and usually signifies osteoarthrosis. Multiple clicks during opening indicate perforation of the disk or changes in joint form. Reciprocal clicking means the disk is displaced anteriorly, especially if the mandible shifts near full closure. Clicks associated with painful chewing or intermittent locking are the most bothersome. These clicks and soft crepitation should be considered abnormal, unless they have shown no change in characteristics for at least 5 years and they do not bother the patient or interfere with function.[11]

Diagnostic or *reductive manipulation* is a means of distracting the patient's condyle. The patient is asked to **"bite on a cork"** on the symptomatic side for 5 minutes. The cork is removed, and the examiner pushes the mandible inferiorly and posteriorly with one hand at the level of the molars and simultaneously raises the

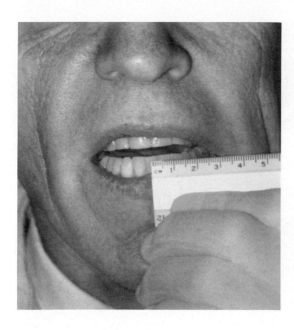

Figure 7-3.
Measurement of laterotrusion is made from the diastema of the maxillary central incisors to the diastema of the mandibular central incisors as the patient moves as far laterally as possible to each side.

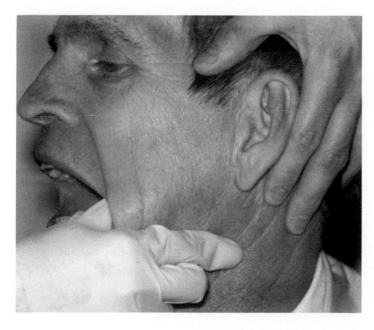

Figure 7-4.
Diagnostic manipulation of the mandible. The examiner grasps the mandible.

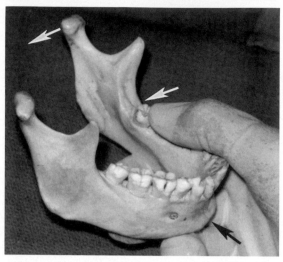

Figure 7-5.
The examiner applies pressure inferiorly in the molar area and superiorly at the chin.

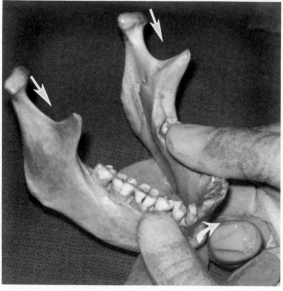

Figure 7-6.
As the patient protrudes the mandible, the examiner distracts it laterally.

chin with the other hand (Fig. 7-4). The patient is asked to "**move the mandible forward and then to the opposite side**" as the examiner distracts the mandible (Figs. 7-5 and 7-6). If the distraction is of recent origin, the force necessary to accomplish disk reduction is minimal.

Significance: This test has diagnostic and treatment value. It identifies acute locking of the joint. Typically, the patient reports with a history of clicking and sudden loss of clicking. After successful manipulation, the AROM should increase immediately to within normal limits.

Masticatory Muscle Palpation

The procedures for muscle palpation have been documented.[12] For the extraoral masticatory muscles, pressure is applied bimanually with the examiner's index and middle fingers. The recommended amount of pressure is 2 lb/in^2, a level that proved useful for examination of these muscles in another study.[8] The amount of pressure can be determined with a pressure algometer or by simulation after practicing palpation on a postal scale with the index finger.

The patient is asked, "**Is there any difference between the two sides?**" If the answer is yes, the patient is asked, "**Does it hurt or is it just uncomfortable?**"

The degree of severity is graded at 0 (no pain), 1 (mild pain), 2 (moderate pain), or 3 (severe pain), based on the patient's verbal and nonverbal responses to the pressure. Severity applies to tenderness involving bodily withdrawal or eye-wincing responses. The examiner follows the routine for palpation described below and in Table 7-5.

In palpation of the *masseter*, both the superficial head and the deep head originate from the zygomatic arch and have fibers inserting on the ramus of the mandible (Figs. 7-7). The superficial head lies more anteriorly; it is easily palpated when the patient is asked to "**clench the teeth.**" The deep head lies posteriorly and is palpated in the depression about 10 mm anterior to the tragus.

The *temporalis* is located along the side of the head and can be elevated by asking the patient to "**clench the teeth**" (Fig. 7-8). Anterior fibers are palpated as they originate on the lateral surface of the skull and insert on the coronoid process and anterior border of the mandible. Middle and posterior fibers are palpated by asking the patient to "**close on the back teeth and pull the mandible backward.**"

The *digastric* region is palpated by pressing the little finger upward parallel to the ramus of the mandible (Fig. 7-9). The muscle originates from the mastoid notch and is joined at the hyoid bone by a tendinous sheath. Palpation of the posterior fibers of the digastric muscle is more appropriately designated palpation of the *stylohyoid* region because the examiner is unsure of what is being palpated.

The insertion of the *medial pterygoid* near the inferior angle of the mandible allows extraoral palpation. An index finger placed below the angle is pushed slightly upward

Table 7-5

Palpation of Masticatory Muscles and TMJ

Region	Right		Left	
	Pos.	*Neg.*	*Pos.*	*Neg.*
Extraoral Jaw				
Superficial masseter	___	___	___	___
Deep masseter	___	___	___	___
Anterior temporal	___	___	___	___
Middle temporal	___	___	___	___
Posterior temporal	___	___	___	___
Posterior digastric	___	___	___	___
Medial pterygoid	___	___	___	___
Intraoral Jaw				
Insertion temporal	___	___	___	___
Pterygoid complex	___	___	___	___
TMJ				
Lateral capsule	___	___	___	___
Posterior capsule	___	___	___	___
Superior capsule	___	___	___	___

Severity scale: 0 = no pain, 1 = mild pain, 2 = moderate pain, 3 = severe pain.

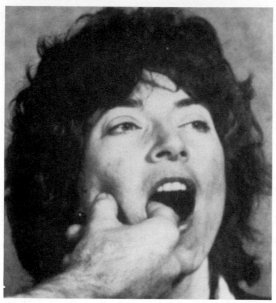

Figure 7-7.
Intraoral and extraoral palpation of the masseter muscle. (Abbott DM, Bush FM, Butler JH. Principles of occlusion, 3rd ed. Chapel Hill, NC: Health Sciences Consortium, 1980.)

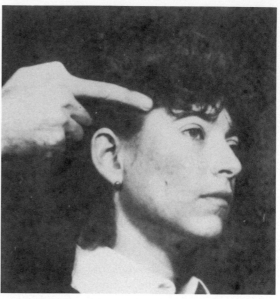

Figure 7-8.
Palpation of the temporalis muscle. (Abbott DM, Bush FM, Butler JH. Principles of occlusion, 3rd ed. Chapel Hill, NC: Health Sciences Consortium, 1980.)

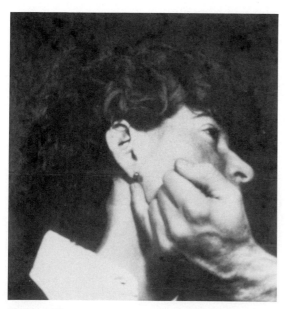

Figure 7-9.
Palpation of the digastric muscle. (Abbott DM, Bush FM, Butler JH. Principles of occlusion, 3rd ed. Chapel Hill, NC: Health Sciences Consortium, 1980.)

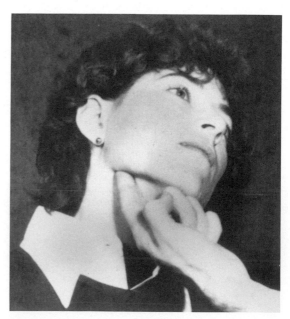

Figure 7-10.
Palpation of the medial pterygoid muscle. (Abbott DM, Bush FM, Butler JH. Principles of occlusion, 3rd ed. Chapel Hill, NC: Health Sciences Consortium, 1980.)

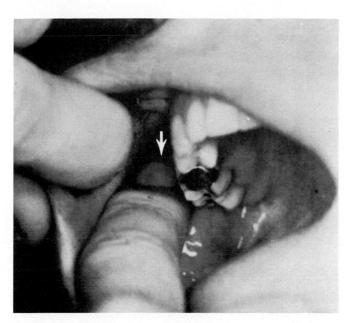

Figure 7-11.
Palpation of the temporalis tendon region.
Pressure is applied upward in the vestibule
(arrow; Abbott DM, Bush FM, Butler JH.
Principles of occlusion, 3rd ed. Chapel Hill, NC:
Health Sciences Consortium, 1980.)

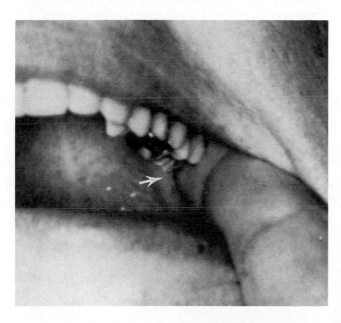

Figure 7-12.
Palpation of the pterygoid region. Pressure is applied
upward and inward (arrow; Abbott DM, Bush FM,
Butler JH. Principles of occlusion, 3rd ed. Chapel
Hill, NC: Health Sciences Consortium, 1980.)

and medially (Fig. 7-10). Simultaneous intraoral palpation is done by placing the other index finger in the retromyohyoid fossa on the same side. Because of overlap with other muscles in this region, the palpation should be designated palpation of the *suprahyoid* region.

In palpation of the *temporalis tendon*, the patient is asked to **"open the mouth."** The index finger is pushed posterosuperiorly into the upper vestibule lateral to the maxillary tuberosity (Fig. 7-11). The finger is moved along the coronoid process.

In palpating the *pterygoids*, the index finger is placed in the upper vestibule at a 45° angle to the sagittal plane (Fig. 7-12). The finger is moved distally to the tuberosity, and pressure is applied in a downward and medial direction toward the tongue. Because the heads of the lateral and medial pterygoids originate near one another at the pterygoid plates, the region should be designated the *pterygoid* region.

    Significance: Although there is a tendency to overinterpret findings of widespread tenderness, the referral pattern of pain elicited by palpation should be outlined. This mapping adds credence to the diagnosis of palpable trigger points producing localized and referred pain. The presence of numerous tender muscles may be used to augment a diagnosis of myofascial pain exclusive of true joint pain or to confirm a diagnosis of simultaneous joint-related and muscle-related disorders.

TMJ Palpation

The patient is asked to **"open slightly."** Pressure of 2 lbs/in^2 is applied bimanually with the index fingers along the lateral poles of the condyles (Fig. 7-13). A similar amount of pressure is applied to the superior surface along the fossae. The finger is moved toward the ear to palpate the posterior capsule. Tenderness of the meatus is detected by placing the little finger in the auditory meatus and pulling forward with slight pressure (Fig. 7-14).

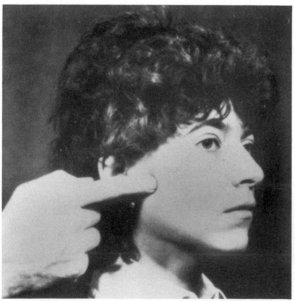

Figure 7-13.
Palpation of the lateral pole of the condyle. (Abbott DM, Bush FM, Butler JH. Principles of occlusion, 3rd ed. Chapel Hill, NC: Health Sciences Consortium, 1980.)

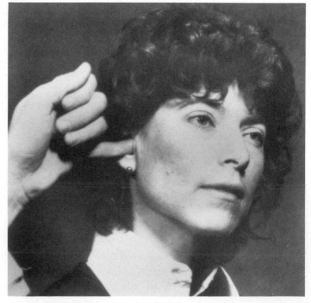

Figure 7-14.
Palpation of the condyle by means of the external auditory meatus. (Abbott DM, Bush FM, Butler JH. Principles of occlusion, 3rd ed. Chapel Hill, NC: Health Sciences Consortium, 1980.)

Significance: Without associated tenderness of the masticatory muscles, tenderness in the joint identifies inflammation. A check should be made for swelling and temperature change, which augment a diagnosis of true joint pathology.

Craniocervical Evaluation

Because the relation between TMD symptoms and craniocervical symptoms is unclear, craniocervical status should be evaluated along with symptoms of TMD.

The range of motion for the neck is tested following movement (Table 7-6). The patient is asked to perform a series of neck and head exercises while standing in an upright position. The minimal limits for normal ranges of motion given here are accepted from published standards.[10,13] The limits accepted for impairment are described in degrees as the patient moves as far as possible in each direction.

Flexion is recorded as the patient is asked to **"touch the chin to the chest,"** starting with the head held in a vertical, neutral position (0°). The examiner judges the limitation from a sagittal position (Fig. 7-15). The minimum for acceptable normal motion is 60°. At less than 60°, there is impairment.

Extension is recorded as the patient is asked to **"move the top of the head backward"** from the neutral position. Judgment is made from a sagittal position (see Fig. 7-15). The minimum for normal motion is 75°. For both flexion and extension, the patient should be able to move a minimum of 135° (60° + 75°).

Rotation is recorded as the patient is asked to **"turn the nose toward the right and then toward the left shoulder."** Judgment is made from a superior or anterior position (Fig. 7-16). The minimum for normal motion is 80° in each direction or 160° to the right and then to the left.

Table 7-6
Physical Tests for Craniocervical Function*

Activity	Normal	Impaired	Comment
Flexion	____	____ (<60°)	_____
Extension	____	____ (<75°)	_____
Rotation	____	____ (<80°)	_____
Side bending	____	____ (<45°)	_____
Cervical sounds	____	____	_____
Cervical tenderness	____	____	_____
Bony process palpation	____	____	_____
Craniocervical posture	____	____	_____
Neurosensory changes	____	____	_____

Modified from Clark GT. Examining temporomandibular disorder patients for craniocervical dysfunction. J Craniomand Pract 1984;2:55–63. Craniocervical limits for health and impairment are borrowed with permission from American Medical Association. AMA guides to evaluation of permanent impairment, 3rd ed. Chicago: AMA, 1990.

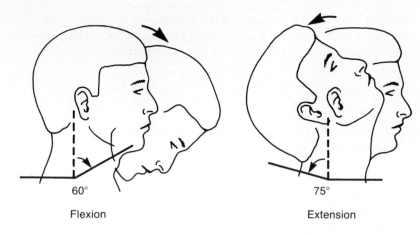

Figure 7-15.
Test for flexion–extension of the neck with neutral position at center. (Modified from Guides to evaluation of permanent impairment, 3rd rev ed. Copyright 1990, American Medical Association, Chicago, IL.)

60° Flexion

75° Extension

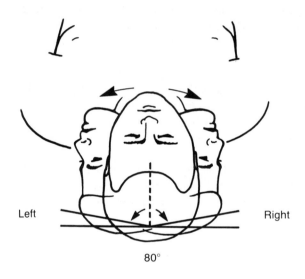

Figure 7-16.
Test for rotation of the neck with neutral position at center and after left and right movements. (Modified from Guides to the evaluation of permanent impairment, (3rd rev ed. Copyright 1990, American Medical Association, Chicago, IL.)

Left   Right

80°

Side-bending or *lateral flexion* is recorded as the patient is asked to **"tilt the side of the head toward the right and then to the left shoulder"** (Fig. 7-17). The minimum for normal motion is 45° in each direction or 90° to the right and left.

Cervical sounds are recorded if the noise can be reproduced by movement. The patient is asked to **"turn the head to each side."** If noise is present, the location, type (eg, clicking, popping, or crepitus), and degree of associated discomfort are recorded.

Cervical tenderness is checked bilaterally with index finger pressure of about 7 lbs/in^2, a level that proved useful in one study.[10] This level can be judged from palpation with a pressure algometer or by simulating the pressure after practicing palpation on a postal scale. Palpation should include the anterior, lateral, and posterior cervical regions (Table 7-7). Muscles are palpated from origin to insertion.

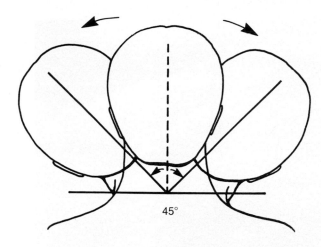

45°

Figure 7-17.
Test for lateral flexion of the neck with neutral position at center and after left and right movements. (Modified from Guides to the evaluation of permanent impairment, 3rd rev ed. Copyright 1990, American Medical Association, Chicago, IL.)

1. The *anterior cervical region* includes the clavicular and sternal parts of the sternocleidomastoid (SCM) and longus colli muscles (Fig. 7-18). The patient is asked **"to rotate the head to each side."** Each SCM is palpated on the side opposite the direction that the nose is turned. The longus colli muscle is palpated by moving the thyroid cartilage medially and palpating deeply toward the cervical spine.
2. The *lateral cervical region* includes the scalenus (Fig. 7-19), the upper part of the levator scapulae, and the splenius capitis. The scalenus passes posterior to the SCM, and fibers radiate in an superoinferior direction. Palpation extends to the transverse process of the cervical spine at the level of the first and second

Table 7-7
Palpation of Muscle and Bony Regions of the Neck

| | Right | | Left | |
Region	Pos.	Neg.	Pos.	Neg.
Anterior Cervical				
Sternocleidomastoid	——	——	——	——
Longus colli	——	——	——	——
Lateral Cervical				
Scalenus	——	——	——	——
Levator scapula	——	——	——	——
Splenius capitis	——	——	——	——
Posterior Cervical				
Trapezius	——	——		
Vertebral				
Cervical vertebra 1	——	——		
Cervical vertebra 2	——	——		
Cervical vertebra 3	——	——		
Cervical vertebra 4	——	——		
Cervical vertebra 5	——	——		
Cervical vertebra 6	——	——		
Cervical vertebra 7	——	——		
Thoracic vertebra 1	——	——		

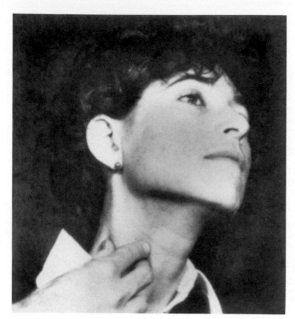

Figure 7-18.
Palpation of the sternocleidomastoid muscle.

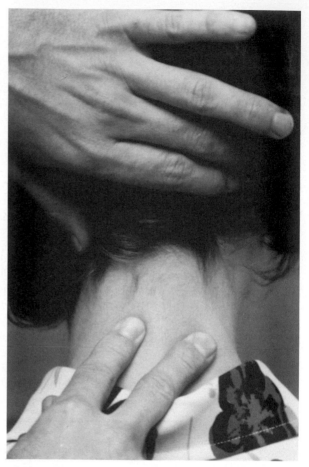

Figure 7-19.
Palpation of the lateral cervical region.

ribs. The splenius capitis and the levator scapulae are palpated by pressing posterosuperiorly from the scalenus muscle.

3. The *posterior cervical region* includes the lower part of the levator scapulae and the upper trapezius. These muscles are palpated from the acromion process to its origin in the base of the skull and the lateral cervical spine (Fig. 7-20).

Vertebral processes are palpated from the lateral process of the first cervical vertebra and extending through the second thoracic vertebra. The lateral processes of the first cervical vertebra are palpated anterior to the mastoid process and toward the distal part of the mandible.

Craniocervical posture is evaluated from sagittal, anterior, and posterior directions to the clinician. Postural deviations such as forward or posterior head position, unequal shoulder height, and scoliosis are recorded.

Neurosensory changes include areas of numbness, tingling, or pronounced sensitivity. They are palpated to confirm location, pattern of radiation, and intensity in the neck, shoulder, arm, hands, and fingers.

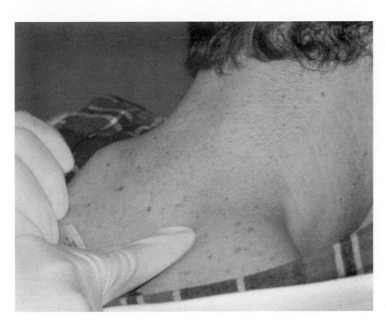

Figure 7-20.
Palpation of the upper part of the trapezius muscle.

Significance: Overt mechanical problems in the neck and shoulder girdle compromise successful treatment of TMD complaints.

Loading Tests

Placement of the mandible under a load may aid in deciding whether the complaint originates from the masticatory muscles or from the TMJs (Table 7-8). This testing is not recommended for routine screening purposes.

In *resistance testing*, the patient is asked to **"open the width of an index finger."** The examiner supports the patient's head with one hand and pulls the mandible inferiorly with the other hand. The patient is asked to **"resist the pull"** (Fig. 7-21). If pain develops at the site of the initial complaint, a positive response is recorded.

Significance: Complaints correlated with resistance most likely involve the muscles responsible for jaw opening, if no joint movement occurs. This test has less value for the interpretation of referred pain.

Bitestick testing is done to put the masticatory muscles and TMJs under load. For testing of muscles, the bitestick is placed between the molars on the ipsilateral, symptomatic side. The patient is asked to **"close firmly against it."** This action may produce pain within the elevator muscles. If the pain is ameliorated, the lateral pterygoid muscle may be involved. For testing of TMJs, closure against the bitestick on the asymptomatic side aggravates the pain on the contralateral side (Fig. 7-22). Ipsilateral biting relieves the pain.

Significance: To differentiate joint pain from muscle pain, bitestick testing must be supplemented with findings of palpable tenderness and with the patient's report of the pain site.

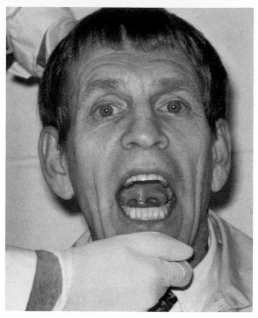

Figure 7-21.
Resistance test for status of jaw-opening muscles.

Table 7-8
Resistance, Bitestick, and Elevator Muscle Tests

Test	Pos.	Neg.
Resistance	——	——
Bitestick (muscle)	——	——
Bitestick (TMJ)	——	——
Closure—clench	——	——
Masseter function	——	——

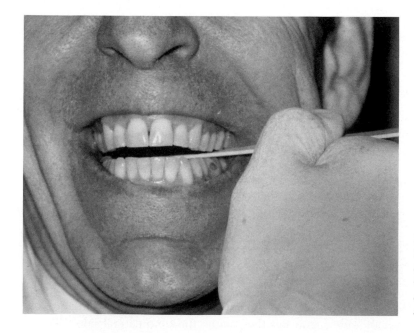

Figure 7-22.
Bitestick test on left side. TMJ pain is confirmed if relief occurs on the ipsilateral side. Biting on the contralateral side causes pain in the symptomatic joint.

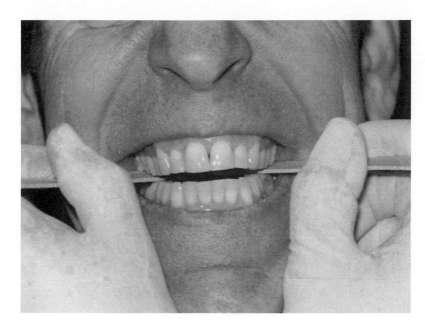

Figure 7-23.
Test for elevator muscle function.

Elevator Muscle Function

In tests of the *closure–clench* function, individuals with healthy jaw mechanics should be able to close the teeth to a stable jaw position. For this test, the patient is asked to **"clench the teeth hard for 60 seconds."** Clenching at maximal intercuspation may provoke fatigue or painful contraction of the symptomatic elevator muscles (see Table 7-8).

To test *masseter function*, the patient is asked to **"close the teeth against tongue depressors"** placed bilaterally between the molars (Fig. 7-23). The pressure may ameliorate the pain.

Significance: These tests may aid in diagnosis of pain of the elevator muscles. The findings are compared with palpation data and the patient's identification of the painful site to confirm the diagnosis.

Occlusal Analysis

No definitive relation has been established between occlusion and TMD symptoms. Logic dictates that patients should have a stable jaw position at maximal intercuspation and be free of major cuspal interferences during excursive jaw movements. Dental wear and fractures should be assessed to determine the effect on occlusal stability.[12] This information is recorded on the occlusal findings form (Table 7-9).

Intercuspal Position

The teeth should be checked for firmness of contact at full intercuspation. The firmness is checked with occlusal registration strips or with thin articulating paper.

Table 7-9
The Occlusal Findings Form

Position	Tooth															
Intercuspal	1	2	3	4	5	6	7	8	9	10	11	12	13	14	15	16
	32	31	30	29	28	17	26	25	24	23	22	21	20	19	18	17
Retruded	1	2	3	4	5	6	7	8	9	10	11	12	13	14	15	16
	32	31	30	29	28	27	26	25	24	23	22	21	20	19	18	17
Lateral R	1	2	3	4	5	6	7	8	9	10	11	12	13	14	15	16
	32	31	30	29	28	27	26	25	24	23	22	21	20	19	18	17
Lateral L	1	2	3	4	5	6	7	8	9	10	11	12	13	14	15	16
	32	31	30	29	28	27	26	25	24	23	22	21	20	19	18	17
Protruded	1	2	3	4	5	6	7	8	9	10	11	12	13	14	15	16
	32	31	30	29	28	27	26	25	24	23	22	21	20	19	18	17
Wear	1	2	3	4	5	6	7	8	9	10	11	12	13	14	15	16
	32	31	30	29	28	27	26	25	24	23	22	21	20	19	18	17

Retruded contact position to intercuspal position slide

Right _____ mm   Forward _____ mm
Left _____ mm   Upward _____ mm

Modified from Bush FM, Abbott DM, Butler JH. Occlusal adjustment of natural dentition. In Hardin JF (ed). Clark's clinical dentistry. Philadelphia: JB Lippincott, 1988:40:1.

Gross Occlusal Interferences

Gross interferences are identified with the strips or with paper. If found to deflect the mandible significantly during opening or closing or during excursive movements, they are charted.

Dental Wear

Excessive dental wear as indicated by thinned or crazed enamel of the anterior teeth and wear facets or cupping of the molars are charted.

Movement Between Retruded Contact Position and Intercuspal Position

The "slide" or movement between retruded contact position and intercuspal position is negligible in most dentitions. If this movement is more than 2 mm in lateral, anterior–posterior, and inferior–superior directions, the finding may be important enough to chart.

Significance: Examination of the occlusion may provide insight into certain complaints. Recurrent tooth fractures and bruxism are reflective of the overall health of the masticatory system. Parafunctional habits contribute to deterioration of the dentition and may compromise function of the masticatory muscles and TMJs.

Diagnostic Blocking and Analgesic Spraying

Blocking or analgesic spraying with vapocoolant agents may help determine whether the pain complaint is of dental/osseous origin or from another source. Before blocking is attempted, the pattern of pain referral needs to be evaluated. For osseous/dental pathology, this pattern can be traced from published figures.[14,15] The patient is asked to **"point to the painful area."** The examiner marks the area on the appropriate figure (Figs. 7-24 through 7-29). Checks along the referral zone may confirm the site of the pathology.

There are several contraindications to the blocking of stellate ganglia, myofascial trigger points, and occipital nerves. Each requires expertise beyond the training of the general practitioner and is usually performed by an anesthesiologist or neurolo-

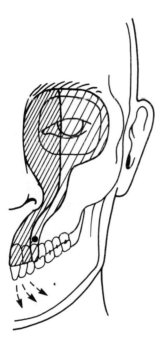

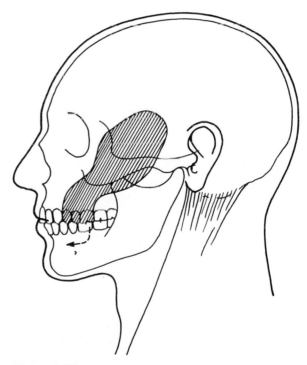

Figure 7-24.
Pain distribution pattern for pathosis associated with the maxillary anterior teeth. The major path for incisors extends to the supraorbital rim. The small black dot over the left canine shows the location of pathosis. The shaded area indicates the upward pattern of referred pain. The dotted arrow line represents pain distributions of lesser frequency or intensity. (Ratner EG, Person P, Kleinman DJ, Shklar G, Socransky SS. Jawbone cavities and trigeminal and atypical facial neuralgias. Oral Surg Oral Med Oral Pathol 1979;48:3.)

Figure 7-25.
Pain distribution pattern for pathosis associated with maxillary premolar and first molar teeth. The major path terminates diffusely in the temporal region. A minor referral pattern extends to the mandibular canine region. (Ratner EG, Person P, Kleinman DJ, Shklar G, Socransky SS. Jawbone cavities and trigeminal and atypical facial neuralgias. Oral Surg Oral Med Oral Pathol 1979;48:3.)

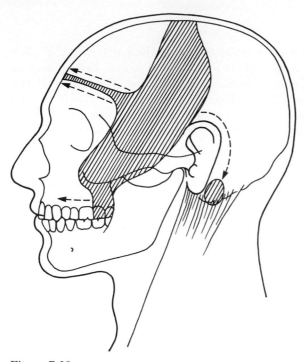

Figure 7-26.
Pain distribution pattern for pathosis associated with maxillary second and third molar teeth. The major path extends along the zygoma to the vertex. Minor referral areas include the front of the skull, the postauricular and canine areas, and possibly the anteriolateral surface of the tongue. (Ratner EG, Person P, Kleinman DJ, Shklar G, Socransky SS. Jawbone cavities and trigeminal and atypical facial neuralgias. Oral Surg Oral Med Oral Pathol 1979;48:3.)

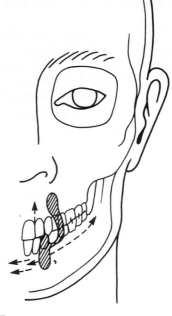

Figure 7-27.
Pain distribution pattern for pathosis associated with mandibular anterior teeth. The major path for incisors includes the opposing maxillary incisors. A minor referral pattern may occur horizontally across the midline. The major path for the canine terminates in the maxillary first premolar region. Minor referral may extend along the entire mandible on the same side. (Ratner EG, Person P, Kleinman DJ, Shklar G, Socransky SS. Jawbone cavities and trigeminal and atypical facial neuralgias. Oral Surg Oral Med Oral Pathol 1979;48:3.)

gist. Still, the generalist should be familiar with each to discuss their use with the patient and the referral clinician (Table 7-10).

Dental Blocks

After the patient localizes the painful site, the examiner can mark an X on the appropriate figure and follow the distribution pattern of referral (see Figs. 7-24 through 7-29). The maxillary zones to be blocked are the anterior superior alveolar, middle superior alveolar, and posterior superior alveolar zones. The mandibular zones to be blocked are the inferior alveolar and long buccal zones.

Injection with 3% mepivacaine is recommended because of the short duration of action. Because some mandibular gingiva or mucosa may not become totally numb, direct infiltration into these alternate hypersensitive zones may be necessary to obtain "full terminus."[15]

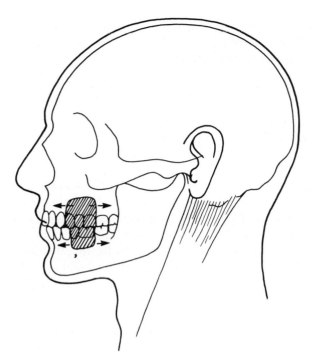

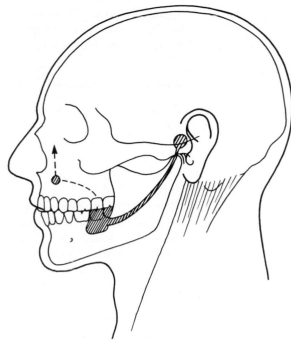

Figure 7-28.
Pain distribution pattern for pathosis associated with mandibular premolar and first molar teeth. The major paths extend vertically to the opposing maxillary teeth. Horizontal components vary in frequency of occurrence and extent of referral. (Ratner EG, Person P, Kleinman DJ, Shklar G, Socransky SS. Jawbone cavities and trigeminal and atypical facial neuralgias. Oral Surg Oral Med Oral Pathol 1979;48:3.)

Figure 7-29.
Pain distribution pattern for pathosis associated with mandibular second and third molar teeth. The main path extends to the temporomandibular joint. Pain is rarely referred to opposing teeth. A minor component may extend to the maxillary anterior region, if both dental and bony pathosis exist. (Ratner EG, Person P, Kleinman DJ, Shklar G, Socransky SS. Jawbone cavities and trigeminal and atypical facial neuralgias. Oral Surg Oral Med Oral Pathol 1979;48:3.)

Table 7-10

Diagnostic Analgesic Blocking and Spraying of Tissues

Dental blocks
Vapocoolant sprays
Myofascial trigger point blocks
Auriculotemporal nerve block
Stellate ganglion block
Occipital nerve block

Significance: If localized and referred pain are eliminated by zone blocking, tooth or bone pain is confirmed. If the referred pain persists after dental blocking to "full terminus," another source should be suspected.

Vapocoolant Sprays

Perception of painful impulses is negated by application of these sprays. The sprays act as counter irritants and promote local anesthesia. Examples include fluoromethane and ethyl chloride. *Caveat:* ethyl chloride is highly flammable.

Usually sprays are used before analgesic blocking. Application should be explained to the patient before use. A short burst of mist is applied to the patient's forearm to demonstrate the product. For spraying the TMJs, the patient's eyes are covered and external auditory meatus blocked (Fig. 7-30). The mist is directed at a 45° angle to the surface to be sprayed. It should be moved frequently to avoid frosting the skin. After application, the patient is asked to **"open as wide as possible"** and then to **"move the mandible to each side as far as possible."** Measurements are made as the patient opens fully and then moves to the right and to the left.

Significance: The benefits of vapocoolant sprays include relief of muscle splinting, improvement in voluntary opening, and confirmation of locked TMJs. If improvement of more than 2 mm occurs in maximal opening and lateral movements, the problem is most likely muscle related. If little to no improvement occurs, the problem is most likely joint related.

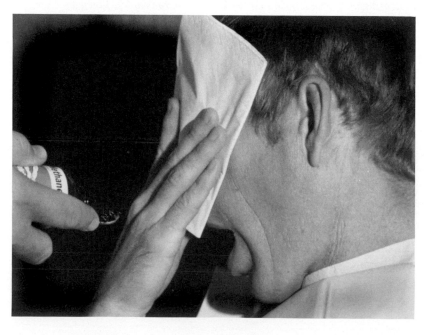

Figure 7-30.
Application of vapocoolant spray to test for voluntary opening. The spray is moved continually along the TMJ area to avoid frosting the skin.

Myofascial Trigger Point Blocks

Muscles difficult to palpate are typically chosen for injection. These include the deep head of the masseter and the lateral and medial pterygoids. The recommended anesthetic is 1% procaine without epinephrine.

Techniques for the injection of different muscles, including the masseter, temporalis, lateral and medial pterygoids, are described in Figures 7-31 through 7-34.[16,17]

Significance: Local injection may relieve pain from specific groups of muscles. Repetitive injections into different groups is unwarranted. Acute inflammatory reaction and muscle necrosis occur after injection, and regeneration requires up to 45 days.[18] Persistent soreness may result.

Auriculotemporal Nerve Block

Blocking of the auriculotemporal nerve may reveal if the pain is totally within the joint. A technique for injection has been described.[19] The examiner palpates the head and neck of the condyle. Ethyl chloride is sprayed on the site to achieve surface

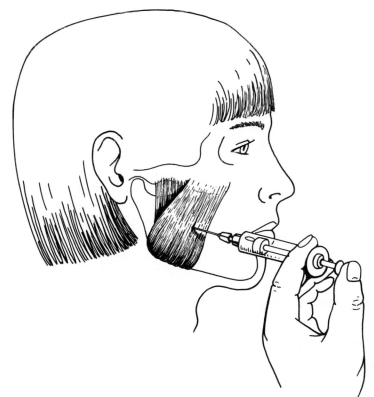

Figure 7-31.
Injection of the masseter muscle. The needle pierces the midbody and passes at several angles to reach both deep and superficial layers of muscle. After aspiration of each layer, the anesthetic solution is injected as the needle is withdrawn. (Alling CC III, Mahan PE. Facial pain, 2nd ed. Philadelphia: Lea & Febiger, 1977.)

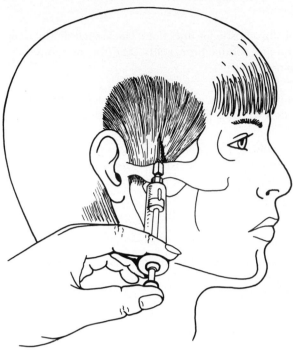

Figure 7-32.
Injection of the temporalis muscle. After aspiration at each point (X) above the zygoma, the anesthetic solution is delivered slowly. (Alling CC III, Mahan PE. Facial pain, 2nd ed. Philadelphia: Lea & Febiger, 1977.)

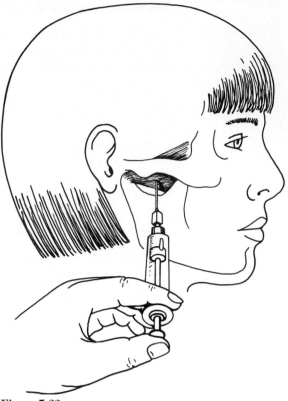

Figure 7-33.
Injection of the lateral pterygoid muscle. The needle enters across the sigmoid notch and is directed upward and inward to about 35 to 40 mm. After aspiration, the anesthetic solution is slowly deposited. (Alling CC III, Mahan PE. Facial pain, 2nd ed. Philadelphia: Lea & Febiger, 1977.)

anesthesia. A dental aspirating syringe with a long needle is used to deliver 0.2 mL of 2% lidocaine with 1:100,000 epinephrine subcutaneously at the junction of the tragus and lobule (Fig. 7-35). Without infiltration, the needle is pushed through the parotid gland 1 cm anterior and medial to the posterior surface of the condylar neck. The remaining anesthetic is injected at this site. Analgesia occurs within 5 minutes and lasts up to 1.5 hours.

Significance: Abolition of pain confirms joint derangement.

Stellate (Cervicothoracic) Ganglion Block

Stellate ganglion blocking may confirm that the orofacial pain is mediated by afferent sympathetic fibers. The stellate ganglion is formed by fusion of the inferior cervical and first thoracic ganglia.

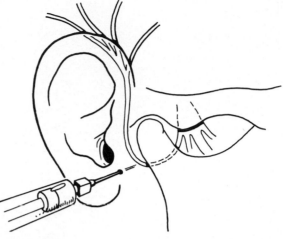

Figure 7-35.
Injection of the auriculotemporal nerve. The anesthetic solution is injected posterior to the neck of the condyle. (Donlon WC, Truta MP, Eversole LR. A modified auriculotemporal nerve block for regional anesthesia of the temporomandibular joint. J Oral Maxillofac Surg 1984;42:544.)

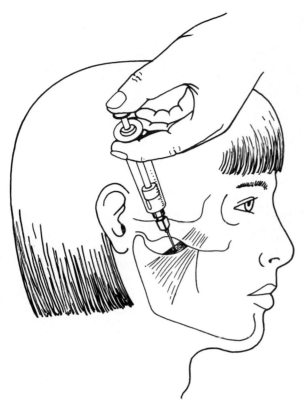

Figure 7-34.
Injection of the medial pterygoid muscle. The needle enters across the sigmoid notch and is directed downward and inward to about 40 mm. After aspiration, the anesthetic solution is slowly deposited. (Alling CC III, Mahan PE. Facial pain, 2nd ed. Philadelphia: Lea & Febiger, 1977.)

A modification of the original technique has been described.[20] The lateral surface of the cricoid cartilage is the site of delivery (Fig. 7-36). The needle is positioned in a vertical–dorsal direction to a depth of 2 to 3.5 cm. until the transverse process of C6 is located. It is then withdrawn about 2 mm, followed by aspiration, and 5 mL of 1% mepivacaine is injected (Fig. 7-37).

Significance: Sympathetic fibers are known vasoconstrictors. Blocking of the ganglion enhances dilation and increases circulation to the head. Pain of vascular origin in the trigeminal complex is arrested by blocking. Because autonomic changes have been observed in cases of reflex sympathetic dystrophy, the pain of this disorder and similarly related burning pains may be relieved.

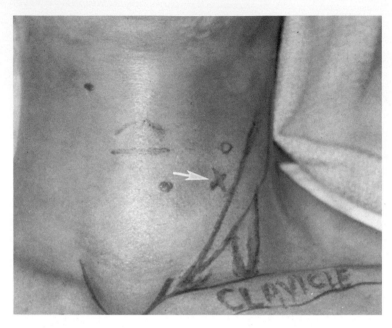

Figure 7-36.
Arrow indicates the injection site (X) for the stellate ganglion block. (Courtesy of Robert Campbell, Virginia Commonwealth University, Richmond, VA.)

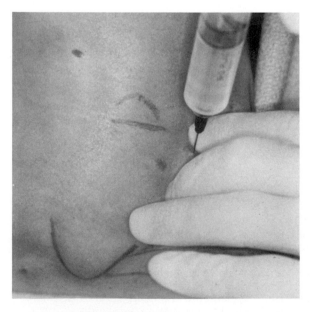

Figure 7-37.
Delivery of anesthetic solution for the stellate ganglion block. (Courtesy of Robert Campbell, Virginia Commonwealth University, Richmond, VA.)

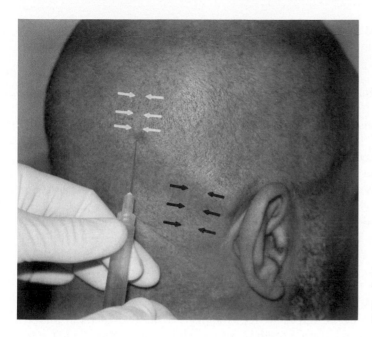

Figure 7-38.
White arrows indicate the injection site for the greater occipital nerve. Dark arrows indicate the injection site for lesser occipital nerve.

Occipital Nerve Block

Blocking the occipital nerve may relieve neuralgia caused by degenerative changes in the upper cervical nerves or by muscular tension. Simultaneous injection of myofascial trigger points may improve outcome.

Needle entry for the occipitalis major nerve is made 3 cm laterally from the occipital protuberance (Fig. 7-38) of the linea nuchae.[17] The occipitalis minor nerve is located posterosuperiorly to the mastoid process and 2.5 cm lateral from this site. Two to 10 mL of 1% mepivacaine is injected once the needle tip strikes bone.

Significance: Abolition of occipital pain may distinguish the complaint from TMD pain.

Collateral Examination

Dental Condition

Because some TMD-like symptoms overlap dental symptoms, the dentition and related soft and hard tissues should be checked for pathology. Significant findings are recorded in the progress notes.

Visual inspection should follow the same routine from patient to patient (see Table 7-2). Missing, broken, and carious teeth and the distribution of plaque should be documented.

Exploration of pits and fissures with an explorer may detect caries. Insertion of the explorer is at a 90° angle with the occlusal surface. Resistance on withdrawal indicates possible caries.

Bursts of air into occlusal sulci or the apical third of the tooth may trigger pain. Rubbing the explorer tip along the gingival third of the tooth may cause wincing or withdrawal. Usually this implies cemental hypersensitivity.

Percussion testing is accomplished by tapping on the teeth with a mirror handle. The patient is asked, **"Is the tapping painful?"** The occlusion sounds clear if the teeth are healthy and dull if unhealthy. Painful response to tapping needs further evaluation.

Mobility testing is done by pushing against the facial surface of the teeth lingually with the blunt end of a mirror handle and bracing the lingual surface with the tip of another mirror handle. The degree of mobility is graded: 0, no mobility; 1, mobility = 1 mm horizontal; 2, mobility = 2mm horizontal; 3, mobility = 1 mm vertical, direction, respectively.

Thermal sensitivity should be checked. Ice is applied to individual teeth under a rubber dam if the response between teeth is questionable. Application of a hot gutta-percha point to a moistened tooth may evoke pain. Positive response confirms pulpal inflammation.

Vitality testing with an electric pulp tester should be done on teeth for which pathology is suspected. The tooth is isolated under a rubber dam or with cotton rolls and then air dried. Toothpaste is used to make contact between the tip of the electrode and the gingival third of the tooth free of restoration. No contact must occur with the gingiva. The patient is asked to **"raise the hand once the sensation occurs."** Testing requires an adequate control. An unrestored, similar tooth of the contralateral side can be used. Positive or negative responses are recorded.

Transillumination can be used to check for caries. If the fiberoptic light is of sufficient intensity, apical pathology may be detected.

Bitesticks may be useful for identification of fractured teeth. Placement of a narrow tip of the stick on specific cusps and asking the patient to **"close the teeth together"** may elicit the pain. Visual inspection or exploration with the explorer tip may reveal the fracture.

Probing of the periodontium is done to record sulcular depth and pattern of bone loss. Three recordings—mesiobuccal, midbuccal, and distolingual–are made around each tooth. Sulcular depths greater than 4 mm require further evaluation.

Palpation of the gingiva, tongue, and other oral soft tissues must be done carefully. Any anatomic landmark viewed suspiciously needs to be compressed with an index finger or between the fingers. Palpation of alveolar ridges may elicit pain or tenderness.

Significance: Undetected caries or periodontal problems are often confused with TMD symptoms.

Swallowing

If swallowing is difficult, the floor of the mouth, tongue, and pharynx should be examined. Palpation of the larynx may reveal tenderness along the thyroid or cricoid cartilages (Fig. 7-39). The thyroid cartilage lies inferior to the hyoid bone but superiolateral to the cricoid cartilage. The latter abuts with the trachea and is covered laterally by the thyroid gland (Fig. 7-40).

Provocation of the tonsillar area with a cotton swab may trigger the pain. The patient is asked to **"turn the head and neck to the side opposite the side with the complaint."** This movement may provoke the pain. Palpation of the site may create a feeling of a lump in the throat.

Significance: Occasionally, postnasal drip from the sinuses produces excessive swallowing and fatigue of the muscles of the throat. Pain evoked by probing with the swab may trigger an episode of glossopharyngeal neuralgia. Pain and discomfort that results from turning the head and neck may be caused by Eagle's syndrome, which is associated with elongation of the stylohyoid process or calcification of the stylohyoid ligament. If no other reasons are found for recurrent pain on swallowing or palpation, the patient should be referred an otolaryngologist.

Sinuses

Nasal and paranasal sinuses should be evaluated for presence of pain, tenderness, and pathology. Fortunately, most tumors of paranasal sinuses are benign polyps and osteomas.[21]

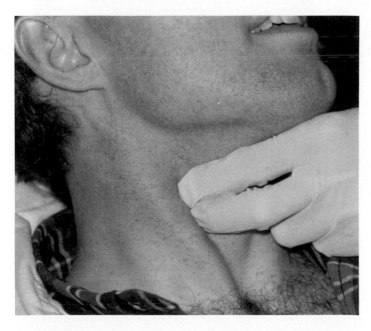

Figure 7-39.
Palpation of the larynx.

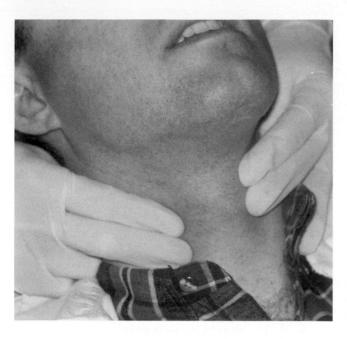

Figure 7-40.
Palpation of the junction of the thyroid gland and cricoid cartilage with the trachea.

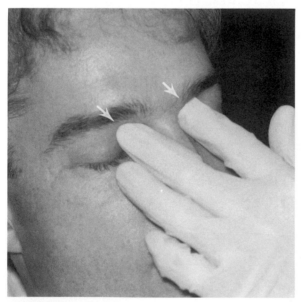

Figure 7-41.
Palpation of the frontal sinuses.

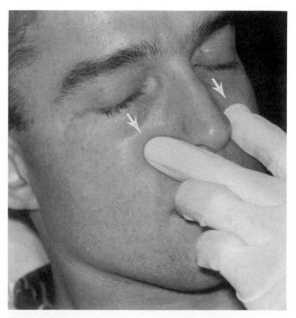

Figure 7-42.
Palpation of the maxillary sinuses.

Palpation of the *nasal sinus* is done by applying gentle pressure with an index finger on one side of the nose and the thumb on the other side.

The *frontal sinus* is palpated by applying gentle pressure with an index finger superiorly positioned at the inner canthus of the eye and pushing likewise with the middle finger on the other side (Fig. 7-41). Percussion with the index finger may provoke the pain. Transillumination can be done by directing a fiberoptic light in a darkened room against the overlying skin of the sinus.

Palpation of the *maxillary sinus* is done by applying gentle pressure with an index finger superiorly positioned below the rim of the orbit at the level of the nostrils and pushing the middle finger likewise on the other side (Fig. 7-42). Percussion with the index finger may provoke the pain. Transillumination can be accomplished by directing the light beam against the hard palate.

Significance: Pain of the nasal sinus has dull, burning characteristics. Little pain emanates from the paranasal sinuses unless major inflammation exists. Some pain has been described as deep, aching, and nonpulsatile.[21] Most tumors are painless unless malignant invasion of nerve occurs. Often, confirmation of problem depends on radiographic findings. Magnetic resonance imaging provides the greatest resolution of these areas.[21]

Salivary Glands

Because of their proximity to the TMJs, the major salivary glands should be palpated for tenderness. Salivary flow from their respective ducts is checked for normality.

Stensen's duct of the *parotid gland* opens through the buccinator muscle into the upper oral vestibule near the second molar (Fig. 7-43). The gland lies lateral to

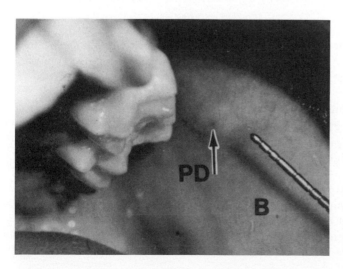

Figure 7-43.
Opening of parotid duct (PD) along the buccal mucosa (B) near the second molar. (Bush FM, Abbott DM, Butler JH. Fundamentals of occlusion, 2nd ed. Chapel Hill, NC: Health Sciences Consortium, 1980.)

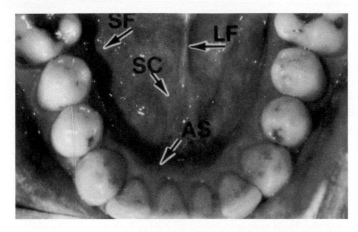

Figure 7-44.
Opening of the submandibular duct at the salivary caranculus (SC), sublingual fold (SF), lingual frenulum (LF), and alveololingual sulcus (AS). (Bush FM, Abbott DM, Butler JH. Fundamentals of occlusion, 2nd ed. Chapel Hill, NC: Health Sciences Consortium, 1980.)

the masseter muscle, superiorly to the posterior digastric muscle, and abuts with the SCM inferiorly.

The *submandibular* gland is separated from the parotid gland by the stylomandibular ligament. It lies below the body of the mandible at the junction of the posterior and anterior digastric muscles. Numerous small muscles form the remaining boundaries. Wharton's duct opens at the salivary caruncle, an elevated area lateral to the lingual frenum (Fig. 7-44).

Significance: Because the glands may become obstructed, infected, or subject to neoplasia, they should be examined if there are complaints of xerostomia, sialorrhea, or pain. Radiography may be necessary to rule out the presence or absence of stones.

Lymph Nodes

Regions of lymph nodes in and around the TMJs should be visually inspected and palpated (Table 7-11). Nodes are either superficial or deep, depending on location. The superficial nodes form a chain associated with the external jugular vein. The deep nodes form the largest and most prominent group.

A routine for palpation follows anatomic triangles of the neck (Fig. 7-45).[22] Palpation of the anterior chain is begun along the SCM (Fig. 7-46). Other areas include the posterior chain and the supraclavicular (Fig. 7-47), submandibular (Fig. 7-48), submental (Fig. 7-49), and suboccipital nodes (Fig. 7-50).

Significance: Patients often mistake tenderness on palpation of certain masticatory muscles as swollen lymph nodes. Generalized lymphadenopathy, caused by viruses or bacteria, has other dominant features (eg, history of fever). If doubt exists, biopsy of the node may be necessary.

(text continues on p. 272)

Table 7-11
Lymph Nodes and Site of Palpation

Nodes	Site of Palpation
Superficial	
TMJ area	
Anterior auricular	Preauricular
Parotid	Anterior to auricular
Retroauricular	Posterior to earlobe
Face and skull	
Buccal	Cheek
Mandibular	Inferior ramus
Infraorbital	Beneath eye
Occipital	Base of skull
Neck	
Submental	Beneath chin
Submandibular	Inferior ramus
External jugular	Lateral to sternocleidomastoid
Anterior jugular	Medial to sternocleidomastoid
Deep	
Cervical—Superior and Inferior	
Parotid	Anterior to auricular
Retropharyngeal	Posterior to sternocleidomastoid
Jugulodigastric	Posterior digastric
Jugulo-omohyoid	Omohyoid

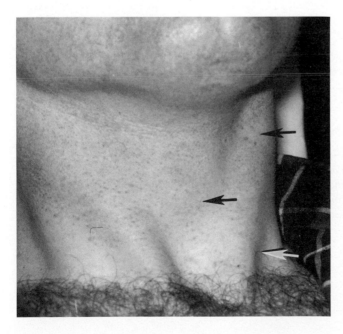

Figure 7-45.
Anterior and posterior triangles of the neck showing the sternocleidomastoid muscle (upper arrow), *the anterior triangle* (middle arrow), *and the posterior triangle* (lower arrow).

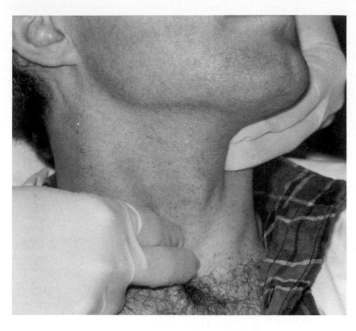

Figure 7-46.
Palpation of lymph nodes of the anterior chain along the sternocleidomastoid muscle.

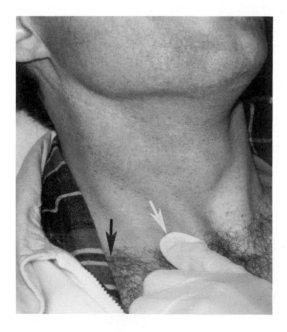

Figure 7-47.
Palpation of lymph nodes of the posterior chain along the sternocleidomastoid muscle (white arrow). *Region for palpation of the subclavicular lymph nodes* (dark arrow).

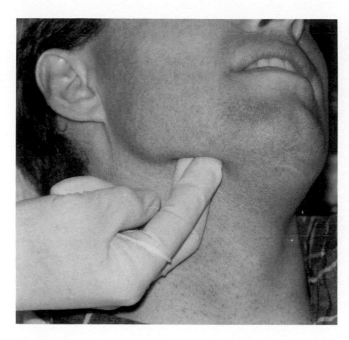

Figure 7-48.
Palpation of submandibular lymph nodes.

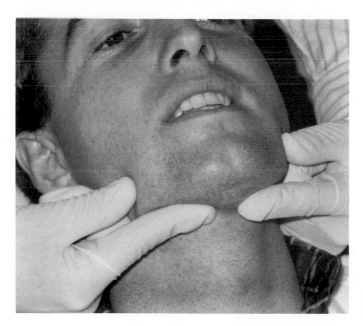

Figure 7-49.
Palpation of submental lymph nodes.

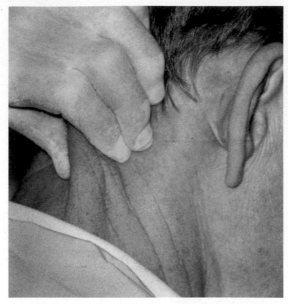

Figure 7-50.
Palpation of suboccipital lymph nodes.

Cranial Nerves

The purpose is to supply diagnostic information about the functional status of specific cranial nerves. The patient is asked to respond to a series of facial and head movements outlined below. The clinician observes and listens to responses during this performance. The tests are simple to conduct, but they are not definitive for abnormality (Table 7-12).

Separate checks are made of the three branches of the *trigeminal nerve*. For testing the sensory branches, the patient is asked to **"respond yes or no"** to the sensation of light touch tested by dragging a wisp of cotton along the brow (V1), upper lip (V2), and lower lip (V3). These same areas are then pricked with a sharply pointed object (Figs. 7-51 through 7-53). For testing of the motor branch, the patient is asked to **"open and close the mouth and protrude to the right and to the left with the lips closed"** (Fig. 7-54).

The motor branch of the *facial nerve* is tested by asking the patient to **"wrinkle the forehead and pucker the lips"** (Fig. 7-55). The sensory branch involves the sensation of taste. Most patients recognize this loss quickly.

For the *glossopharyngeal-vagus nerves*, the patient's gag reflex is tested as the clinician stimulates the patient's soft palate with a cotton-tipped applicator (Fig. 7-56). The patient is also asked to **"swallow water."** The inability to gag or cough during swallowing suggests derangement.

Table 7-12
Tests for Specific Cranial Nerve Functions

Trigeminal nerve
    V_1 sensory branch
    V_2 sensory branch
    V_3 sensory branch
    V_3 motor branch
Facial nerve
    Motor branch
Glossopharyngeal–vagus nerve
Spinal accessory nerve
Hypoglossal nerve

In testing of the *spinal accessory nerve*, the patient is asked to **"shrug the shoulders and turn the head"** (Fig. 7-57). This motion activates the trapezius and SCM muscles. Inability to turn suggests limitation.

In tests of the *hypoglossal nerve*, the patient is asked to **"protrude the tongue as straight as possible"** (Fig. 7-58). Lateral deviation suggests derangement.

Significance: There is a tendency to overinterpret mild deviations in normal movements. The clinician should be guided by the anatomic pattern of change described by the patient.

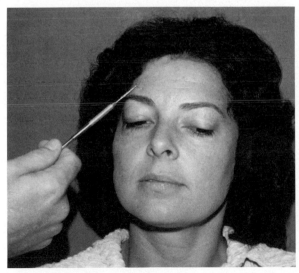

Figure 7-51.
Light prick of forehead to test the sensory branch (V1) of the trigeminal nerve. (Abbott DH, Bush FM, Butler JH. Principles of occlusion, 3rd ed. Chapel Hill, NC: Health Sciences Consortium, 1980.)

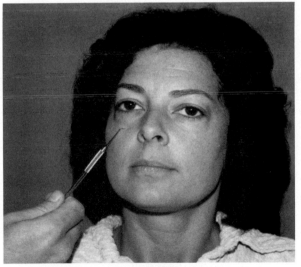

Figure 7-52.
Light prick of the cheek to test the sensory branch (V2) of the trigeminal nerve. (Abbott DH, Bush FM, Butler JH. Principles of occlusion, 3rd ed. Chapel Hill, NC: Health Sciences Consortium, 1980.)

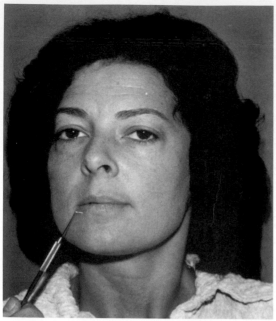

Figure 7-53.
Light prick of the lower lip to test the sensory branch (V3) of the trigeminal nerve. (Abbott DH, Bush FM, Butler JH. Principles of occlusion, 3rd ed. Chapel Hill, NC: Health Sciences Consortium, 1980.)

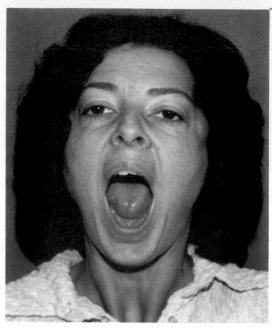

Figure 7-54.
Opening the mouth to test the motor branch of the trigeminal nerve. (Abbott DH, Bush FM, Butler JH. Principles of occlusion, 3rd ed. Chapel Hill, NC: Health Sciences Consortium, 1980.)

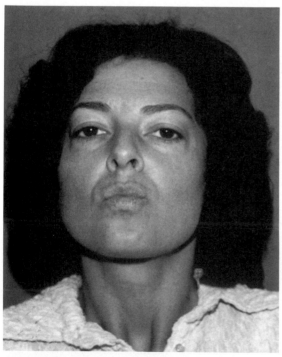

Figure 7-55.
Puckering the lips to test the motor branch of the facial nerve. (Abbott DH, Bush FM, Butler JH. Principles of occlusion, 3rd ed. Chapel Hill, NC: Health Sciences Consortium, 1980.)

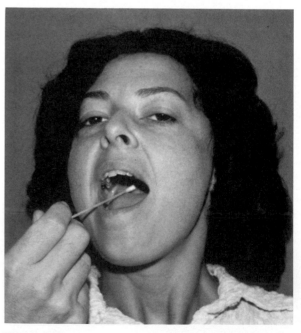

Figure 7-56.
Stimulation of the soft palate with a cotton-tipped applicator to test the glossopharyngeal and vagus nerves. (Abbott DH, Bush FM, Butler JH. Principles of occlusion, 3rd ed. Chapel Hill, NC: Health Sciences Consortium, 1980.)

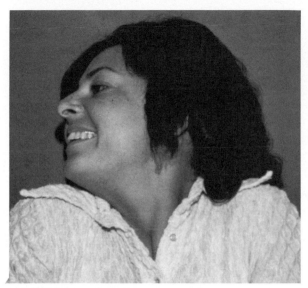

Figure 7-57.
Shrugging the shoulders and turning the head to test the spinal accesory nerve. (Abbott DH, Bush FM, Butler JH. Principles of occlusion, 3rd ed. Chapel Hill, NC: Health Sciences Consortium, 1980.)

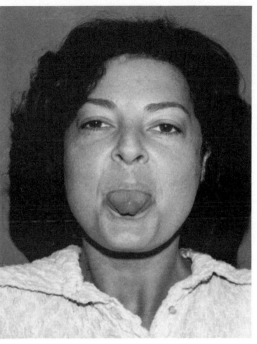

Figure 7-58.
Protruding the tongue to test the hypoglossal nerve. (Abbott DH, Bush FM, Butler JH. Principles of occlusion, 3rd ed. Chapel Hill, NC: Health Sciences Consortium, 1980.)

Radiography

In addition to case history and objective clinical findings, analysis of anatomic contours observed from radiographs can provide useful information about the TMJs (Table 7-13). Conventional radiography, tomography, and bone scanning can furnish evidence of osseous disease unavailable from clinical findings. Newer technology such as magnetic resonance imaging has vastly improved the visibility of soft tissue anatomy. Still, none of these techniques has proved reliable for definitive diagnosis of TMD.

The advantages and disadvantages of different radiographic techniques must be weighed in terms of costs, risks, and need for patient evaluation and treatment. The clinician may need to rely on them to maintain quality assurance, confirm diagnosis, and avoid problems with litigation.

Conventional Radiography

Because of location of the TMJs, radiography of the joints is difficult for the clinician. Techniques commonly used by clinicians for screening are transcranial and panoramic projections.

Table 7-13
Radiographic and Imaging Techniques Used
for Evaluation of Head and Neck Anatomy

Transcranial
Panoramic
Anterior–posterior (transorbital)
Submentovertex
Tomography
  Classical
  Computed
Bone scintigraphy
Arthrography
Magnetic resonance imaging

Transcranial projections provide a lateral view of the TMJs. They show only the laterosuperior border of the condyle and the lateral surface of the glenoid fossa (Fig. 7-59). The radiographic beam is directed from the opposite side of the skull and passes across the superior surface of the petrous bone. Because of this obstacle, the superior border of the condyle between the lateral and medial poles cannot be seen.

Much has been said about the radiographic position of the condyle with respect to the fossa and abnormality within the joint. Sufficient reliability has never been established to prove diagnostic value.[23]

  Significance: Fixed positioners are available to assist in alignment of the cone with the joint.[22] They permit multiple exposures of the condyle without changing head positions. Unfortunately, the site where most osseous changes occur cannot be obtained. Spicules and erosion of the laterosuperior surface of the condyle can be seen.

Panoramic analysis with the mandible in open and closed positions allows for bilateral viewing of condyle–fossa relation. Because of rotational capabilities, panoramic radiographic units permit an oblique anteroposterior view of the joint. Two different views can be obtained for each joint on the same radiograph (Fig. 7-60). Although uncommon, occasional bilateral degeneration occurs as found in this patient with rheumatoid arthritis (Fig. 7-61).

  Significance: These radiographs are useful to rule out gross intraosseous disease from dental disease.[24] No correlation has been found between joint appearance and signs and symptoms of TMD.[25]

With *anterior–posterior* (or transorbital) projection, both condyles can be viewed simultaneously (Fig. 7-62).

  Significance: The size and shape of each condyle, particularly the medial and lateral surfaces, can be viewed within the glenoid fossa.

In the *submentovertex* view, as in the anterior–posterior view, the condyles can be viewed inferiorly (Fig. 7-63).

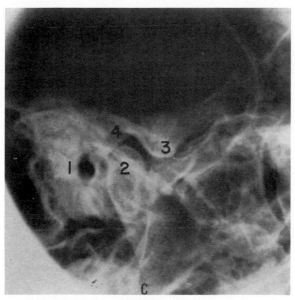

Figure 7-59.
Transcranial radiograph of normal right TMJ showing the external auditory meatus (1), the condyle (2), the articular eminence (3), and the glenoid fossa (4). Note the convex, superior surface of the condyle. A degenerated condyle may show areas of erosion or appear flattened. (Langland OE, Sippy FH, Langlais RP. Texbook of dental radiology. Springfield, IL: Charles C. Thomas, 1984:527.)

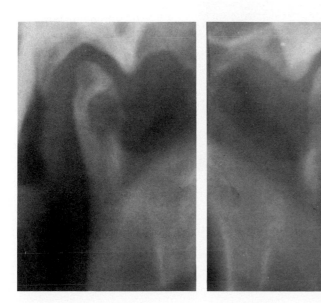

Figure 7-60.
Panoramic view of an elongated condyle within normal limits on the patient's left and an abnormal condyle with a cyst on the patient's right.

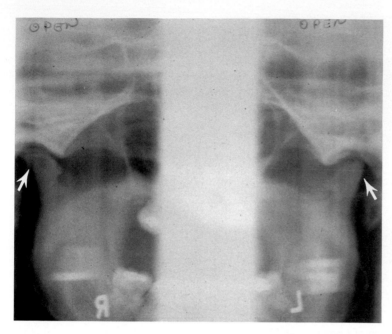

Figure 7-61.
Panoramic view of degenerated condyles of a patient with rheumatoid arthritis. Arrows indicate the flattened anterior surface on the patient's right side and the "moth-eaten" condyle on the patient's left side.

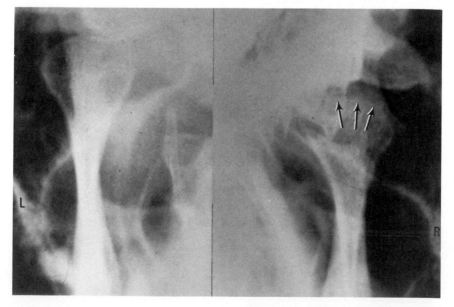

Figure 7-62.
Anterior–posterior view of a left condyle that is within normal limits. The right condyle shows resorption of bone (arrows). (Langland OE, Sippy FH, Langlais RP. Textbook of dental radiology, 2nd ed. Springfield, IL: Charles C. Thomas, 1984:542.)

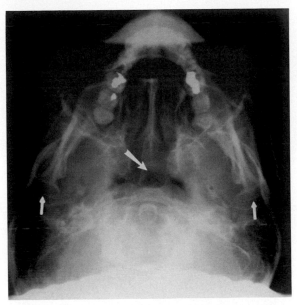

Figure 7-63.
Submentovertex (basilar) view of condyles. Note that the medial surfaces, which are often difficult to observe, are within normal limits (small arrows). The sphenoidal sinuses lie posterior to the hard palate and equidistant between the condyles (large arrow). Just anterior are the ethmoidal sinuses.

Significance: This view allows determination of the horizontal condylar angles. Visualization of the sinuses and zygomatic arches makes this view valuable.

Tomography

Tomography is a specialized technique that allows detailed images of structures lying in a predetermined plane, while blurring or eliminating details of unwanted structures in other planes.

Classic tomography involves taking several exposures of a selected area at arbitrary intervals or sections. Blurring occurs in the focal plane, obscuring some desired anatomic detail. Unlike transcranial radiography, lateral, central, and medial parts of the joint can be seen on separate images (Figs. 7-64 and 7-65).

Computed tomography (CT) scanning represents an improvement over the classic technique. It permits scanning of a well-defined area of detail, which minimizes the effect of superimposition (Figs. 7-66 through 7-68). The computer analyses x-ray absorptions at many different points and converts them into an image on a video screen.

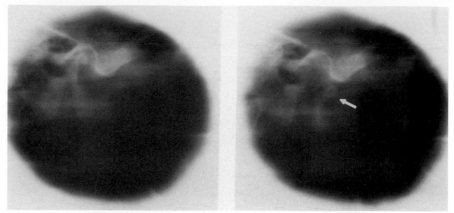

Figure 7-64.
Tomographic radiograph of TMJs with the condyle situated in the glenoid fossa on the left panel and the translated condyle beneath the eminence on the right panel. Although the condyle appears small, a determination of abnormality cannot be confirmed from these lateral views.

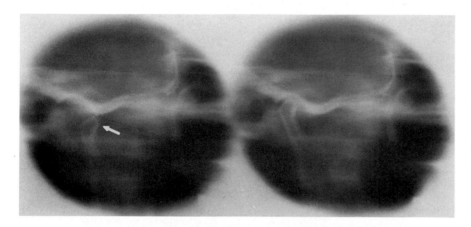

Figure 7-65.
Tomographic radiograph of TMJs with the translated condyle beneath the eminence on the left panel and the condyle situated in the glenoid fossa on the right panel. The flattened superior surface in the left panel suggests degenerative joint disease but may represent an alteration in form.

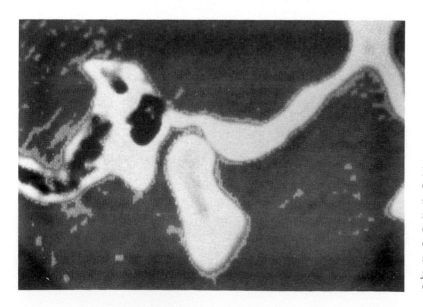

Figure 7-66.
Computed tomography of a right TMJ within normal limits. The mandible is in the closed position. (Cohen HR, Silver CM, Schatz SL, Motamed MM. Correlation of sagittal computed tomography of the temporomandibular joint with surgical findings. J Craniomandib Pract 1985;3:351.)

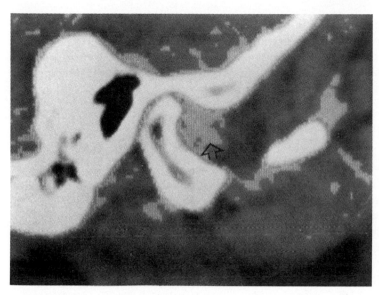

Figure 7-67.
Computed tomography of a right TMJ. Arrow indicates displacement of the disk anterior to the condyle. (Cohen HR, Silver CM, Schatz SL, Motamed MM. Correlation of sagittal computed tomography of the temporomandibular joint with surgical findings. J Craniomandib Pract 1985;3:351.)

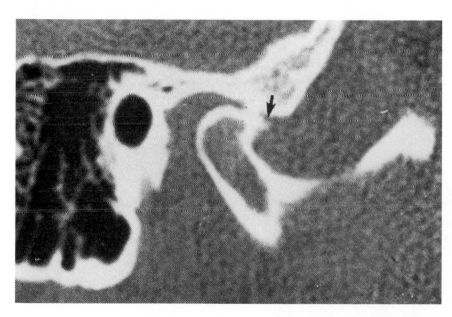

Figure 7-68.
Computed tomography of the right TMJ. Arrow indicates an osteophyte on the anterior surface of the condyle. (Cohen HR, Silver CM, Schatz SL, Motamed MM. Correlation of sagittal computed tomography of the temporomandibular joint with surgical findings. J Craniomandib Pract 1985;3:351.)

Significance: Condylar erosion and osteophytic changes can be seen with more detail than with conventional radiography. An advantage is gross determination of the condyle–disk relation without using invasive means. Because the head is placed in a scanner gantry during CT scanning, some patients may become claustrophobic. Reassurance may be needed.

Arthrography

Arthrography involves the injection of contrast medium into the synovial cavities followed by radiography of the injected site.[26] Usually a fluoroscopic evaluation is done with the contrast medium. The medium is injected into the lower synovial cavity. Patients are asked to open and close the mandible. This movement changes the shape of the contrast medium. Serial radiographs are made, resulting in a series of arthrograms (Figs. 7-69 through 7-74).

Significance: Arthrography is an invasive procedure and should be weighed against clinical findings. The position and shape of the disk can be seen relative to the condyle and eminence at various positions. Perforations in the disk or its attachments can be seen readily.[27]

Magnetic Resonance Imaging

In magnetic resonance imaging (MRI), as in CT scanning, radiant energy is beamed into the patient. Unlike the x-rays of CT, radiofrequency waves provide the energy in MRI. Waves are beamed into magnetic fields, and a receiver coil measures the

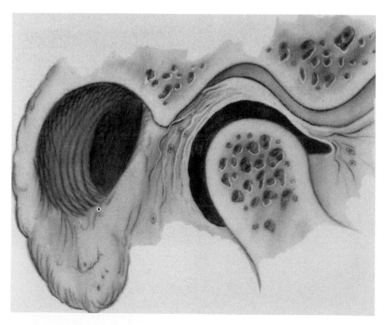

Figure 7-69.
Drawing of arthrogram of normal right side TMJ with the jaw in closed-mouth position. (Dolwick MF, Sanders B. TMJ internal derangement and arthrosis. St. Louis: CV Mosby, 1985:89.)

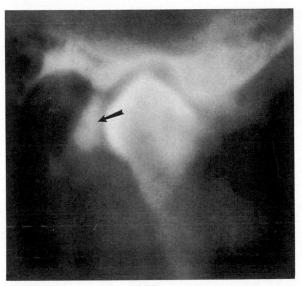

Figure 7-70.
Arthrogram of Figure 7-69. Note the teardrop shape of the lower synovial cavity after injection with contrast medium (arrow). (Dolwick MF, Sanders B. TMJ internal derangement and arthrosis. St. Louis: CV Mosby, 1985:89.)

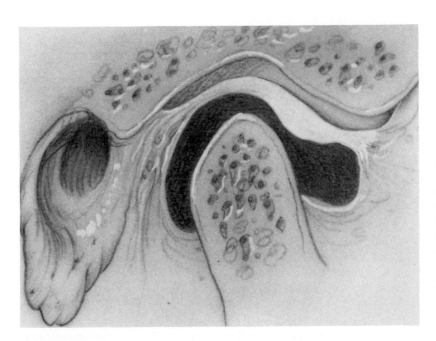

Figure 7-71.
Drawing of arthrogram of TMJ with anteriorly displaced disk. Compared with the normal shape in Figure 7-69, the lower joint space has changed shape anteriorly (arrow). Note that the disk is pushed anteriorly as the condyle translates slightly. (Dolwick MF, Sanders B. TMJ internal derangement and arthrosis. St. Louis: CV Mosby, 1985.)

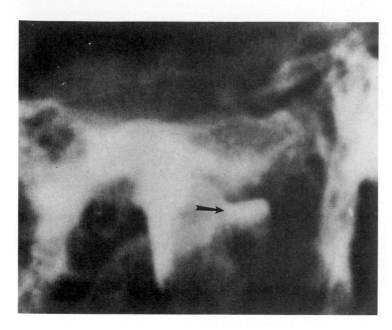

Figure 7-72.
Arthrogram of Figure 7-71. Note that the disk fails to reduce to the position in Figure x-xx. (Dolwick MF, Sanders B. TMJ internal derangement and arthrosis. St. Louis: CV Mosby, 1985:113.)

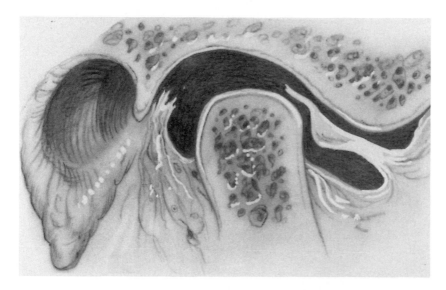

Figure 7-73.
Drawing of arthrogram of TMJ with perforation of disk. The disk is separated with loose bodies. (Dolwick MF, Sanders B. TMJ internal derangement and arthrosis. St. Louis: CV Mosby, 1985:123.)

energy released. A unique feature of MRI is its ability to differentiate small differences between tissues. Resolution is so high that injuries and diseases affecting a tendon, ligament, and cartilage can be detected. A computer uses this information and constructs an image on the video screen. It is possible to see two- or three-dimensional images of the joint's interior (Figs. 7-75 through 7-78).

Significance: It has been claimed that disks displaced anteriorly can be differentiated from normal variants.[28] But the general usefulness of MRI in the assessment

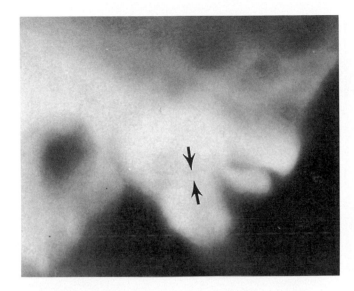

Figure 7-74.
Arthrogram of Figure 7-73. Both joint spaces are filled with the contrast medium, obscuring individual cavities (arrows). (Dolwick MF, Sanders B. TMJ internal derangement and arthrosis. St. Louis: CV Mosby, 1985:123.)

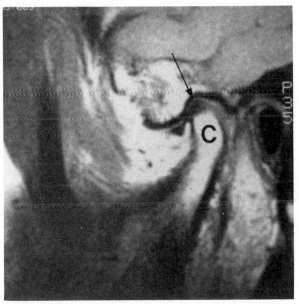

Figure 7-75.
MRI scan of normal left TMJ showing the condyle (C). Note the biconcave appearance (arrow) of a normally positioned disk. (Schellhas KP, Fritts HM, Heithoff KB, Jahn JA, Wilkes CH, Molie MR. Temporomandibular joint: MR fast. J Craniomandib Pract 1988;6:209.)

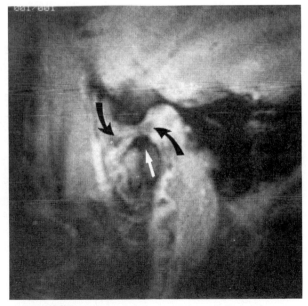

Figure 7-76.
MRI scan of abnormal left TMJ. The disk is displaced anteriorly. The small arrow indicates condylar marrow with hypointensity characteristic of avascular necrosis. (Schellhas KP, Fritts HM, Heithoff KB, Jahn JA, Wilkes CH, Molie MR. Temporomandibular joint: MR fast. J Craniomandib Pract 1988;6:209.)

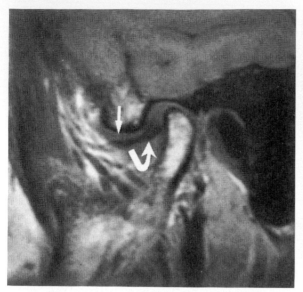

Figure 7-77.
MRI scan of abnormal left TMJ showing effusion above the disk (small arrow) *and disk deformity* (large arrow). *(Schellhas KP, Fritts HM, Heithoff KB, Jahn JA, Wilkes CH, Molie MR. Temporomandibular joint: MR fast. J Craniomandib Pract 1988;6:209.)*

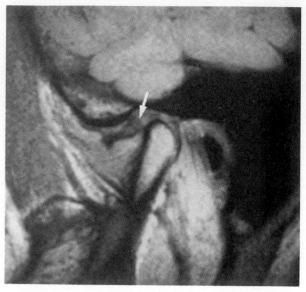

Figure 7-78.
MRI scan of abnormal left TMJ showing myxogenous degeneration. (Schellhas KP, Fritts HM, Heithoff KB, Jahn JA, Wilkes CH, Molie MR. Temporomandibular joint: MR fast. J Craniomandib Pract 1988;6:209.)

of TMD has been questioned. Studies on TMD patients indicate that the MRI appearance has little or no bearing on subjective and objective outcome of treatment.[29]

No injection of contrast material or x-rays is necessary, and no short-term side effects have been found. MRI was as accurate as arthrography and more accurate than tomography in correlating with surgical findings of TMD cases.[27] This feature makes it preferable to either CT or arthrography for diagnostic and surgical purposes. Because the body must remain motionless inside of the magnetic tunnel for 30 to 45 minutes, claustrophobic or anxious patients may require reassurance.

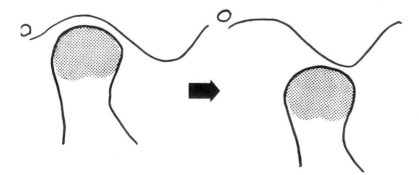

Figure 7-79.
Osteogenic activity in the condyle at the closed and open jaw positions. (Alexander JM, Bloom CY, Fratkin MJ. Image patterns of radionuclide bone scintigraphy of the temporomandibular joint. In Hjorting-Hansen E [ed]. Oral and maxillofacial surgery. Proceedings of the 8th International Conference on Oral and Maxillofacial Surgery. Carol Stream, IL: Quintessence, 1985:651.)

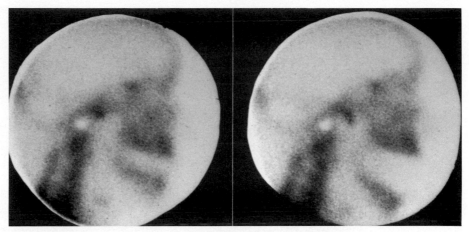

Figure 7-80.
Scintiscan of osteogenic activity in the condyle at the closed and open positions. (Alexander JM, Bloom CY, Fratkin MJ. Image patterns of radionuclide bone scintigraphy of the temporomandibular joint. In Hjorting-Hansen E [ed]. Oral and maxillofacial surgery. Proceedings of the 8th International Conference on Oral and Maxillofacial Surgery. Carol Stream, IL: Quintessence, 1985:651.)

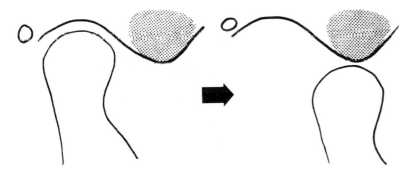

Figure 7-81.
Osteogenic activity in the glenoid fossa at the closed and open jaw positions. (Alexander JM, Bloom CY, Fratkin MJ. Image patterns of radionuclide bone scintigraphy of the temporomandibular joint. In Hjorting-Hansen E [ed]. Oral and maxillofacial surgery. Proceedings of the 8th International Conference on Oral and Maxillofacial Surgery. Carol Stream, IL: Quintessence, 1985:651.)

Bone Scintigraphy

Another radiologic technique useful in evaluating TMD is radionuclide bone scintigraphy. Scanning with technetium diphosphonates produces a functional display of bony metabolism and improves interpretation of joint pathology. Uptake of technetium is thought to provide a sensitive indicator of adaptive changes in the bone.[30]

A small amount of technetium methyl diphosphonate is given by intravenous injection. Images of the head and neck are obtained about 3 hours after injection, using a conventional gamma scintillation camera. The scan shows uptake of technetium where the bone undergoes osteogenic activity (Figs. 7-79 through 7-84).

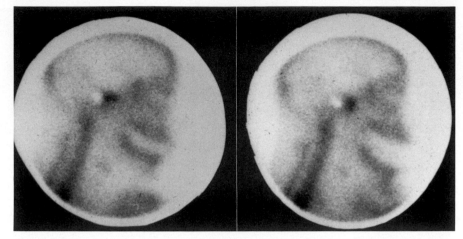

Figure 7-82.
Scintiscan of osteogenic activity in the glenoid fossa at the closed and open jaw positions. (Alexander JM, Bloom CY, Fratkin MJ. Image patterns of radionuclide bone scintigraphy of the temporomandibular joint. In Hjorting-Hansen E [ed]. Oral and maxillofacial surgery. Proceedings of the 8th International Conference on Oral and Maxillofacial Surgery. Carol Stream, IL: Quintessence, 1985:651.)

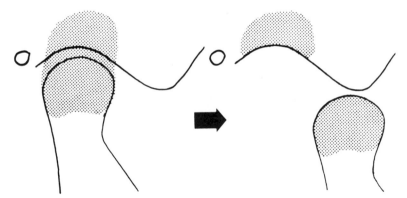

Figure 7-83.
Osteogenic activity in the condyle and the glenoid fossa at the closed and open jaw positions. (Alexander JM, Bloom CY, Fratkin MJ. Image patterns of radionuclide bone scintigraphy of the temporomandibular joint. In Hjorting-Hansen E [ed]. Oral and maxillofacial surgery. Proceedings of the 8th International Conference on Oral and Maxillofacial Surgery. Carol Stream, IL: Quintessence, 1985:651.)

Significance: The role of bone scanning in clinical practice has not been established.[31] No significant association was found between the symptomatic side of the TMD complaint and the side with highest uptake of technetium.[25] Still, scintigraphs made with the mandible in open and closed positions permit the examiner to differentiate osteogenic changes in the glenoid fossa from osteogenic changes in the condyle. Another advantage is that uptake in areas of apical pathosis is indicative of dental disease.

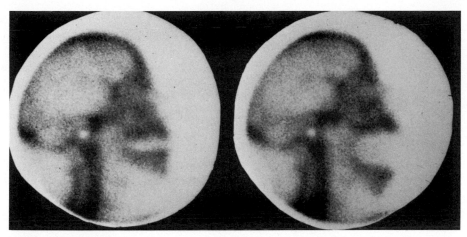

Figure 7-84.
Scintiscan of osteogenic activity in the condyle and the glenoid fossa at the closed and open jaw positions. (Alexander JM, Bloom CY, Fratkin MJ. Image patterns of radionuclide bone scintigraphy of the temporomandibular joint. In Hjorting-Hansen E [ed]. Oral and maxillofacial surgery. Proceedings of the 8th International Conference on Oral and Maxillofacial Surgery. Carol Stream, IL: Quintessence, 1985:651.)

References

1. Helkimo M. Studies on function and dysfunction of the masticatory system. Part II. Index for anamnestic and clinical dysfunction and occlusal state. Swed Dent J 1974;67:101.

2. Solberg WK. Occlusion-related pathosis and its clinical evaluation. In Clark JW (ed). Clinical dentistry, rev ed 2. Philadelphia: JB Lippincott, 1990;35:1.

3. Solberg WK. Temporomandibular disorders: physical tests in diagnosis. Br Dent J 1986;160:273.

4. Solberg WK. Temporomandibular disorders: data collection and examination. Br Dent J 1986;160:317.

5. Clark GT, Seligman DA, Solberg WK, Pullinger AG. Guidelines for the examination and diagnosis of temporomandibular disorders. J Craniomandib Disord 1989;3:7.

6. Fricton JR, Schiffman EL. The craniomandibular index: validity. J Prosthet Dent 1987;58:222.

7. Schiffman EL, Anderson GC, Fricton JR, Lindgren BR. The relationship between level of mandibular pain and dysfunction and stage of temporomandibular joint internal derangement. J Dent Res 1992;71:1812.

8. Truelove EL, Sommers EE, LeResche L, Dworkin SF, Von Korff M. Clinical diagnostic criteria for TMD: New classification permits multiple diagnoses. J Am Dent Assoc 1992;123:47.

9. Clark GT. Examining temporomandibular disorder patients for cranio-cervical dysfunction. J Craniomandib Pract 1984;2:55.

10. Clark GT, Green EM, Dornan MR, Flack VF. Craniocervical dysfunction levels in a patient sample from a temporomandibular joint clinic. J Am Dent Assoc 1987;115:251.

11. Stegenga B, De Bont LGM, Boering G, Van Willigen JD. Tissue responses to degenerative changes in the temporomandibular joint: a review. J Oral Maxillofac Surg 1991;49:1079.

12. Abbott DM, Bush FM, Butler JH. Principles of occlusion, 3rd ed. Chapel Hill, NC: Health Sciences Consortium, 1980.

13. American Medical Association. AMA guides to evaluation of permanent impairment, 3rd ed. Chicago: American Medical Association, 1990:88.

14. Ratner E, Person P, Kleinman DJ, Jawbone cavities and trigeminal and atypical facial neuralgias. Oral Surg Oral Med Oral Pathol 1979;48:3.

15. McMahon RE, Adams W, Spolnik KJ. Diagnostic anesthesia for referred trigeminal pain, part 2. Compendium 1992;13:980.

16. Bell WE. Management of masticatory pain. In Alling CC III, Mahan PE. Facial pain, 2nd ed. Philadelphia: Lea & Febiger, 1977:181.

17. Flöter TH. Blocks in the area of the head. In Zenz M, Hoester W, Niesel H Chr, Kreuscher H (eds), translated by DeKornfeld TJ. Regional anesthesia, 2nd ed. St. Louis: Mosby Year Book, 1990:240.

18. Dolwick MF, Bush FM, Seibel HR, Burke GW Jr. Degenerative changes in masseter muscle following injection of lidocaine: a histochemical study. J Dent Res 1977;11:1395.

19. Donlon WC, Truta MP, Eversole LR. A modified auriculotemporal nerve block for regional anaesthesia of the temporomandibular joint. J Oral Maxillofac Surg 1984;42:544.

20. Hankemeier U. Sympathetic blockade. In Zenz M, Hoester W, Niesel H Chr, Kreuscher H (eds), translated by DeKornfeld TJ. Regional anesthesia, 2nd ed. St. Louis: Mosby Year Book, 1990:223.

21. Schor DI. Headache and facial pain–the role of the paranasal sinuses: a literature review. J Craniomandib Pract 1993;11:36.

22. Langland OE, Sippy FH, Langlais RP. Textbook of dental radiology, 2nd ed, Springfield, IL: Charles C. Thomas, 1984.

23. Blaschke DD. Radiology of the temporomandibular joint: current status of transcranial, tomographic, and arthrographic procedures. In Laskin D, Greenfield W, Gale E, et al (eds). The President's Conference on the Examination, Diagnosis and Management of Temporomandibular Disorders. Chicago: American Dental Association, 1983:64

24. Seals RR, Williams EO, Jones JD. Panoramic radiographs: necessary for edentulous patients? J Am Dent Assoc 1992;123:74.

25. Bush FM, Harrington WG, Harkins SW. Interexaminer comparison of bone scintigraphy and panoramic radiography of temporomandibular joints: correlation with signs and symptoms. J Prosthet Dent 1992;67:246.

26. Dolwick MF, Sanders B. TMJ internal derangement and arthrosis: surgical atlas. St. Louis: CV Mosby, 1985.

27. Donlon WC, Moon KL. Comparison of magnetic resonance imaging, arthrotomography and clinical and surgical findings in temporomandibular joint internal derangements. Oral Surg Oral Med Oral Pathol 1987;64:2.

28. Conway WF, Hayes CW, Campbell RL. Dynamic magnetic resonance imaging

of temporomandibular joint using flash sequences. J Oral Maxillofac Surg 1988;46:930.

29. Weissman JL, Rudy TE, Curtin HD, Zaki HS. MR findings and treatment outcome in TMD patients. J Dent Res 1993;72(Abstract 709):192.

30. Alexander JM, Bloom CY, Fratkin MJ. Image patterns of radionuclide bone scintigraphy of the temporomandibular joint. In Hjorting-Hansen E (ed). Oral and maxillofacial surgery. Proceedings of the 8th International Conference on Oral and Maxillofacial Surgery. Carol Stream, IL: Quintessence, 1985:651.

31. Fogelman I. Bone scanning and photon absorptionmetry in metabolic bone disease. Baillieres Clin Endocrinol Metab 1986;2:59.

The Temporomandibular Joint and Related Orofacial Disorders,
by Francis M. Bush and M. Franklin Dolwick.
J.B. Lippincott Company, Philadelphia, © 1995.

8

Practical Guide to Differential Diagnosis

Differential diagnosis of conditions that may cause chronic pain in the mandible, cranium, and neck involves a broad range of disorders. In most instances, the site of the complaint can be traced to a specific anatomic site, but frequent overlap in symptoms with other disorders confounds diagnosis, confusing even the expert diagnostician. Often this enigma is compounded by a suspected psychological basis for the presence or continuance of pain.

Among the many painful orofacial conditions confounding diagnosis of TMD are those arising from the masticatory muscle, followed by those with dental and sinus-related origins. Although these latter two nonarticular conditions often result in acute pain, they tend, if persistent, to mimic TMD pain and may produce limited joint movement. Otic and neurologic diseases, pain of intracranial origin, headache, sympathetic fiber-mediated pain, and neoplasms also may produce symptoms resembling TMD symptoms.

Differentiating these mimicking disorders from TMD relies on the general acceptance of terms and meanings associated with signs and symptoms. These descriptors and their definitions must be continually evaluated to improve validity and reliability. Acceptance of these descriptions will help to develop a diagnostic classification that can identify specific disorders.

In contrast to the vast diagnostic literature on headache, no fully validated classification is available to differentiate TMD from overlapping disorders or forms of TMD from one another. Classifications that have been attempted include the following: painful disorders of the head and neck;[1–9] myofascial pain from mimicking disorders;[10] head and neck fibromyalgia from temporomandibular arthralgia;[11] internal derangements from muscular disorders;[12–14] and types of internal derangements.[15,16]

Other useful literature discusses sinus and nasal disorders,[17–20] dental problems,[21] headache,[22–24] auditory disorders,[25,26] and infratemporal space pathosis.[27] The different psychological factors involved in chronic pain,[28–30] including chronic TMD pain,[31] allow for further diagnostic distinction.

It can be difficult to make a positive decision about whether a disorder represents a separate condition. Warning signs may be few, nonspecific, and appear late in the disease. In usual practice, the diagnostic decision relies on both anamnestic and clinical results. From existing findings, a system of algorithms can be developed permitting clinicians to differentiate TM disorders from one another and from overlapping disorders. Although not every clinician will agree with certain descriptive features of TMD or disorders mimicking TMD, clinicians need a practical system to communicate with one another, with the patient, and with insurance carriers.

The following algorithms are designed to assist in classifying similar disorders. Each provides a set of instructions for discerning disorders in a limited number of steps. Although the algorithms should not be considered definitive, they are representative benchmarks for keying problems or disorders from one another. The algorithms focus on diagnostic features of specific anatomic sites (eg, TMJ, masticatory muscle, nerve, tooth, and head) and on nonarticular disorders mimicking TMD. These are followed by algorithms for psychological disorders that may be related to TMD.

ALGORITHM FOR KEYING TMJ PROBLEMS

1. Sounds present after jaw movement . . . 2
   Loss of sounds or no history of recent sounds . . . 9
2. Reciprocal clicking or popping, passive stretch ≥35 mm . . . 3
   Other sounds, passive stretch ≥35 mm . . . 4
3. Sounds during range of movement . . . **Disk displacement with reduction (type I)**
   Sounds with episodic catching . . . **Disk displacement with reduction (type II)**
4. Crepitus or hard grating, report of pain or no pain . . . 5
   Crepitus present or absent, pain acute . . . 6
5. Report of pain (inflammatory phase), radiologic evidence of bony change . . . **Arthritis with arthralgia (degenerative joint disease [DJD] with pain)**
   No report of pain (noninflammatory phase), radiologic evidence of bony change . . . **Arthrosis (DJD without pain)**
6. Signs of inflammation in other joints, positive serologic test, radiologic evidence of bony change . . . **Polyarthritis (rheumatoid)**
   No inflammation in other joints, negative serology . . . 7
7. Localized pain on palpation, pain on function, pain during assisted jaw opening, possible swelling . . . **Synovitis or capsulitis**
   Rarely localized pain . . . 8
8. Excessive range of motion (translation), ability to close mandible without assistance . . . **Hypermobility**
   Excessive range of motion, inability to close mandible without assistance . . . **Dislocation**

9. Loss of sounds coincides with unilateral deviation . . . 10

   No recent sounds . . . 11

10. Sudden loss of sounds coincides with decreased translation of ipsilateral condyle, opening 25 mm or less . . . **Disk displacement without reduction, acute form**

    Loss of sounds greater than 6 months duration, coincides with decreased translation, opening 25 mm or less . . . **Disk displacement without reduction, chronic form**

11. Radiologic evidence of osseous change . . . 12

    Without osseous change . . . 13

12. Recent enlargement of condyle or bony destruction, positive bone scan . . . **Neoplasm**

    Bony proliferation limiting translation of ipsilateral condyle, negative bone scan . . . **Bony ankylosis**

13. Contralateral movement <7 mm . . . **Fibrous ankylosis**

    Contralateral movement ≥7 mm . . . **Normal**

ALGORITHM FOR KEYING MUSCLE PROBLEMS

1. Report of orofacial pain . . . 2

   Orofacial pain rarely reported . . . 6

2. Dull ache at static jaw position, stiffness on function . . . 3

   Fluctuant pain in morning or evening, or acute pain . . . 4

3. Pain on palpation in two or more muscles (masseter, temporalis, pterygoid origin, suprahyoid, and styloid regions), and a rating of 2 or more on a 0 to 3 scale in no more than a single muscle . . . **Myalgia I or masticatory fibromyalgia (mild form)**

   Pain on palpation in two or more muscles (as above) with pain rated 2 or more in two or more muscles . . . **Myalgia II or masticatory fibromyalgia (moderate or severe form)**

4. Myalgia I and II plus localized tenderness in firm bands of muscle in posterior neck or shoulder, restricted opening improved 4 mm or more by manual assistance . . . **Myofascial pain (generalized fibromyalgia)**

   None of above, but report of acute pain . . . 5

5. Acute tenderness of entire muscle, possible swelling, positive inflammatory findings on biopsy . . . **Myositis**

   Continuous contraction (fasciculation), localized, positive findings on electromyogram . . . **Myospasm**

6. Rigidity of several jaw muscles to manual manipulation . . . **Reflex splinting**

   No rigidity . . . 7

7. Unyielding resistance to passive stretch . . . **Contracture**

   No such resistance . . . 8

8. Enlargement of muscle, localized . . . 9

   Without enlargement . . . 10

9. Uncontrolled growth, recent origin, confirmation by magnetic resonance imaging (MRI), positive biopsy . . . **Neoplasm**

Grossly enlarged muscle, related to functional activity of jaw, negative MRI report or biopsy . . . **Hypertrophy**

10. None of the above features . . . **Normal**

ALGORITHM FOR KEYING DENTAL PROBLEMS MIMICKING TMD

1. Toothache caused by obvious dentino-enamel defect . . . 2
   No obvious dentino-enamel defect . . . 6
2. Carious defect identified visually or radiologically, short, sharp shock evoked by heat, cold, or air, relieved by sedative filling . . . **Odontalgia**
   Acute ache of variable intensity, sensitivity to cold and percussion variable, not relieved by periodontal curettage . . . 3
3. Mild, vague discomfort of pulpitis, slight sensitivity to cold, disappears within 24 to 48 hours . . . **Incipient acute pulpalgia**
   Persistent pain, slight or no sensitivity to percussion, sensitive to cold . . . 4
4. Persistent nagging or boring pain that originates spontaneously, tolerable but aggravated by cold . . . **Moderate acute pulpalgia**
   History of periapical abscess or painful to pressure . . . 5
5. Particularly painful to pressure, throbbing pain relieved by cold, may not be relieved by local anesthesia, usually periapical radiolucency . . . **Advanced acute pulpalgia**
   Diffuse radiating pain, often beginning as acute apical abscess, relieved by local anesthesia . . . **Chronic pulpalgia**
6. Gingival inflammation or abscess along lateral surface of tooth, radiolucency lateral if present, pain relieved by infiltration of local anesthesia or by curettage . . . 7
   Not as above . . . 8
7. Abscess, swelling, and possible suppuration . . . **Periodontal abscess**
   Localized inflammation around partially erupted teeth, usually molars . . . **Pericoronitis**
8. History of trauma, unexplained ache, or lancinating pain of abrupt onset during mastication, may not be identified clinically or radiologically . . . **Cracked tooth**
   Not as above . . . **Normal or consider pain of another location**

ALGORITHM FOR KEYING PROBLEMS OF HEADACHE

1. Well-defined symptoms preceding unilateral head pain . . . 2
   Less well-defined symptoms, unilateral or bilateral head or neck pain . . . 4
2. Throbbing pain, gastrointestinal disturbance, blurred vision, no rhinorrhea . . . 3
   Mild to moderate pain, no gastrointestinal disturbance or blurred vision . . . 5
3. Dull pain, visual, motor, or sensory symptoms, behavioral disturbance, alterations in consciousness . . . **Migraine with aura (classic)**
   Mood changes, autonomic disturbances, psychological phenomenon, food cravings . . . **Migraine without aura (common)**

4. Tightness, tenderness in suboccipital muscles, sustained contraction of neck muscles, pain fluctuating during the day, precipitated by fatigue . . . **Tension-type headache**

Steady ache, lower part of orbit or maxillary area, no infection . . . **Atypical facial pain**

5. Boring, burning, or severe periorbital pain; attacks lasting 15 minutes to 3 hours, occurring in clusters for weeks and then disappearing; ptosis in 25% to 30% of patients . . . **Cluster**

Not as above . . . 6

6. Seizures, loss of neurologic function or consciousness, mental changes . . . **Intracranial vascular, infection, or tumor headaches**

Not as above . . . 7

7. Localized pain mimicking migraine, occurring on a daily basis, associated with trauma . . . **Trauma headache**

Not associated with trauma . . . 8

8. Headache associated with substances (eg, caffeine, alcohol, tobacco, and drugs) or their withdrawal . . . **Withdrawal headache**

Not as above . . . **Referral to neurologist**

ALGORITHM FOR KEYING NEURAL PROBLEMS MIMICKING TMD

1. Pain paroxysmal . . . 2

Pain continuous . . . 6

2. Sharp, stabbing, or shooting pain following nerve distribution . . . 3

Not as above . . . 6

3. Electric-like bursts of pain of short duration, unilateral, trigger zone in lips or cheek, usually eliminated by nerve V block . . . **Trigeminal neuralgia**

Not localized to lips or cheek, not eliminated by nerve block . . . 4

4. Pain or altered sensitivity along the skin in the temporal, zygomatic, cervicofacial, and chin areas and in the anterior two-thirds of tongue, possible altered taste sensitivity (both usually eliminated by nerve VII block) . . . **Facial nerve neuralgia**

Pain localized to throat . . . 5

5. Pain provoked by swallowing or chewing, trigger zone in tonsillar or posterior pharyngeal area, normal radiology of styloid process . . . **Glossopharyngeal neuralgia**

Pain provoked by turning of head, radiologic evidence of elongated styloid process . . . **Eagle's syndrome**

6. History of nerve trauma to face . . . 7

Without history of facial trauma, but history of trauma to extremity . . . 8

7. Dull ache in tooth after root canal therapy or extraction, radiation to adjacent tissues, negative radiology, usually relieved by local anesthesia . . . **Atypical odontalgia**

Pain rarely localized to surgical site or fracture . . . **Traumatic neuroma**

8. Dull, burning pain, history of varicella-zoster virus . . . 9

Without history of varicella-zoster virus . . . 10

9. Dysesthesia, pain along nerve followed by vesicles (shingles) on nose or face . . . **Postherpetic neuralgia**

    Rare vesicles in auditory canal, followed by severe lancinating pain in canal, possible nerve VII palsy . . . **Geniculate neuralgia**

10. Rare, severe hyperpathy on moving or touching the skin, disuse atrophy of limb, early relief with sympathetic ganglion block . . . **Reflex sympathetic dystrophy (causalgia)**

    None of above . . . normal or seek neurologic consultation

ALGORITHM FOR KEYING LESS COMMON DISORDERS MIMICKING TMD

1. Vague headache or intense pressure in frontal, maxillary, ethmoid, or sphenoid cavities following infection, pain increased by lowering the head, intact tympanum, opacification of the antrum radiographically if severe . . . **Sinusitis**

    Not as above . . . 2

2. Infection in middle ear, ear pain, inflamed tympanum, fluid behind tympanum confirmed by tympanometry or air insufflation into auditory meatus . . . **Otitis media**

    Not as above . . . 3

3. Unilateral, nonspecific postnasal irritation and obstruction, restricted movement of soft palate, sudden hearing loss, posterior triangle adenopathy limiting mastication . . . . . . **Nasopharyngeal carcinoma**

    Not in pharynx . . . 4

4. Unilateral or bilateral ear pain, skin sensitivity, long-standing hearing loss confirmed by audiogram, vertigo exacerbated by head movement . . . **Acoustic neuroma**

    No hearing loss or vertigo . . . 5

5. Swelling, redness, and tenderness over gland, suppuration from duct, pain worst when eating . . . **Parotitis**

    Tenderness over temples, constant throbbing pain, elevated erythrocyte sedimentation rate, arterial pathology confirmed by biopsy . . . **Giant cell (temporal) arteritis**

ALGORITHM FOR KEYING AXIS I PSYCHOLOGICAL DISORDERS POSSIBLY ASSOCIATED WITH TMD

1. The development of symptoms associated with a physical traumatic event affecting general responsiveness outside the range of human experience . . . **Post-traumatic stress disorder**

    Not trauma-related . . . 2

2. A disturbance usually lasting less than 6 months, but may recur . . . 3

    Excessive fear, worry, or concern . . . 5

3. Mood disturbance lasting at least 2 weeks with loss of interest or pleasure in all activities . . . **Depression (major)**

    Depressed mood lasting for 6 months or more . . . 4

4. One or more depressive episodes accompanied by manic episodes . . . **Bipolar disorder**

   Depressed mood for most of day and for more days than not for at least 2 years . . . **Dysthymia**

5. Maladaptive reaction to identifiable psychosocial stressors occurring within 3 months after onset . . . **Adjustment disorder**

   Frequent, unrealistic worry . . . 6

6. Discrete periods of intense fear or discomfort . . . **Panic disorder**

   No fear . . . 7

7. Excessive worry about two or more life circumstances, person is bothered by concerns more days than not . . . **Generalized anxiety disorder**

   Not as above . . . 8

8. Time-consuming obsession or compulsion in functions unrelated to health concerns causing marked distress that interferes with daily activities . . . **Obsessive-compulsive disorder**

   Similar but health-related concerns . . . 9

9. Multiple somatic complaints with no frank physical findings for which medical attention is sought . . . **Somatization disorder**

   Preoccupation with pain in the absence of physical evidence of disease . . . **Somatoform pain disorder**

ALGORITHM FOR KEYING AXIS II PERSONALITY DISORDERS POSSIBLY ASSOCIATED WITH TMD

1. A pervasive pattern of peculiarities of ideation, appearance, and behavior with deficits in interpersonal relatedness . . . **Schizotypal personality disorder**

   No ideation with deficits . . . 2

2. A pattern of excessive emotionality and attention gathering . . . **Histrionic personality disorder**

   No attention gathering . . . 3

3. Social discomfort, fear of negative evaluation, and timidity . . . **Avoidant personality disorder**

   No fear of negative evaluation . . . 4

4. Pattern of passive resistance to demands for adequate social and occupational performance . . . **Passive-aggressive personality disorder**

   No resistance to demands . . . 5

5. Pattern of perfection and inflexibility . . . **Obsessive-compulsive personality disorder**

   No pattern of perfection . . . 6

6. Unwarranted tendency to interpret actions of others as deliberately threatening . . . **Paranoid personality disorder**

   No sense of being threatened . . . 7

7. Pattern of self-defeating behavior . . . **Self-defeating personality disorder**

   Instability of self image, interpersonal relationships, and mood . . . **Borderline personality disorder**

References

1. Fricton JR, Kroening R. Practical differential diagnosis of chronic craniofacial pain. Oral Surg Oral Med Oral Pathol 1982;54:628.
2. Bell WE. Temporomandibular disorders, 2nd ed. Chicago: Year Book, 1986.
3. Fricton JR, Schiffman EL. Reliability of a Craniomandibular Index. J Dent Res 1986;65:1359.
4. Mersky H. Classification of chronic pain: description of chronic pain syndromes and definition of pain terms. Pain Suppl 3. Amsterdam: Elsevier, 1986;S$_1$.
5. Clark GT, Seligman DA, Solberg WK, Pullinger AG. Guidelines for the examination and diagnosis of temporomandibular disorders. J Craniomandib Disord 1989;3:7.
6. McDonald JS, Pensak ML, Phero JC. Differential diagnosis of chronic facial, head, and neck pain conditions, part 1. Am J Otol 1990;11:299.
7. American Academy of Craniomandibular Disorders. Craniomandibular disorders: guidelines for evaluation, diagnosis, and management. Chicago: Quintessence, 1990.
8. Pertes RA, Heir GM. Chronic orofacial pain: a practical approach to differential diagnosis. Dent Clin North Am 1991;35:123.
9. Truelove EL, Sommers EE, LeResche L, Dworkin SF, Von Korff M. Clinical diagnostic criteria for TMD: new classification permits multiple diagnoses. J Am Dent Assoc 1992;123:47.
10. Laskin DM, Block S. Diagnosis and treatment of myofacial pain-dysfunction (MPD) syndrome. J Prosthet Dent 1986;56:75.
11. Truta MP, Santucci ET. Head and neck fibromyalgia and temporomandibular arthralgia. Otolaryngol Clin North Am 1989;22:1159.
12. Eversole LR, Machado L. Temporomandibular joint internal derangements and associated neuromuscular disorders. J Am Dent Assoc 1985;110:69.
13. Bush FM, Whitehill JM, Martelli MF. Pain assessment in temporomandibular disorders. J Craniomandib Pract 1989;72:137.
14. Bush FM, Harrington WG, Harkins SW. Interexaminer comparison of bone scintigraphy and panoramic radiography of temporomandibular joints: correlation with signs and symptoms. J Prosthet Dent 1992;67:246.
15. Butterworth JC, Deardorff WW. Internal derangements: a comment on the need for diagnostic homogeneity. J Craniomandib Disord 2:148.
16. Schiffman E, Anderson G, Fricton J, Buton K, Schellhas K. Diagnostic criteria for intraarticular T. M. disorders. Community Dent Oral Epidemiol 1989;17:252.
17. Rihani A. Maxillary sinusitis as a differential diagnosis in temporomandibular joint pain-dysfunction syndrome. J Prosthet Dent 1985;53:97.
18. Vigneau D, David JM, Calvet H, Pesswey J, Lacomme Y. A propos de 63 tumeurs malignes des fosses nasales et des sinus. Rev Laryngol Otol Rhinol (Bord) 1986;107:373.
19. Friedman WH, Rosenblum BN. Paranasal sinus etiology of headaches and facial pain. Otolaryngol Clin North Am 1989;22:1217.
20. Pincus RL. Nasopharyngeal obstruction. Otolaryngol Clin North Am 1989;22:367.
21. Ingle JI, Beveridge EE. Endodontics, 3rd ed. Philadelphia, Lea & Febiger, 1985.

22. Saper JR. Migraine, migraine variants, and related headaches. Otolaryngol Clin North Am 1989;22:1115.

23. Ryan RE, Jr, Ryan RE, Sr. Cluster headaches. Otolaryngol Clin North Am 1989;22:1131.

24. Olesen J. The classification and diagnosis of headache disorders. In Headache: assessment and management. Refresher Course Syllabus. Seattle: International Association for the Study of Pain, 1993:107.

25. German DS. Acoustic neuroma confused with TMD. J Am Dent Assoc 1991;122:59–60.

26. Selesnick SH, Jackler RK. Clinical manifestations and audiologic diagnosis of acoustic neuromas. Otolaryngol Clin North Am 1992;25:521–551.

27. Keith DA, Glyman ML. Intratemporal space pathosis mimicking TMJ disorders. J Am Dent Assoc 1991;122:59.

28. American Psychiatric Association. Diagnostic and statistical manual of mental disorders, 3rd rev ed. Washington, DC: American Psychiatric Association, 1987.

29. American Psychiatric Association. Diagnostic and statistical manual of mental disorders, 4th ed. Washington, DC: American Psychiatric Association, 1994.

30. Reich J, Rosenblatt RM, Tupin J. DSM-III: a new nomenclature for classifying patients with chronic pain. Pain 1983;16:201.

31. Kinney RK, Gatchel RJ, Ellis E, Holt C. Major psychological disorders in chronic TMD patients: implications for successful management. J Am Dent Assoc 1992;123:49.

The Temporomandibular Joint and Related Orofacial Disorders,
by Francis M. Bush and M. Franklin Dolwick.
J.B. Lippincott Company, Philadelphia, © 1995.

9

Conservative Treatment

O pinions about the treatment of TMD are as controversial as beliefs about the etiology of TMD and the technical aids used to diagnose this disorder. Traditional methods have focused on correcting functional bite disharmonies or anatomic malalignments. Present trends favor TMD as a musculoskeletal disorder that is treatable with simple procedures.

By and large, there are insufficient data to permit comparison of different therapies and thus to establish a priority for their use. Many treatments routinely prescribed today for musculoskeletal disorders have never been tested clinically for safety or effectiveness. Therefore, the management of TMD should begin with conservative, reversible measures and escalate slowly to irreversible procedures if necessary (Table 9-1).

A sampling of 472 dentists of the American Equilibration Society showed that the most common treatments for TMD were intraoral appliance (84%), occlusal adjustment (45%), nutrition (40%), relaxation and stress management (40%), physiotherapy (37%), and counseling (36%).[1] Differences existed between general dentists and dental specialists for some lesser used treatments.

Another survey of dentists' knowledge and beliefs indicates the lack of uniformity about the kind of treatment needed (Table 9-2).[2] Using the opinions of a selected panel of TMD "experts," a higher percentage of dental specialists concurred with the experts than did general dentists. Usually, the percentages for the specialists were lower than for the experts. This trend existed among responses for which no statistical differences were found between generalists and specialists (Table 9-3). The authors attributed some differences to outright disagreement with expert opinion or to the uncertainty of specialists and general dentists about specific issues.

Table 9-1

Treatment Continuum for Orofacial Pain

Lowest Risk, Self-Help Measures	Minimum Risk, Conservative Therapies	Invasive Procedures	
		Moderate Risk	*High Risk*
Home care	Medications Oral appliance Physical therapy Manual therapy Exercises Relaxation Biofeedback Support groups Counseling/psychotherapy	Acupuncture Nerve blocks Chemical injections Occlusal rehabilitation	Nerve destructive agents Surgery

Table 9-2

Statistically Significant Differences ($P \leq 0.05$) in Opinions of General Dentists and Dental Specialists Regarding TMD Treatment. Opinions of Experts Used as the Basis for Comparison.

Treatment	Experts Disagreeing With Statement (%)	Concurring With Experts (%)	
		General Dentists	*Dental Specialists*
Occlusal adjustment is a useful early modality.	85	30	43
Orthodontics prevents TMD.	77	14	35
Orthodontics resolves TMD in patients with skeletal malocclusions.	92	29	50
Tomographic evidence and crepitus indicate need for treatment	77	25	40
All individuals with clicking need treatment.	100	93	98
PRN narcotics are treatment of choice for severe TMD pain.	93	42	56
Antidepressants are never indicated for TMD.	88	50	62
Extensive prior history of treatment failure is usually indication for surgery.	100	70	80

Modified from Le Resche L, Truelove EL, Dworkin SF. Temporomandibular disorders: a survey of dentists' knowledge and beliefs. J Am Dent Assoc 1993;124:90.

Table 9-3
Nonstatistical Differences ($P \geq 0.05$) in Opinions of General Dentists and Dental Specialists Regarding Treatment. Opinions of Experts Used as Basis for Comparison.

Treatment	Experts' Opinion (%)	Concurring With Experts (%)	
		General Dentists	*Dental Specialists*
Disagreement			
Mandibular repositioning splints are more effective than maxillary splints.	90	45	43
Progressive muscle relaxation is not an effective treatment.	82	62	62
Agreement			
Ice packs or heat packs and passive muscle stretching are good early treatments.	100	74	70
Biofeedback can be useful treatment.	77	50	58
Stress management is indicated for many patients.	100	91	89
Behavior modification treatments are appropriate for chronic pain.	88	80	82

Modified from Le Resche L, Truelove EL, Dworkin, SF. Temporomandibular disorders: a survey of dentists' knowledge and beliefs. J Am Dent Assoc 1993;124:90.

Treatment or Referral?

Practitioners face the problem of treating or referring patients with TMD. There is no ready solution about the direction to take. If initial management is directed to control of pain, improved function can be expected to follow.[3] For successful management of pain, the practitioner needs to know a spectrum of pharmacologic, anesthetic, psychiatric, noninvasive, and psychological approaches.[4] Few solo practitioners possess this expertise.

With the best interest of the patient in mind, several guidelines are recommended for practitioners. If the patient can be treated more effectively by someone else, referral should be the choice. If the clinician elects to manage acute pain, mild to moderate improvement can be expected within 1 week to 10 days. For treatment of chronic complaints, if no improvement occurs by 2 months, a change in treatment strategy or a referral is in order.

The next question is to whom you should refer the patient. If health problems other than TMD compromise treatment, these should be managed by the patient's primary care physician. For confusing clinical findings, other specialists may be consulted. If the magnitude of the patient's problem is vast, pain management should be handled in a multidisciplinary pain center. These centers have sufficient equipment and the personnel with skills to diagnose and treat complex head and neck complaints. Comprehensive care can be achieved with optional modalities unavailable to many solo practitioners.

Letter of Referral

A letter of referral to another clinician should precede the initial visit made by the patient. The following information is helpful to the receiving clinician:

- The patient's name, address, and phone number should be identified.
- A brief statement should be made about the patient's primary complaint and about the duration and possible etiology.
- Clinical findings should be addressed. Remarks should be made about previous diagnoses and treatments for the condition.
- The clinician's name, address, and phone number should be identified.

For referral to a physical therapist, a prescription with at least a minimum of information is necessary (Fig. 9-1).

- Identification of the patient
- Written instructions with the clinician's signature
- Diagnostic impression
- Identification of the anatomic areas to be treated
- Kind of treatment
- Number and duration of treatment
- Expectation of a written post-treatment report sent to the clinician.

Treatment Guidelines and Goals

In treating the TMD patient, the primary goals are to:

1. Achieve normal jaw function.
2. Reduce or eliminate pain.
3. Encourage a return to normal activities of daily living.
4. Reduce long-term health care use.

Other important goals are to:

5. Improve the patients' understanding of the complaint.
6. Improve the patients' management of the complaint.
7. Eliminate unhelpful thinking about the complaint.
8. Increase the patients' confidence in his or her ability to function and cope.
9. Reduce or eliminate powerful medications.

TEMPOROMANDIBULAR JOINT – OROFACIAL PAIN CENTER
VIRGINIA COMMONWEALTH UNIVERSITY

P.O Box 566 MCV Station   (804)7869651   Richmond, VA 23298

Name *J. M. Jones*   Date   *9/30/93*

Address *16 N. 5th St., Richmond, Va 23298*

Diagnosis: Left masseter muscle soreness
Treatment: Please apply dexamethasone cream
iontophoretically to the left masseter muscle region.
Treat at 1.5mA for 5–6 min. positive and 10–12
min. negative at 3–7 day intervals for a month.

Please provide a written post-treatment
report upon completion of treatment.

5076   *Francis M Bush DMD*

Clinician's number   Clinician's signature

Figure 9-1.
Sample of a prescription submitted to the physical therapist authorizing treatment of a patient.

Clinician–Patient Relationship

Success in managing TMD requires an ongoing assessment of the patient's complaint. Patients need to form a healing partnership with the clinician. Once management begins, the clinician should discuss treatment issues with the patient.

Clinicians should ensure patients a place in the "communications loop." They should encourage patients to ask questions and voice concerns. Each question, complaint, or request requires consideration and an appropriate response. Clinicians should educate patients about the most appropriate means of meeting their needs rather than dictating to them. Family members may request information about the patient's diagnosis or condition; if these requests are made, the patient should be present to maintain the bounds of privacy. Patients or family members may also ask about appropriate credentials of the practitioner and other health care workers.

It may be necessary to offer specific explanations about certain symptoms. With acute complaints, the clinician should pay attention to sensory components of the patient's pain.[5] For example, patients want to know if the intensity or frequency of the pain will increase or decrease. They may ask if the pain will move to another location. With chronic complaints, the clinician should address psychosocial and behavioral factors that affect the patient.

Frequently, patients want to know about the long-term progression of their disorder. Conclusions drawn about the progression of painful conditions are informative. An account of 55 untreated patients suffering with TMJ osteoarthritis showed that joint pain had nearly disappeared by 9 months.[6] A period of discomfort characterized by joint crepitus burned out by 2 to 3 years. This finding differs from a report of the progression of myofascial pain of the masticatory muscles. Evidence indicates that the condition is not self-limiting, may increase in severity, and may lead to joint problems. An examination conducted by an examiner blind to the status of the masticatory muscles in 25 patients suffering with myofascial pain and in a control sample of 25 healthy subjects showed that muscular tenderness persisted after 3 years.[7] Finally, if the pattern of TMD pain follows the evolution of other chronic musculoskeletal pains, it can be expected to persist in slightly less than two thirds of individuals and disappear in one third.[8] Patients need to be informed that none of the patterns of response is absolute.

The clinician should inform the patient that it is possible to use noninvasive procedures to avoid rather than treat pain (see Table 9-1). The value of noninvasive management should be explained fully to the patient.

The patient should be given a concise explanation of the recommended procedure. Details should include a discussion of the procedure's purpose (ie, why it is necessary), what is expected of the patient, what the patient might expect, approximate time of response or result, and the patient's right to refuse treatment. Simple diagrams of procedures are often helpful.

The facts about controversial treatments should be provided. The clinician should make an effort to correct any misinformation, particularly when the procedure's efficacy has not been established. An explanation of the therapy should be based on a consensus of research findings and on the clinical experience of practitioners in the field. Reassurance about treatment safety is a must. Patients should not be subjected to any unnecessary treatment.

The clinician may have to tell patients that successful management requires medication. Although some patients refuse medications, relief can be achieved in a high percentage of patients by dosing "around the clock." The problem for the clinician is in choosing the appropriate medication. The problem for the patient is compliance.

Significance: No one is capable of managing someone else's pain. Patients must learn this early in treatment. Practitioners can only assist patients to come to terms with untoward physiologic and emotional reactions that affect them.

Conservative Program of Home Care

Although patients can receive instructions from the clinician by telephone, they can obtain more useful information by visiting the clinician. Therapy described only in verbal terms frequently limits success. Patients need a written reminder of what is expected at the office visit. To avoid misinterpretation, this information should be spelled out, in writing, in words that the patient understands. Sticky notes can be placed in convenient areas around the patient's home as reminders.

Patient compliance is a must. Patients should be made aware of the need to take responsibility for treating their complaints. Research findings confirm that most

TMD discomfort arises from muscle-based pain. In a study of 295 TMD patients who visited a private practice, 87% were classified as suffering from myogenous pain.[9] This finding agrees with the occurrence of muscular pain found among patients admitted to TMD clinics around the world. Thus, therapy should focus on obtaining relief of muscular pain.

Home care practices have proved effective in management of TMD. Nearly three fourths of patients managed for 2 years obtained total resolution or improvement in their condition with simple therapies.[9] Some home care practices are discussed below.[3,9,10]

Reassurance

Patients should be reassured that most acute TMD symptoms are self-limiting. Self recognition of the physical basis for muscle symptoms is difficult. Typically, acute muscle complaints last 7 to 10 days. Exacerbations may recur periodically, but once pain diminishes, normal function should return.

Placebo Effect

A placebo is a form of therapy given for suggestive effect. Some symptoms may be relieved by rendering harmless therapy to the patient. A healthy physiologic response may result from the patient's enthusiasm and desire for cure, from the clinician's enthusiasm and desire to please the patient, or from an unexpected side reaction.[11]

Rest and Diet

A diet of soft foods can be recommended, particularly if there is acute pain. It should be continued for as long as 2 weeks.

Avoidance of excessive caffeine, sugar, and alcohol may help. These substances change the patient's daily mood. Although not proved convincingly, mood swings tend to intensify pain.

A regular sleep schedule of at least 7 hours a night should be followed. An orthopedic pillow may relieve neck complaints. Sleeping on the back helps if the patient has jaw pain. Placing a sore jaw against a hard surface tends to worsen the pain during sleep.

Relaxation

Patients should be instructed to control excessive oral habits. This awareness of bruxism can be taught by asking patients to "feel" their tight jaw muscles once the teeth are clenched. A conscious effort should be made to keep their teeth apart.

A program involving "deep breathing" may benefit the patient. Clinicians should instruct the patient to practice this exercise for 3 to 5 minutes every hour, particularly during painful episodes.

Avoidance

There should be no "overuse" of the jaw, including excessive talking on the telephone, yawning, choir singing, or playing of wind instruments. Rapid, jerky stretching movements of the jaw should be avoided. Once the acute pain diminishes, a few stretching exercises can be performed.

Active Range of Motion

Individuals with healthy TMJs can achieve "three finger" opening of the mouth. An inability to perform this "check" indicates limitation on opening. Restriction may result from muscle or joint dysfunction, or both.

For this check, the patient is instructed to open the mouth as wide as possible. The index, middle and fourth digits are aligned adjacent to one another and inserted perpendicular to the lips between the upper and lower central incisors. This check, and moving the mandible to the right, left, forward, and backward can be done twice weekly, 6 times for each movement.[12]

Use of Heat

Moist heat from a heating pad, hot water bottle, Hydrocollator, or hot pack placed on sore muscles of the jaw has proved effective in relieving jaw pain. Moist heat delivered by a heating pad for 6 weeks reduced painful jaw symptoms by about 35% in 19 of 27 TMD patients, whereas a 4% reduction in symptoms occurred in the remaining 8 untreated patients during this period.[13] Application of moist heat on the jaw (20 minutes, 2 to 3 times daily) increased mouth opening up to 9 mm after 12 days of treatment in 55 patients with progressive degeneration of the TMJ.[14] At the final evaluation, 31% required no further treatment.

Moist heat can be delivered according to following recipe:[15]

1. Damp washcloth—next to skin
2. Plastic wrap
3. Dry towel—four layers
4. Heating pad
5. Duration: 20 minutes, 2 to 3 times a day at temperature tolerance

Use of Ice

Ice can be applied directly to the skin or applied with a separating medium between the skin and ice. Application of ice directly exceeds the efficacy of an ice pack in reducing skin temperature.[16] Tolerance to ice improves after a few applications.

Ice from water frozen in a paper cup can be applied in a massaging manner across an affected area. If an ice pack is chosen, the following alcohol ice-pack recipe has been recommended.[15]

1. 1/2 cup rubbing alcohol
2. 1 cup water

3. Pour into a pint-size reclosable plastic bag and freeze
4. Place ice pack on top of moist towel against the skin
5. Duration: 20 minutes, 2 to 3 times a day at temperature tolerance

Stretching and Massage

Most patients fail to stretch on a regular basis. Muscle flexibility is achieved by stretching the muscle to its normal length. Like muscles of other joints, muscles of the TMJ region shorten if they are not stretched properly. Limited motion of the jaw can ensue. In the presence of pain, the restriction worsens the outcome.

Gentle massage of tender muscles before stretching often aids in relief of pain. Massage and stretching are more tolerable after use of heat and ice. Cold water packs coupled with stretching of the jaw and the neck proved effective as a short-term intervention for relief in 10 TMD patients.[17] Comparison of pre- and post-treatment ratings showed that self-report of pain was significantly reduced after 2 weeks of treatment. No significant effect was found for tenderness of muscles to palpation or for range of motion.

Medications

The patient's history in use of medication provides the clinician more complete understanding of the complaint. Most have some history involving over-the-counter analgesics. Many have discovered that TMD pain responds poorly to these analgesics when no other form of treatment has been rendered.

Significance: This conservative program of home care may have the following results: (1) improvement in symptoms with no other treatment needed; (2) no change in symptoms and continuation of the same treatment; or (3) marked increase in symptoms with other treatment needed.

Optional Therapies

If home care management proves ineffective, the patient may require specific advice and special care other from health care practitioners. To obtain a successful outcome, more complex medications and accessory therapies such as intraoral appliances, physiotherapy, behavioral modification, and occlusal and surgical treatments may be needed.[18,19] Evidence for and against many common therapies is discussed below.

Medications

Orofacial pain may be severe and require specific medications (Table 9-4). Acute therapy is aimed at stopping the symptoms or reducing the discomfort of an attack. Medication should be given as early as possible as the initial treatment approach. Once selected, the medication should be prescribed in the optimal formulation for each patient. Care is needed to explain the distinction between acute and prophylactic medication to avoid unwarranted side effects.

Table 9-4
Medications Commonly Used in the Treatment of Orofacial Pain

Medication	Dosage/Schedule	Effect
Anti-inflammatories		
Ibuprofen	200–400 mg q 4–6 h	Analgesic, antipyretic, antiprostaglandin, limited relief of muscular pain
Meclofenamate	200 mg/d	
Salicylate	500–1000 mg/d	
Naproxen	500 mg initial q 12 h	
	250 mg subsequent	
Anxiolytics		
Diazepam	2–10 mg q 6 h	Sedation, psychological dependency
Lorazepam	0.5–3 mg q 6–12 h	
Alprazolam	0.25 mg q 6 h	
Antiheadache		
Sumatriptan	6 mg (s.c.) maximum twice/ 24 h	Acute attack, possible cardiac side effects
	100 mg q 8 h	Prophylactic for migraine
Propanolol	40 mg q 6–8 h	Prophylactic for migraine
100% oxygen	71 min/mask/15 min	Acute attack prophylactic for cluster
Methysergide	2 mg q 8–12 h	
Antidepressants		
Amitriptyline	25 mg q 8 h	Sedation, analgesia, drying effects
Doxepin	25 mg q 8 h	
Cyclobenzaprine	10 mg q 12 h	Analgesia poor, muscle relaxation
Muscle Relaxants		
Carisoprodol	350 mg q 6 h	Sedation, no direct muscle relaxation
Methocarbamol	1.5 g q 6 h initial	
	1.0 g q 6 h subsequent	
Anticonvulsants*		
Baclofen	40–80 mg/d	Relief of neurogenic pain, trigeminal neuralgia
Carbamazepine	400–1200 mg/d	
Phenytoin	300–600 mg/d	
Antihistamines		
Diphenhydramine	25–50 mg q 6–8 h	Drying, sedation, drowsiness, coordination decreased

Adapted from Physicians' desk reference. Oradell, NJ: Medical Economics, 1993.

*After Merrill RL, Graff-Radford SB. Trigeminal neuralgia: how to rule out the wrong treatment. J Am Dent Assoc 1992;123:63.

Once acute relief is obtained, the patient should be given the option of prophylactic management. Some patients assume a cure once mild relief occurs and may stop the medication. If other therapies have failed to provide lasting relief, a program of polymedication may be required.

A recent study of 109 patients treated by medications for chronic pain showed that 56% of compliant patients achieved relief, whereas 75% of noncompliant patients had no change in pain severity.[20] Compliant patients were more satisfied with outcome than noncompliant patients.

Muscular Pain

Acute muscular pain responds poorly to most analgesics, yet they are the medication most frequently prescribed by both general dentists and dental specialists.[1] About 39% of dentists prescribe anti-inflammatory medication. Combination treatment with an anxiolytic agent has been suggested to improve relief, but no definitive superiority has been demonstrated by taking both simultaneously.[21] If sedation is desired, a low dose of diphenylhydramine may be substituted for the muscle relaxant.

For generalized myofascial pain, a tricyclic antidepressant (eg, amitriptyline) taken at a low dosage produces analgesia. Few dentists prescribe antidepressants. A survey of dentists showed that about 9% prescribe antidepressants for TMD.[1] If prescribed, patients tend to associate the antidepressant with the stigma of having a psychiatric disorder. They may consider it a permanent reminder of a chronic illness that they view as a weakness. Reassurance may be necessary because many patients are reluctant to take even the lowest dose recommended.

Amitriptyline has proved effective in treating patients with widespread myofascial pain, termed *fibromyalgia*. A study of 23 double-blind, randomized, cross-over trials showed that this medication was 74% effective in final management.[22] The effect was evident within 2 weeks of therapy. Conclusions were based on findings of a symptom questionnaire and count of tender points. The medication was so effective that 35% of the cases were able to discontinue its use. Other evidence points to the benefit of this therapy. Four of 8 myofascial pain dysfunction patients who were unresponsive to biofeedback training achieved remission of symptoms by the second week of antidepressant therapy.[23]

For patients suffering from chronic somatoform pain, decreased pain intensity and increased level of activity may result from using amitriptyline.[24] The effects of medication were less predictable if patients required psychotherapy. Side effects of amitriptyline include dry mouth, weight gain, and sedation. Patients should be encouraged to drink plenty of water and to chew sugarless gum or eat candy. Although improvement may be expected within 2 weeks, up to 8 weeks may be needed for some patients to gain relief.

Schedule: The dosage schedule for amitriptyline is 10 mg/night for 3 days, increasing the dose to 20 mg/night for 3 days, to 25 mg/night for 3 days, and up to 50 mg/night for 3 days, as needed.[23]

Polyarthritic Disease

For treatment of generalized osteoarthritis, nonsteroidal anti-inflammatory drugs (NSAIDs) have proved useful agents despite their possible deleterious effects on joint loading and metabolism of cartilage.[25] NSAIDs may be coupled with an antidepressant, but combining medications makes it difficult to discern individual efficacy.

Ibuprofen appears moderately effective as an antiarthritic for TMD. In a double-blind study of 14 TMD patients treated for 6 weeks with 1600 mg/day of ibuprofen and 14 TMD patients treated by placebo, 64% of those receiving ibuprofen had complete remission of symptoms, whereas 42% of those receiving placebo had a similar result.[26]

Headache

Many medications are available for treating headache. Some are more effective against one form of headache than another. Sumatriptan, a self-injectable, may provide sudden relief for emergency treatment of migraine and cluster headache.[27,28] Because the side effects include transient elevation in blood pressure and decreased heart rate, the initial dose of 6 mg subcutaneously should be given in the clinician's office. A maximum dose of 2 injections/day with a 1-hour interval between injections is recommended. Sumatriptan may be taken prophylactically. No major side effects were found after use for 11 months.[29] Propanolol is a useful alternative.

A comparative study of 20 patients with headache and TMD pain showed that meclofenamate reduced pain significantly more than placebo treatment.[30] This double-blind, cross-over study with a washout period showed that subjects in pain had fewer painful days, shorter duration of pain, and a lower number of hyperthermic zones while using this medication.

Among 100 patients with chronic headache, 55 had significant TMD pain.[31] The authors hypothesized a relation between headache and pain localized in the masticatory muscles. Half of the patients were treated by a dentist and half by a neurologist. Headache intensity and medication use dropped significantly in the half treated by dentists.

Dental Pain

If routine dental treatment fails to relieve the patient's pain, a medicament strategy devised for the management of acute dental pain may prove helpful (Fig. 9-2).[32] This strategy may aid in the management of other acute forms of orofacial pain. If treatment of mild pain fails, major episodes are managed by more potent and alternate medications. Certain medications require special consideration and need to be discussed with the patient. Codeine has limited effectiveness in oral pain. About three fourths of patients taking oxycodone experience dizziness, nausea, and drowsiness.

Sinus Inflammation

Symptoms similar to dental pain may result from sinusitis. This complaint is over-diagnosed as a source of orofacial pain. Furthermore, idiopathic headache is often

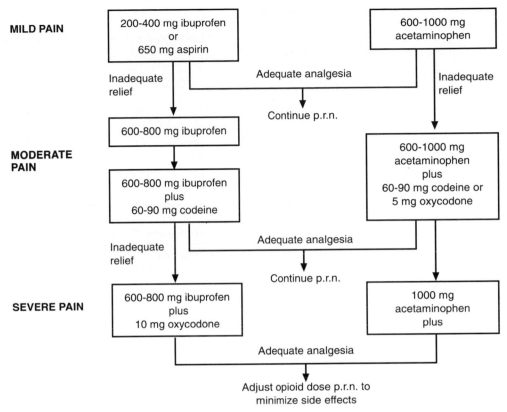

Figure 9-2.
Therapeutic strategy for management of acute dental pain. (Dionne RA. New approaches to preventing and treating postoperative pain. J Am Dent Assoc 1992;123:27.)

termed *sinus headache*. This latter description has not been classified by the Headache Classification Committee of the International Headache Society.[33] Patients with frank sinusitis may be referred to an ear, nose, and throat specialist, who will most likely prescribe some combination of antibiotics, analgesics, and decongestants.

Trigeminal Neuralgia

Some relief from neuropathic pain may be achieved with baclofen or carbamazepine. Baclofen is the first choice.[34] Treatment with carbamazepine requires initial medical laboratory work, including complete blood count, differential leukocyte count, and sedimentation rate, and liver function tests. Periodic follow-ups are necessary. The treatment of more complex cases should be conducted in a multidisciplinary setting.

Some symptoms of trigeminal neuralgia may be confused with TMD or dental pains. Studies conducted on 61 patients diagnosed with pretrigeminal or trigeminal neuralgia revealed that 61% had initial dental pain before the neuropathy was diagnosed.[34]

Intraoral Appliances

Various intraoral appliances have proved useful for diagnostic and therapeutic purposes (Table 9-5).

Diagnosis

Bruxism can be demonstrated to the patient by showing tooth wear on the appliance. The duration of parafunctional contact may reach 4 hours/day with a clench force of up to 975 lb.[35] This biting strength contrasts sharply with the duration of functional contact of the teeth of 4 to 10 minutes/day with a force of 20 to 40 lb. The presence versus absence of jaw pain can be demonstrated by an appliance.

Table 9-5

Common Types of Intraoral Appliances Used in the Treatment of TMD

Name	Construction	Purpose	Problems
Flat, full coverage	Acrylic resin; upper or lower; anterior guidance in lateroprotrusive motions; made at retruded jaw position	Relief of jaw pain, bruxism	Bulky—limits tongue, difficulty speaking
Bite plane, anterior	Acrylic resin; upper; anterior guidance	Relief of jaw pain, bruxism; change positional sense	If worn continuously, may cause eruption of posterior teeth
Bite plane, posterior (MORA)*	Acrylic resin; lower; lingual bar connects posterior segments	Relief of jaw pain, bruxism; increase strength and athletic performance; restore vertical dimension	If worn continuously, may cause eruption of anterior teeth
Repositioning splint	Acrylic resin; upper or lower	Guide mandible to anterior position; recapture disk dislocation	If worn continuously, may cause eruption of unopposed teeth or condylar remodeling
Pivot splint covers one or more posterior teeth	Acrylic resin; unilateral or bilateral	Unload or stretch TMJ	If worn continuously, may cause eruption of unopposed teeth
Soft splint, full coverage	Resilent material; upper or lower	Relief of jaw pain, bruxism	May increase muscle activity as teeth touch resilent surface; difficult to adjust
Hydrostatic, full coverage	Resilent material; thin-walled fluid cell	Allows muscles to reposition mandible	Difficult to make and maintain
Plastic tapered cylinder†	Acrylic resin, placed between anterior teeth	Limited opening, activates depressor muscles	Limited to dentulous patients

After Abbott DM, Bush FM, Butler JH. Occlusal appliances. In Clark JW (ed). Clinical dentistry. Philadelphia: Harper & Row, 1987; and Boero RP. The physiology of splint therapy: a literature review. Angle Orthod 1989;59:165.

*Mandibular orthopedic repositioning applicance.
†Lund TW, Cohen JI. Trismus appliances and indications for their use. Quintessence International 1993;24:275.

Therapeutic Benefits

The use of appliances has been recommended after surgery of the TMJ and in the treatment of fibromyalgia of the masticatory muscles, arthralgia, and disk displacement with or without reduction.[36]

Most appliances delivered by practitioners can help the patient avoid tooth wear and fracture. Clinical evidence shows their value in maintaining the health of teeth.[37] Appliances are indicated when there is a need to:

1. Remove occlusal prematurities temporarily.
2. Reduce traumatic forces from occlusion.
3. Prevent occlusal wear or enamel fracture.
4. Maintain loose teeth in a stable position.
5. Aid in establishment of an optimal occlusal pattern and vertical dimension before definitive restorative and prosthetic procedures.

Management of Pain

Certain orofacial pains are relieved by appliances, although the reason for relief is uncertain. The effects may be central, peripheral, or both. Information is too equivocal to support either hypothesis fully.

The presence of central effects is supported by early and more recent findings. There is a nonspecific placebo effect from wearing an appliance, which suggests that the mind affects outcome. A 25% reduction in symptoms was found in TMD patients who wore a placebo splint that covered only the palate.[38] Efficacy can be measured only after it exceeds this 25% reduction. Recent evidence for a central effect is based on the memory of patients for pain. TMD patients' ratings of pain relief obtained after wearing appliances correlated with rate of change in memory, thus showing a central effect. They did not correlate with either pain intensity or pain unpleasantness.[39]

The argument for peripheral effects relates to relief from muscular or joint complaints. Insertion of an appliance often reduces the abnormal muscle activity associated with bruxism or alters the rhythm of excessive masticatory muscle activity. Another argument is that the "bite-raising" effect allows passive stretching of muscle fibers.

A further opinion is that insertion alters the disk–condyle relation, leading to condylar shift at the most anteroposterior "therapeutic" position within the articular fossae. Presumably, this change reduces resting or functional pain, lessens joint sounds, or unlocks restrictive jaw motions.

Design

Different designs have been developed with the aim of achieving specific outcomes (see Table 9-5).[37,40,41] Appliances have been designed either for full or partial coverage. The latter covers either the anterior or the posterior teeth. Evidence for and against their usefulness is discussed.

FULL ARCH APPLIANCES. Flat, full arch appliances are referred to as *stabilization appliances* (Figs. 9-3 and 9-4). Several studies show improvement in painful symptoms from 30% to 90% after their use.[42–45] A recent study showed more than half of 30 TMD patients had complete relief of pain after 1 month of appliance therapy.[43] Joint sounds improved by 78%, and limitation of mandibular movement by 68%. After 13 weeks of wearing the appliance, TMJ pain improved by 70%. Shoulder and neck pain improved by 76% and 52%, respectively.

Electromyographic studies of the anterior temporalis and masseter muscles in 26 myogenous patients showed that wearing a full arch, flat appliance decreased the activity of the temporalis fibers immediately and that this decrease continued for 1 month.[46] Initial improvement occurred to a lesser extent in the masseter muscle.[46,47] Some worsening of pain was associated with minor occlusal interferences; it was eliminated by correcting the occlusal surface.[47]

Full arch appliances proved as effective as a combination of biofeedback and stress management in relieving pain and depression in sample of 58 TMD patients.[48] Assessment was made by self-report of pain and by checking pain on palpation of masticatory muscles after 6 weeks of treatment. A 6-month follow-up of treated patients revealed that neither post-treatment depression scores nor pain measures were significantly different from pretreatment scores. Treatment with biofeedback and stress management reduced depression, but no changes were found for pain measures. A combination of appliance, biofeedback, and stress management effectively relieved pain and depression. These findings on improvement in muscle and pain contrast sharply with other studies.

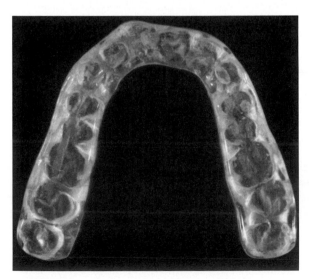

Figure 9-3.
Flat, full arch appliance used to treat TMD. This appliance is recommended for most complaints.

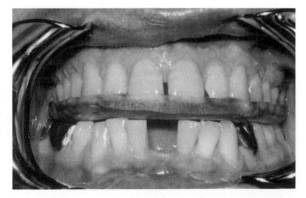

Figure 9-4.
Frontal view of a flat, full arch appliance seated on the maxillary teeth. The border surrounding the anterior teeth may be removed for aesthetic reasons.

A different outcome was reported among 10 patients treated with a flat appliance and 10 treated with a mandibular repositioning appliance.[49] Based on the Helkimo dysfunction index, no significant change in functional, TMJ, or muscle pain was found after wearing the flat appliance. Reciprocal clicking was not reduced in 8 patients. With the repositioning appliance, TMJ and muscle pain improved significantly. Eight of the subjects had no reciprocal sounds at the end of the 90-day treatment period. Another study of 51 TMD patients found that flat appliances were no better than no treatment for TM disk displacement without reduction.[50]

Pro: When a flat appliance can be shown to reduce symptoms significantly, it should be the appliance of choice.[51] Reduction in temporalis muscle activity can be expected based on findings of two studies.[46,52] If no improvement occurs within 2 months, another strategy is necessary.

If properly adjusted, full arch, flat appliances prevent the overeruption of teeth. They can be adapted to complete dentures by use of ball clasps.[36] They can be coupled with a biofeedback and stress management program to alleviate pain and depression in some patients.

Con: The timing of appliance use[53] and proper adjustment[47] affect the outcome. Patient compliance is less likely during an acute episode of pain and is poor if the appliance is ill-fitting.

PARTIAL COVERAGE APPLIANCES. These appliances cover either the anterior or posterior teeth.

An anterior appliance is easy to deliver and adjust (Figs. 9-5 through Fig 9-7), but impressions and mounted dental casts are required for construction. For emergencies, a simple anterior appliance can be constructed by forming uncured acrylic resin into a block. The patient is instructed to retrude the mandible and to open about 10 mm. The "doughy" block is positioned so that about 3 mm of the resin overlaps each of the mandibular and the maxillary incisors. The patient holds this mold with tooth indentations until nearly set. The mold is removed and additional resin is added as needed. The block is cured in warm water, then adjusted and polished. Presumably, tense muscles relax when the patient wears the block. This emergency appliance has been termed an *anterior jig* or *deprogrammer*.

In posterior, partial coverage appliances, a hard acrylic resin covers only the posterior teeth (Figs. 9-8 and 9-9). Some practitioners add excess resin to the bases, thereby increasing the vertical dimension of occlusion.

Pro: Partial coverage appliances are easier to deliver and adjust than flat, full arch appliances.

Con: They can lead to altered occlusions if worn continually (Figs. 9-10 and 9-11). Patients must be warned to wear them either during the night *or* during the day, but never night *and* day. Practitioners should not recommend these appliances routinely.

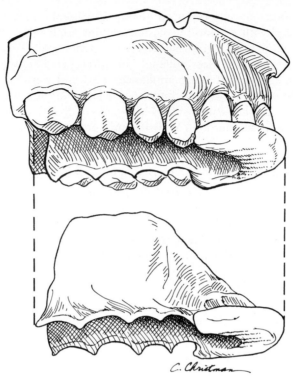

Figure 9-5.
*An anterior, partial coverage used to treat TMD.
(Abbott DM, Bush FM, Butler JH. Occlusal
appliances. In Clark's clinical dentistry. Philadelphia:
Harper & Row, 1987:1.)*

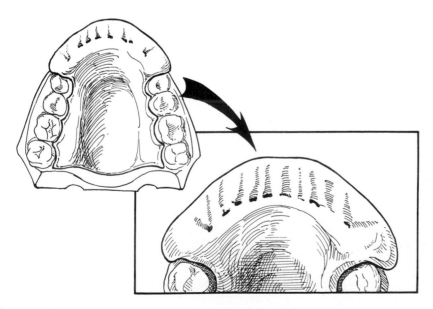

Figure 9-6.
*An anterior, partial coverage
appliance used to treat TMD.
Centric contacts are identified by
the darkest markings on the occlusal
surface, lateral contacts by canine-
guided markings, and straight
protrusive contacts by incisor
markings. (Abbott DM, Bush FM,
Butler JH. Occlusal appliances. In
Clark's clinical dentistry.
Philadelphia: Harper & Row,
1987:1.)*

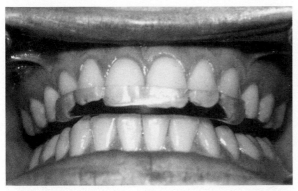

Figure 9-7.
Frontal view of an anterior, partial coverage appliance seated on the maxillary anterior teeth. The absence of posterior contact may contribute to over-eruption of posterior teeth if the appliance is worn continually.

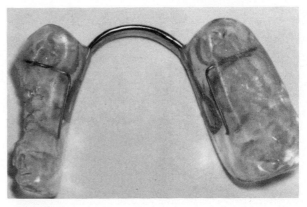

Figure 9-8.
Posterior, partial coverage appliance used to treat TMD. This appliance is often termed a MORA (mandibular orthopedic repositioning appliance).

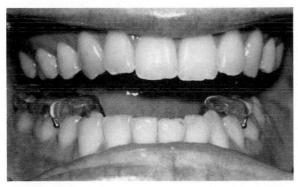

Figure 9-9.
Posterior, partial coverage appliance seated on the mandibular teeth. The absence of anterior contact may contribute to over-eruption if the appliance is worn continually.

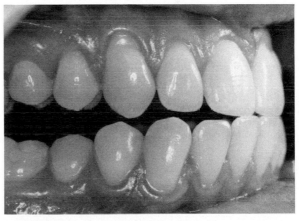

Figure 9-10.
Lateral view of a posterior open bite that resulted from wearing a posterior, partial coverage appliance continually for approximately 1 year. This iatrogenic occlusion could have been avoided by substituting a flat, full arch appliance.

MANDIBULAR REPOSITIONING. This appliance was designed to produce mandibular protrusion (Figs. 9-12 and 9-13). The claim is that an anteriorly displaced disk can be recaptured to a "therapeutic," concentric position between the condylar head and the articular fossa. Although pain may be reduced and recapture may occur, the outcome is unpredictable. Joints sounds may return. Even in selected patients, the elimination of sounds does not mean successful recapture.[54] Among 72 TMD patients with suspected clicking, only 53 had reducing disks. Just 41 were considered suitable candidates for protrusive appliances.

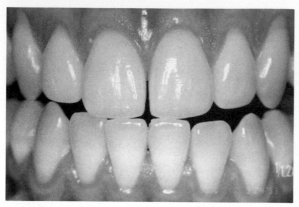

Figure 9-11.
Frontal view of the anterior contact that resulted from wearing a posterior, partial coverage appliance continually for approximately 1 year.

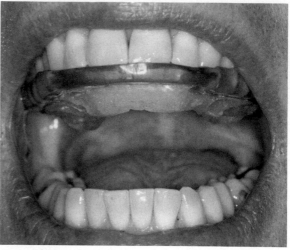

Figure 9-12.
Frontal view of an anterior repositioning appliance designed to "recapture" an anteriorly displaced disk. This one was modified from a flat, full arch appliance. Self-curing resin was added to form a ramp on the lingual surface, which forced the mandible into a protruded position.

Furthermore, studies with direct sagittal computed tomography found that 41.8% of disks were not recaptured, even though sounds were eliminated.[55] In another study of 40 patients treated for 2 months with this appliance, 80% had no joint sounds or pain. At a follow-up about 2½ years later, three fourths were without joint pain, but one third had return of joint sounds.[56]

As a plausible alternative to surgery for diskal displacement, protrusive appliances have been suggested for elimination of joint sounds.[57] Once the therapeutic position is reached, the plan is to restore the occlusion at that position. Some clinicians have considered this form of treatment inappropriate. Mandibular repositioning appliances should not be used to justify other reconstructive repositioning therapies.[58]

Attempts to correlate specific diskal disorders with joint pain have been unsuccessful. Clinical and arthrographic evaluation of 222 TM joints showed that neither pain location (front of the ear, temporal region, or neck) nor pain intensity correlated with specific disk disorders.[59] Ear pain was more common among cases with disk disorders without reduction and among otherwise normal individuals than in patients with reducing disk disorders.

Pro: There are scattered reports that repositioning appliances relieve painful symptoms in some patients.

Con: Evidence is insufficient to prove that disks can be recaptured or that joint sounds can be permanently eliminated. One must continually guard against occlusal

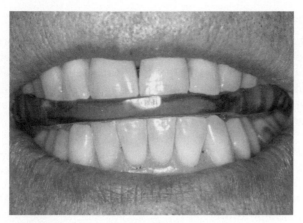

Figure 9-13.
Frontal view of an anterior repositioning appliance showing the end-to-end position of the anterior teeth when the mandible was forced protrusively.

alterations.[60] Dental intrusion was found in 3 cases[61] and extrusion and intrusion in another 3 cases.[60] Occlusal changes can be managed by gradual modification of the appliance. The modification was done 2 months after the patients wore the appliance.[56] This form of management is too difficult for most clinicians.

SOFT APPLIANCE. Improvement in symptoms was found in 84% of 26 TMD patients wearing a water-filled appliance that allowed the muscles to reposition the mandible.[62] A heat-processed latex rubber appliance with a flat occlusal table lessened symptoms in 74% of 19 TMD patients treated for 6 weeks.[63]

Another study found a minor change in joint sounds when a soft appliance was used. Four of 42 TMD patients had no clicking 10 to 20 days after treatment.[64] A few occlusal changes, and intrusion of molars and premolars, were observed in 28 patients. Still other studies have reported occlusal alterations. Nearly all 10 TMD patients lost occlusal contacts after wearing soft splints for as little as 7 hours.[65]

Pro: Soft appliances are just as effective as hard acrylic appliances in reducing symptoms. They can be worn safely for 2 weeks or less in emergencies.

Con: After brief wear, a soft appliance should be replaced with a heat-cured resin appliance to avoid possible occlusal alteration.

Patients should be informed about appropriate wear and care. Recommendations should include:

1. Period of wear—nightly/daily/all the time except to eat.
2. Relief of symptoms may require 2, 4, or 6 weeks/months
3. Cleaning with a brush after each period of wear
4. Warning of possible altered occlusion if worn continually.
5. Need for periodic follow-up to check the status of the appliance and the occlusion.

Vapocoolant Spray

A vapocoolant spray (fluoromethane or ethyl chloride) can be prescribed for muscular complaints. It acts as a counterirritant that inhibits the conduction of pain impulses. Relief may occur from brief anesthesia of trigger points, but the complete physiologic effect is unknown.[66] Speculation is that spraying activates A-delta fibers, closing the gate within the spinal cord and thus reducing the C-fiber activity responsible for chronic pain.

Schedule: The spray is delivered from a 4-oz bottle for 2 minutes, 3 times daily. The tissue is allowed to warm to room temperature between applications. Once applied, manual massage of the tissue can be tolerated and provides further relief. No heat should be applied to the sprayed region because the skin remains hypersensitive for nearly an hour afterwards.

Pro: The spray can be used to assist in jaw opening for the short-term.

Con: Long-term effects have not been determined.

Manual Massage, Myofascial Release, and Acupressure

Information is scant about the benefits of massage on the masticatory muscles of TMD patients. There is ample opportunity to test this treatment. Pericranial muscular tenderness was a common finding in 62 patients with myofascial pain, 63 patients with TMJ internal derangement, and 56 headache patients.[67] Patients in these groups had significantly more pericranial and neck muscular tenderness than asymptomatic individuals. The authors hypothesized that tenderness leads to craniofacial pain and that improvement follows after the tenderness is treated.

A massage therapy widely practiced around the world is termed *myofascial release*. The assumption is that the fascia forms a web connecting the cranium and sacrum to the brain and spinal cord.[68] Fascia invests every structure that connects to the spinal dura. Presumably, restriction of fascial mobility exerts deleterious effects on the dura, disrupting the craniosacral rhythm. A disturbance of rhythm results in somatic pain and dysfunction. Treatment is aimed at restoring rhythm and normal fascial mobility. The patient dictates which direction the therapist pushes and pulls the muscle.

The general opinion is that pressure to specific points reduces fatigue and stimulates production of endorphins, which block pain. Sufficient pressure must be applied to loosen tense muscles. Lack of pressure is one of the most common faults hindering successful outcome. Pressure can be applied in several different ways.[69]

Straight-on pressure is applied with a single finger or knuckle (comparable to shiatsu massage). For localized tenderness around the TMJ, the rubber eraser (the flatter the better) of a pencil can be applied in a straight-on manner and then rotated in a circular motion, moving the muscle beneath the skin.

For tenderness in the temporal region, straight-on pressure is applied with the one or two fingers or knuckles flat against the head and moving in small circles.

For tenderness in the neck, shoulder, or upper back, pressure from the thumb or finger is applied in a straight-on manner. Sustained pressure to a localized area can be done by placing a tennis or golf ball between the tender area and a hard surface such as the floor.

In the *compass maneuver*, the affected area is visualized as a compass. Pressure is applied with the finder beginning at the center and pushing in north, east, south, and west directions.

Roller technique therapy consists of forming a fist and rolling the knuckles along tender areas. The latter procedure is particularly useful for tenderness of the head, where curved contours of the skull limit therapy.

The flexibility of tissue in some regions allows for kneading of the muscles. For generalized tenderness in the neck, shoulder, or upper back, the muscles can be kneaded.

Schedule: Any of these procedures are done for 3 to 5 minutes once or twice daily.

Pro: Because frequent treatment is required to effect improvement, myofascial release or manual manipulation most likely helps only in the short term.

Con: The concept remains speculative. Practitioners have termed outcomes as successful based on patient testimonials.

Exercises and Muscle Strengthening

To strengthen a muscle, one must exercise it regularly. Muscle endurance is accomplished by adding repetition and frequency to an exercise. Muscle integrity is maintained by keeping the muscle strengthened throughout its arc of motion. To strengthen a muscle to its full capacity on demand, resistance must be added to exercise to add power to the muscle.

A program of appropriately planned exercises may provide symptomatic relief. Active and passive range of jaw motion exercises were used successfully to reduce pain intensity and improve mouth opening in 6 TMD patients.[70] Patients were instructed in exercises twice a week for 6 weeks.

Other claims support the usefulness of exercises as part of a multidisciplinary program. One such study of 30 patients with mixed forms of head and neck pain found an 87% recovery rate at the time of discharge and 83% at a 6-month follow-up.[71]

Improvement has been found even among more debilitated patients with TMD. Among 28 patients with rheumatoid arthritis and 34 patients with ankylosing spondylitis, short-term effects were obtained with a stomatognathic physical training program.[72] Joint mobility improved in both groups after 3 weeks of training, and the clinical scores improved in patients with rheumatoid arthritis. Measures exceeded scores of controls. Recommended forms of exercise are discussed below.

Jaw Exercises

Strengthening of the jaw muscles can be accomplished by isometric or isotonic exercise. Examples of isometric exercise are rhythmic stabilization and massed practice therapy.

RHYTHMIC STABILIZATION (OR REFLEXIVE INHIBITION). The patient attempts mandibular movement as the therapist resists the force with a hand beneath. The patient opens about 10 mm, and the force is applied. Lateral and protrusive motions are done in the same way. This exercise can be done solely by the patient. The patient places one hand behind the head and pushes the jaw against an opposing fist beneath the chin.

This exercise produced a 30% reduction of pain intensity in 11 TMD patients treated at two sessions with an interval of 21 days between sessions.[17]

MASSED PRACTICE THERAPY. The patient clenches tightly for 5 seconds and then relaxes the jaw for 5 seconds. This exercise proved useful in management of bruxism in 33 individuals with almost 80% success.[73]

Schedule: 5 repetitions 6 times daily for 2 to 4 weeks.

Examples of isotonic jaw exercises are active stretch and retrusion exercises.

ACTIVE STRETCH. The patient is taught with the aid of a hand mirror to open symmetrically and then to translate the mandible in a straight pattern.

RETRUSION. The patient is taught with the aid of a hand mirror to pull the jaw posteriorly. The patient learns to flex and relax the suprahyoid muscles by feeling changes along the throat.

Mobilization

Tongue depressors can be used to improve the jaw opening in patients with limited function (Fig. 9-14). With extreme care under emergency conditions, a mouth gag retractor may be substituted to prop the jaws open gradually.

TONGUE DEPRESSOR. The patient's opening is measured at the central incisors. Several depressors are bound with masking tape to fit the opening (see Fig. 9-13). Then single depressors are added to tolerance. As the stretch improves the opening, more depressors can be added. The patient holds the depressors in the mouth for about 5 minutes. The depressors are removed and the mandible is stretched in all directions.

Schedule: The exercise is performed 5 to 10 minutes daily in the morning and evening until normal opening is attained.

For patients who have experienced recent TMJ surgery, two other forms of mobilization have been recommended.[74]

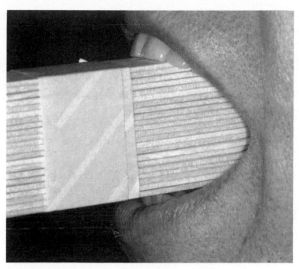

Figure 9-14.
Tongue depressors wrapped with masking tape can be used to stretch the jaw opening.

LONG-AXIS DISTRACTION. The therapist stabilizes the chin of the patient with an index or middle finger, then presses inferiorly with the thumb on the lower molars distracting the mandible in a forward direction.

Schedule: 10 seconds, 3 to 5 times each session.

OVERPRESSURE WITH OPENING. The patient is asked to open the mouth as wide as possible. The therapist presses inferiorly again in the lower molar region, stabilizing the chin with an index or middle finger.

Schedule: 10 seconds, 1 to 3 times each session.

Neck and Head Exercises

Several head and neck exercises have been recommended.[75,76]

CHIN TUCK. The patient is instructed to keep the ears over the shoulders and obtain a neutral position for the head and neck. Practice of this postural routine helps the patient avoid strained neck muscles that may develop when the head is protruded.

EXTENSION–FLEXION. The patient touches the chin to the chest and then pulls the head backwards. An *axial extension* can be done by having the patient place their hands flat across the back of the neck and gently pulling the neck forward while nodding the head in a forward direction.[74]

LATERAL. The patient touches the chin to each shoulder without raising the shoulder.

TILT. The patient moves the right ear towards the right shoulder and then moves the left ear towards the left shoulder.

SHRUG. The patient submerges the head down into the shoulders.

Schedule: Each exercise can be done 5 to 6 times daily for 6 repetitions[75,77,78] at the most convenient time.

Pro: These stretching exercises probably improve and maintain short-term flexibility.

Con: Further research with matched controls is needed to verify long-term efficacy.

Cervical Traction

Because neck pain frequently accompanies jaw pain, therapists often apply traction to the occipital region to reduce neck pain or relax the cervical musculature (see Fig. 9-14).

Selected studies fail to confirm the efficacy of this modality. No relaxation was found after study of the myoelectric activity of the upper trapezius muscle in 12 patients treated with traction for cervical spine disorders.[79] Traction used as part of an active program of physical therapy was less beneficial than a molded collar with slight flexion in the treatment of 135 adults with soft tissue neck injuries caused from motor vehicle accidents.[80] Another report was unable to establish efficacy of traction in the management of neck pain.[81]

If used in conjunction with other treatment for a jaw disorder, care must be taken to avoid excess force on the joint. Mechanical force applied to the mandible that is delivered vertically by some units may irritate a painful jaw.[82] The recommended head strap angle is 45° to 60° to the horizontal plane, with the patient's body in a supine position (Fig. 9-15). This position reduces the pressure on the chin strap and thus the force against the jaw.

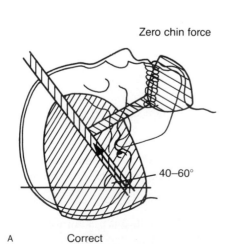

Zero chin force

40–60°

A   Correct

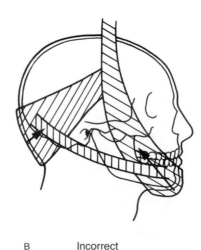

B   Incorrect

Figure 9-15.
Correct placement (A) and incorrect placement (B) of the strap used for cervical traction. (Danzig WN, Van Dyke AR. Physical therapy as an adjunct to temporomandibular joint therapy. J Prosthet Dent 1983;49:96.)

Schedule: 5 to 10 lb for 15 minutes daily initially, increased to tolerance.

Pro: This stretching exercise may be mildly useful for treating neck pain in the short-term. The effect may be no greater than the placebo response.

Con: A long-term program needs to be conducted to fully evaluate efficacy.

Physiotherapy

Physiotherapy includes a host of special therapies with the purpose of reducing musculoskeletal pain and improve function. An enlightening review of procedures that may assist in management of specific TMD complaints is available.[83]

Electrical Stimulation

Many forms of electrical stimulation have been used in the treatment of TMD. The efficacy of some therapies, namely ultrasound (US) and transelectrical nerve stimulation (TENS), has not been proven.[84] A summary reported that convincing evidence is lacking about the efficacy of US in the treatment of musculoskeletal disorders.[81] Some studies have been criticized for a tendency to overinterpret clinical success and specific therapeutic effects, partly as a result of technical difficulties and lack of appropriate controls. There is also difficulty in determining whether an effect is a therapeutic or placebo response. Despite these limitations, some clinicians have been unable to conclude that physiotherapy has no beneficial effect.[81]

Ultrasound

Ultrasound is based on a piezo electrical effect that produces acoustic energy at an ultrasonic range.[85,86] Effects are thermal and mechanical vibration (cavitation). Deep heating occurs quickly, presumably leading to increases in blood flow, metabolism, and permeability of the cell membrane. Because circulation is increased, these changes decrease inflammation, increase soft tissue extensibility, and promote healing. Some pain relief occurs from the heating of peripheral nerves and free nerve endings.

Studies reflecting clinical improvement in the range of 20% to 30% can be explained by a placebo effect.[87] The placebo response has been documented in other studies. From a double-blind, cross-over study of 93 patients with different forms of musculoskeletal pain, actual US stimulation produced 46% improvement, whereas the response with placebo was 32%.[88]

Information exists on the treatment of TMD patients with US (see Table 9-4). Evaluation of 100 TMD patients divided into four equal groups showed that subjects obtained more relief when treated with US combined with an intraoral appliance than when US or appliance was used separately or when both were combined with another therapy.[89]

Muscle pain dysfunction (MPD) symptoms were reduced in 23 of 28 patients.[90] Of 19 patients treated with muscle and diskal dysfunction, 18 improved. Of 9 patients treated for diskal dysfunction, 5 improved. In another study, 6 patients reported less pain after twice weekly sessions for 6 weeks.[70]

Ultrasound produced greater relief of pain and tenderness on palpation of the masticatory MPD patients than did muscle relaxers or short wave diathermy.[91] Three groups of 40 patients each received US, short wave diathermy, or muscle relaxers for 2 weeks. Follow-up occurred from 6 to 12 months. Based on a four-point scale for pain, the reduction was US 46%, diathermy 40%, and muscle relaxers 5%. For tenderness on a four-point scale, reduction was US 34%, diathermy 35%, and muscle relaxers 5%.

Ultrasound, superficial heat, and jaw exercises were used to treat half of 58 patients after TMJ surgery.[92] Compared with patients not receiving physical therapy, treated patients had more pain and less voluntary opening during the treatment period. One year later, no difference was found between groups in subjective report or by clinical examination. Statistical analysis showed patients with opening of less than 30 mm postoperatively were more likely to achieve 40 mm opening if they had physical therapy than if they did not. Patients with 30 mm or more opening likewise showed increased tendency to achieve 40 mm if physical therapy was done.

Schedule: 1.0 to 1.5 W/cm^2 for 3 to 5 minutes in the TMJ region and 7 minutes in the cervical region, 2 to 4 times a week for 3 to 4 weeks.[74,82,93]

Pro: Benefits are minimal (about 14% improvement) and are probably of short duration.

Con: More frequent and widespread application may be required to overcome the placebo response.

Transcutaneous Electrical Nerve Stimulation

This modality has been used to control pain (Table 9-6). TENS has been described as working by two different mechanisms. In the first mechanism, electrical energy from a TENS unit alters the gate control of pain transfer. Presumably, stimulation of large fibers that transmit sensations of touch and vibration can close the "gate" in the spinal cord and block the painful signals that travel in smaller and slower fibers. A second mechanism is that TENS promotes the release of brain endorphins that reduce pain.

Recent findings on low back pain reveals the complexity in establishing efficacy. TENS reduced both the ratings for pain intensity and pain unpleasantness and motivational-affective aspects in the short term. However, it is likely that most reduction in the affective dimension is a placebo response.[94]

A claim has been made that TENS treatment of neck and shoulder trigger points significantly reduced myofascial discomfort.[95] Recomputation of the data from this study failed to reveal a statistically significant effect between treated and untreated subjects.[96] This corrected finding agrees with the results of another study in patients treated for head, neck, or facial pain.[97] Only 20% to 25% of these patients obtained good to excellent relief. In one third of patients with facial pain, needle stimulation

Table 9-6
Studies of TENS Therapy in the Symptomatic Relief
of TMD

Patients Improved (%)	No.	Reference
95	21	Wessberg et al, 1981[98]
72	25	Terezhalmy et al, 1982[99]
70	22	Block and Laskin, 1980[26]
70 placebo		
70	40	Gold et al, 1983[101]
60 placebo		
100	3	Clark et al, 1987[102]
70	33	Niv et al, 1989[103]
50, 100 Hz	12	Graff-Radford et al, 1989[104]
30, 100 Hz	12	
30 supp	12	
0, 2 Hz	12	
0, 0 Hz	12	
>50, 100 Hz	16/42	Hansson and Ekblom, 1983[105]
>50, placebo	2/20	
100 Hz	19	Møystad et al, 1991[106]
2 Hz vs placebo*		

*No significant effect of 2 hz versus placebo.
supp, pain suppressor

was more effective than surface stimulation. The needles were inserted paraspinally at the C1 to C2 transverse processes.

The efficacy of standard TENS or high-frequency neural modulation in the treatment of TMD has been reported to range between 30% to 100% (see Table 9-6).[98–106]

Based on a double-blind design, four modes of TENS versus no stimulation were compared in 60 subjects (12 in each group) suffering from myofascial pain, including pain of the temporalis and masseter muscles.[104] Significant pain reduction was attained in the group receiving 100 Hz/250 ms for 10 minutes followed by 100 Hz/50 ms and pain suppressor TENS (see Table 9-6). No pain reduction occurred at 2 Hz/250 ms TENS or for the controls. Tests with a pressure algometer showed no significant difference in trigger-point sensitivity between groups. The authors concluded that high-frequency, high-intensity TENS reduced myofascial pain but had no effect on trigger-point sensitivity.

A double-blind, cross-over study of 19 patients with TMJ rheumatoid arthritis revealed that high-frequency TENS reduced functional pain but had no significant effect on resting pain or tenderness of the masticatory muscles or TMJs.[106] Cathodes were placed over the auriculotemporal nerve and the temporalis muscle. No significant effect was found between low-frequency TENS and placebo treatment.

TENS treatment proved effective in patients with postherpetic neuralgia. Good to excellent relief was obtained in 60% of chronic cases treated with TENS.[97] In another study, a 70% decrease in pain was found in 33 of 97 patients after one or two treatments.[103]

TENS was valuable in reducing pain produced by venipuncture in children.[107] A double-blind study with untreated and placebo controls showed that VAS pain intensity and unpleasantness were lowest for the TENS group (200 Hz/5 ms) and highest for the untreated controls.

Pro: Based on these studies, the effect of TENS probably exceeds the 30% to 40% placebo response for the short term.[94] A high frequency of 100 Hz or greater is more effective than a lower frequency.

Con: Choosing the best site for electrode placement appears to be crucial. Because myofascial pain presents in a diffuse pattern, many muscles may need to be treated over a longer period.

High-Voltage Electrogalvanic Stimulation (HVGS)

Present HVGS units deliver currents of positive and negative polarities. Positive polarity produces a vasoconstrictive effect, whereas negative polarity produces a vasodilatory effect. Typically, positive polarity reduces nerve irritability and negative polarity enhances it. Negative polarity tends to soften tissue and thus seems to reduce regions of muscular tension and trigger points.

Treatment with HVGS relieved pain intensity and improved mouth opening in 8 TMD patients.[70] Patients were treated twice weekly for 6 weeks. HCVG was used in the rehabilitation of 1 patient after TMJ arthroscopy. *Schedule:* 100 pulses per second for 10 to 20 minutes, twice weekly.[74]

An alternate form of this stimulation is inferential current stimulation (ICS), which produces biphasic pulses within the tissue but no skin irritation. Two different currents are applied simultaneously and superimpose as a modified current deep within the tissue. A study using ICS treatment of subjects with recurrent jaw pain did not prove helpful. No significant difference was found in decreasing jaw pain or increasing vertical opening in 20 patients receiving ICS compared with 20 subjects receiving placebo treatment.[108]

Pro: A few studies suggest that HVGS may be valuable for improving mandibular motion.

Con: Because of the lack of appropriate controls and because no effect exceeds placebo response, efficacy must be view cautiously.

Laser Therapy

Laser therapy has been widely publicized for as a treatment for acute and chronic musculoskeletal pain syndromes. Analysis of 36 randomized clinical trials of 1704 patients suggests that the efficacy of laser therapy for these disorders seems only slightly greater than placebo treatment.[109] There may be too many technical variables to confirm benefits.

Other assessments of pain showed no significant difference between 62 patients with chronic fibromyalgia treated at acupuncture points with low-output helium-neon laser therapy than was found for an untreated placebo group.[110] Six treatments of tender points in the neck and the shoulder girdle of 47 female laboratory technicians with low-level laser therapy was not significantly different from six placebo treatments of the same regions.[111] In fact, subjects of a double-blind, cross-over study rated the placebo best. No significant difference was found in the use of analgesics between treated and untreated sessions.

A double-blind, cross-over study of MPD patients treated with infrared laser therapy at 31 active trigger points (including the infraspinatus, levator scapulae, trapezius, extensor carpi radialis, and tibialis anterior) showed an increased pain threshold immediately after treatment.[112] At nonactive trigger points, the effect occurred 15 minutes after laser therapy.

Pro: If masticatory muscles of TMD patients respond to laser therapy as do other bodily muscles, immediate relief can be expected at active trigger points. The effect will likely be of short-term benefit.

Con: The overwhelming difficulty is in treating enough of the active trigger points that refer pain.

Iontophoresis

Iontophoresis transfers ions from a solution through intact skin by passing a DC electrical current between two electrodes.[113] Negative ions are transmitted at the anode and positive ions at the cathode. Examples of negatively ionizing drugs are methylprednisolone and dexamethasone sodium phosphate. These corticosteroids have been indicated for use in reversing acute inflammations of the tendons, ligaments, trigger points, and joints.

Iontophoresis was suggested as a method of treatment for TMD[11] and for postherapeutic neuralgia in 1982. Five patients with different forms of TMD obtained some relief from pain after iontophoresis treatment with corticosteroid.[113]

In a double-blind study of 27 TMD patients with capsulitis and diskal derangement without reduction, dexamethasone sodium and lidocaine delivered by iontophoresis to the TMJ region proved more effective in improving jaw motions than lidocaine only or buffered saline.[114] Jaw opening improved 6 mm, and lateral motion to the nonaffected side improved 1.2 mm. Treatment was 3 times every other day for about 2 weeks.

Schedule: The medicament solution consists of 25 mg methylprednisolone (Solu-Medrol), 2.5 mL 4% lidocaine, 0.5 mL 1/1000 epinephrine. Two to 3 mL of solution delivered with an Iontophor unit (Life Tech, Houston, Texas) are applied to an electrode (Meditrode, Life Tech) over the affected region at a setting of 1.5 mA for 5 to 6 minutes positive and 10 to 12 minutes negative at 3 to 7 day intervals for 2 to 5 weeks.[113] A return electrode is attached to the arm of the same side.

Pro: Clinical evidence shows iontophoresis to be useful for improving jaw function.

Con: More information is needed to confirm long-term effects on pain.

Supportive Counseling and Psychotherapy

Many patients recognize that stress affects their complaints. Among risk factors are major life changes and multiple daily confrontations that trigger unhealthy responses.[115] Some patients have an inadequate support system or are engaged in activities that could undermine treatment. Social support and the learning of coping skills are vital resources for managing physical illness evoked by stress.

Supportive therapy may be given in various ways. The initial focus should center on sympathetic attention and encouragement with regard for physical symptoms and the effects produced by medications or physical modalities. In a multidisciplinary setting, this program proved helpful in management of patients with chronic somatoform pain. Although the average pain intensity or level of productivity did not change, the amount of time patients were in pain decreased significantly.[24]

Often, improvement requires that patients modify their current life study. The practitioner can initiate an awareness of underlying problems. Brief discourse can focus on abrupt emotional reactions or changes in daily living activities that might trigger more muscular tension. Simply having the patient make a list of stressful events and then placing a priority on those that produce the most distress may help. This exercise may identify situations which many individuals take on, but over which they have no control. Most stresses can be managed some of the time. Problems develop when too many stresses overcome the capacity for management.

A program of didactic education relating stress to increased muscle tension and pain coupled with training in cognitive coping skills to control pain has been used successfully with some TMD patients.[48]

Unlike supportive therapy, psychotherapy deals with painful situations and interpersonal experiences. When properly managed, psychotherapy tends to alter the patient's response to pain and level of activity. Treatment of patients suffering with chronic somatoform disorder showed that psychotherapy raised the intensity of pain but improved the overall level of activity.[24] Interventions focused on relating the pain to experiences in medical care or interpersonal conflicts (eg, anger, separation, or abandonment).

Pro: Programs designed to deal with the interpersonal problems of patients are available at multidisciplinary pain centers in university health centers across the United States. Referral should be made to these centers. Additional information about supportive care may be obtained through The TMJ Network, a support system for TMD patients established in 1993 by Ann-Marie C. DePalma (36 Meacham St, Somerville, MA 02145).[116]

Con: Most clinicians lack enough savvy and time to effect significant changes of this sort. Patients should be directed to health professionals capable of managing burdensome daily problems or emotional features involved with pain and suffering. Referral for counseling of TMD patients is not common among dental practitioners. According to a survey of 302 dentists of the American Equilibration Society, one fourth of their patients suffering with MPD were referred for counseling.[1]

Behavioral Modification

Changes in certain behaviors may assist in management of pain and suffering. Methods that have been suggested to lessen anxiety and allow coping with pain include information, distraction, and modeling:[117]

Information: The clinician provides a well-defined description of a given therapy to be used on the patient.

Distraction: The aim is to preoccupy patients with another form of activity. Audio and video programs are examples suitable for diverting attention.

Modeling: Patients are urged to observe the treatment that they will receive being done on a peer individual.

Physiologic Arousal Reduction

Relaxation

Although relaxation therapy is widely extolled as useful for the management of stress,[118] few publications describe its use for TMD pain. Coupled with oral appliance therapy, relaxation therapy led to reduced tenderness of masticatory muscles and a lower level of pain in MPD patients.[119] Palpation and pain scores decreased significantly by 12 weeks in patients wearing oral appliances and receiving instructions to keep the teeth apart and relax the neck. No similar effect was found in 8 TMD patients receiving only appliance therapy.

Progressive Muscle Relaxation

One program of progressive relaxation therapy consists of 20-minute practice sessions in which the therapist instructs the patient to tense the muscles and relax them slowly.[120] Taped instructions about muscular relaxation given to 27 TMD patients showed results comparable to patients treated with biofeedback training.[121]

The benefit of relaxation tapes in the home setting is doubtful. Using tape-recorded instructions, no additional improvement was found in 19 TMD patients treated simultaneously with biofeedback treatment compared with 32 patients receiving only biofeedback therapy.[122]

Paced Respiration

This exercise involves inhaling or exhaling at a predetermined rate. Breathing may be coordinated with repetitive flashing light or sound. Eight inspiratory-expiratory cycles per minute proved more effective than greater cycles. This therapy has been referred to as *autogenic relaxation*.[120] Sessions of 20 minutes focus on an aura of comfort and relaxation.

Stress-Coping Training

This training promotes coping by teaching patients to identify and modulate maladaptive attitudes and expectations that contribute to stress. Comparison of stress-coping training with relaxation training showed that both were equally effective in producing immediate improvement with migraine.[123] After the 3-year follow-up study was completed, stress-coping was recommended for patients who demanded complex solutions.

Pro: Biobehavioral training has potential for relieving TMD suffering. The frequency and intensity of pain during treatment should be recorded daily in the patient's symptom diary.

Con: Repetition is a necessity. Typical length of treatment is at least 6 to 8 sessions. More studies with double-blind design need to be completed to judge individual efficacy.

Hypnosis

The aim of hypnosis is to achieve relaxation and control of physiologic response through increased suggestibility. Hypnotizability implies the capacity to dissociate. Individuals have high or low hypnotic susceptibility. Those with high susceptibility are at significant risk to symptom formation, whereas resistant individuals often delay seeking help until complaints are difficult to manage.[115]

Hypnosis is achieved by induction, either through verbalization or ideo-motor signaling. *Rapid induction* may involve the clinician asking the patient to visualize descending a stairway with several steps. At each step, a suggestion is made to relax. Posthypnotic suggestions are made to continue relaxation. The patient is then asked to describe the experience. *Eye rolling* is a form of self-hypnosis. The patient focuses on a point while holding the chin parallel to the floor. The patient counts to ten and thinks about relaxing at the same time.[120]

Chronic tension headache has been treated successfully with hypnotherapy.[124] A single, blind, time-controlled study revealed significant reductions in the number of headache days, hours, and intensity in 11 headache patients compared with 15 controls. The treatment period was for 3 months. Patients followed a flow-off maneuver in which the headache was expressed as a visual image changed by suggestions.

Few papers describe treating TMD pain with hypnotherapy. Most detail methodology or mention its use with a few cases unresponsive to other forms of therapy.[125–129] A study revealed no significant relation between hypnotizability and weekly pain ratings.[127] No changes were found in prediction of pain reduction when scores were adjusted for other factors.

Pro: If TMD pain mimics tension headache, it may respond successfully to hypnosis.

Con: One problem is in locating qualified hypnotherapists who can effect relaxation in the patient.

Biofeedback

Basically, biofeedback is a form of instrument-aided psychotherapy. The aim is to achieve psychological self-regulation. The procedure involves attaching an electrode to the skin over the muscle and detecting changes in tension. A polygraph is used to record muscular activity, which is displayed on a monitor visible to the patient. Most systems can be adapted for auditory control. Patients are asked to contract then relax the muscle and at the same time to be aware of reactions in the muscle.[130] Increased muscular tension raises the number on the monitor or produces tone of a higher pitch, whereas decreased tension lowers one or the other. By repetitive training, patients are made aware of the relation between muscular tension and pain.

Several TMD studies before 1989 have been criticized because patients were not permitted an adequate period of adaptation or because inappropriate statistical analyses were used.[131] The authors concluded that more research was needed to ascertain if TMD patients evinced symptom-specific psychophysiologic responses.

Review of the literature showed that biofeedback training proved successful in relieving MPD symptoms in 15 of 23 patients.[23] It was effective in reducing mean masseter electromyographic (EMG) levels and symptoms in 16 MPD patients.[132] Compared with 8 MPD subjects not receiving training, 75% of treated patients improved enough that no further treatment was needed after 1 year. Improvement occurred in the amount of mandibular opening, complaint of pain, and tenderness on palpation.

Biofeedback training was used successfully in combination with jaw posturing and with a prosthetic guide to decrease masticatory muscle activity in women with myofascial pain.[133] Holding the mandible at rest position or separating it with a 6.8-mm prosthetic bar augmented the effect of biofeedback treatment.

Comparison of 30 patients with chronic TMD pain versus 90 patients with chronic back pain found that TMD patients were more responsive to biofeedback treatment than back pain patients.[134] Patients completed eight training sessions.

As an add-on therapy, EMG biofeedback has been used successfully to treat subjects with low back complaints.[135] Compared with 30 control subjects, 30 patients with myofascial pain improved the strength of their trunk extensor muscles. The level of pain was not significantly different between treated and untreated subjects after eight sessions over a month.

Biofeedback may be coupled with relaxation training. Long-term efficacy with both has been proved in patients with chronic headache.[136] A study of 12 patients treated by relaxation, 10 by relaxation and EMG biofeedback, and 12 by relaxation and temperature biofeedback showed that less headache activity occurred in the group with EMG treatment than in the other groups when evaluated at 6- and 12-month follow-ups.

The age of the adult patient is not a limiting factor in treatment. Assessment conducted 3 months after frontal biofeedback revealed a reduction in tension headache among 8 sufferers who were 62 years or older.[137] The training program involved 12 sessions. EMG measures for the upper trapezius muscle in patients with cervical neck pain found that patients between 55 and 78 years of age responded similarly to patients between 29 and 48 years of age.[138]

Schedule: 5 minutes no-feedback resting baseline: 20 minutes of biofeedback with a 5 minute no-feedback period, weekly for 6 weeks.[48]

Pro: The more sophisticated systems are adapted to handle eight channels (two EMG panels, two temperature channels, electrodermal response, heart rate, respiratory rate, and continuous blood pressure), so more information can be derived.

Biofeedback is not considered curative for TMD. Opinions of leading clinicians at the 1982 American Dental Association President's Conference on Temporomandibular Disorders described biofeedback as having reasonable scientific support for TMD patients suffering from complaints of the masticatory muscles and for certain patients with chronic discomfort unresponsive to other therapies.

Con: The benefits tend to be transitory.[84] The chief difficulty is an inability to motivate patients.[130] Reinforcement is necessary to achieve an enduring result.

Acupuncture, Needling, and Auriculotherapy

Acupuncture

The lay literature abounds with success stories about acupuncture treatment of generalized muscular and joint pains. The use of acupuncture in treating TMD is limited. Analysis of clinical measures showed that acupuncture performed 3 times over 1 month on 25 TMD patients produced no greater relief of symptoms than 25 patients treated by counseling, occlusal adjustment, muscular exercises for the mandible, or intraoral appliances.[139] A 3-month follow-up showed that neither modality proved superior to the other.

Another study of 110 TMD patients compared the effects of acupuncture to appliance therapy.[140] Nearly equal-sized groups of patients were treated either by acupuncture or by appliance, and a similar number of controls received neither treatment. Relief of pain improved immediately in treated subjects, but no change was found for controls. A 1-year follow-up showed 57% improvement in patients receiving acupuncture and 68% improvement in patients treated with appliances. Muscular tenderness decreased immediately after treatment and remained lower 6 months later. The authors concluded that both therapies produced the same outcome in patients suffering myogenic complaints.

Dry needling has proved effective in the relief of a few patients with postherpetic neuralgia[103] and in other selected patients with localized myofascial pain of the neck.[141] A follow-up 6 months later showed no return of the neck pain.

Method: For treatment of myofascial pain, the muscle is palpated for trigger points. Once the "jump sign" is demonstrated, the area is probed with a 25- to 30-gauge needle,[19,103] which is rotated every few minutes to achieve the desired effect. Spraying the area with vapocoolant mist before needling makes the procedure more comfortable.

Auriculotherapy

There are many anecdotal reports that stimulation of the external ear with a needle or microcurrent alleviates pain at distant sites. The claim is that the therapy elevates the pain threshold and reduces sympathetic tone.

Success with auriculotherapy is doubtful. A comparison of 36 patients with chronic pain showed that the effect was no greater than found in placebo controls.[142] Furthermore, auriculotherapy coupled with TENS failed to produce a significant effect on autonomic functions and on an experimental threshold for pain in other patients.[143]

Pro: Acupuncture and needling appear to offer some benefit in relieving localized regions of pain.

Con: The failure to demonstrate acupuncture as more successful than appliance therapy may relate to the diffuse pattern of pain originating from different sites. The problem is where to begin treatment. Needling an ear is not rational unless one wants an earring.

Chemical Injections

Local Anesthesia

Injection of a local anesthetic into one or more regions of the muscle may produce relief of pain. The procedure for injection of muscle trigger points is to locate the taut band by finger pressure. The patient is asked if "1, 2, or 3" areas hurts the most. The most sensitive area is sprayed with vapocoolant spray because a concentration of local anesthetic even less than used to obtain nerve blocks tends to increase pain. Either chloroprocaine (3%) or procaine (5%) without vasoconstrictors, 0.1 to -0.5 mL, has been recommended.[144,145]

Most dental pain can be blocked effectively after injection of a local anesthetic. Using an intraligamentary syringe, single teeth can be anesthetized, enhancing exact identification of the pain.

Pro: Localized dental pain can be treated effectively once an offending tooth is anesthetized. For diffuse muscle pain, repeated injection may be required to obtain lasting results.

Con: A single injection produces necrosis of muscle. Regeneration may require at least 1 month.

Corticosteroid

Injection of corticosteroids and other agents into joints has produced only short-term results in patients with generalized osteoarthritis.[146] Few studies demonstrate that patients with osteoarthritis improved significantly after injections compared with patients receiving placebo agents.

Other findings are mixed. Improvement has been related to reduced synovitis in the joint. Within a day after injection, 79% of 19 joints in 10 patients with hemophilic arthropathy showed improvement.[147] Two months later, 58% of the patients obtained relief. On the other hand, injections into the synovial fluid of the knee produced no significant benefit in 18% of 102 cases of patients with rheumatoid arthritis, osteoarthritis, or traumatic osteoarthritis.[148]

Long-term follow-up (3 to 15 years) of 93 patients with stenosing tenovaginitus injected with methylprednisolone at 3-week intervals showed that 76% obtained complete relief.[149]

Collectively, these dissimilar findings tend to support the findings obtained with the few TMD patients treated similarly. Recommendation was made that 40 mg of hydrocortisone injected into the upper compartment would afford rapid relief in cases of severe, acute TMJ artharalgia.[85] Single injections of corticosteroid into the TM joint provided complete symptomatic relief in 65% of 46 patients with osteoarthrosis.[6] No additional treatment was required at a follow-up less than 6 months later. Another study showed that intra-articular injections of hydrocortisone into the TMJs of 8 patients provided 2 months relief of pain.[93] In a 2-year parallel study of 15 patients treated with intra-articular injections of corticosteroid and of 18 patients managed with occlusal therapy, injections proved more effective in improving maximum voluntary opening than did the occlusal therapy.[150]

Schedule: 0.5 mL betamethasone (0.6 mg/mL), 0.5 mL lidocaine (10 mg/mL), 1 injection weekly for 3 weeks in the TMJ.[150] No more than 2 to 4 injections per year has been recommended.[25] Based on studies of 50 patients with low back pain, injections are effective only if done by the intra-articular route.[151]

Pro: The few studies on TMD patients suggest that patients receiving corticosteroids within the joints may improve in the short-term.

Con: Side effects can be expected. Corticosteroids tend to remain in connective tissue at the injection site. Among 12 patients, 6 showed a mild reaction, and the attendant tissue was avascular.[152]

Hyaluronate

Presumably because synovial fluid contains sodium hyaluronate, it functions as an intra-articular lubricant. This property offers an opportunity to discover if hyaluronate injections can be used to free intra-articular adhesions. Thus, disk incoordination, particularly in cases of disk displacement without reduction, might improve.

Report of short-term and long-term improvement following intra-articular injections of hyaluronate into the superior joint space has been shown. Comparison of 33 patients with TMJ pain and dysfunction and 24 patients with TMJ arthritis showed decreased symptoms and signs after injection.[152,154] Findings did not differ significantly from patients receiving injections of corticosteroids. A short-term effect was found after pressurized infusion of hyaluronate in 1 patient who had restricted mouth opening.[155]

A study of 121 patients with degenerative joint disease (DJD), displaced disk without reduction (DDN), and displaced disk with reduction (DDR) revealed that the DDR patients received the greatest benefit.[156] Compared with subjects receiving placebo saline solution, about twice as many DDR patients (90% versus 50%) improved after 1% sodium hyaluronate treatment. Few DDR patients treated with hyaluronate relapsed, but 31% relapsed with placebo solution. Patients with DJD did not improve.

The effect of sodium hyaluronate and corticosteroid on papain-induced joint lesions has been studied in the guinea pig knee.[157] Findings showed less deviation in form and granulation tissue after injection, but no overall change in joint severity.

Pro: Injection of hyaluronate may improve early-developing incoordination of the disk.

Con: The disparate findings between patients with different forms of disk derangements suggests that benefit may accrue only to those patients with disks that do not reduce.

Trigeminal Glycerol Gangliolysis

Recalcitrant trigeminal pain, unresponsive to medications, may respond to treatment with glycerol gangliolysis.[158,159] Effectiveness with this procedure has been estimated to range from 89% to 96%. About 7% to 10% of those treated have early recurrence of pain and up to 21% have recurrence later.[158]

The technique requires the expertise of a trained practitioner. After intravenous injection of appropriate sedative, an opaque dye viewed radiographically is used to position a needle in the fluid surrounding the trigeminal nerve (Fig. 9-16). Glycerol (0.5 mL) is injected into the fluid (Fig. 9-17). Some patients obtain relief of pain by 1 day. Relief in others may not occur for 3 weeks. Side effects may include loss of feeling in the face, which usually returns within 3 months.

Other procedures for relief of trigeminal neuralgia are alcohol block, alcohol gangliolysis, neurectomy, radiofrequency gangliolysis, microvascular decompression, rhizotomy, and trigeminal tractotomy.[158] Some are either less predictable or require surgery compared with glycerol gangliolysis. Microvascular decompression involves the surgical removal of dilated vessels surrounding the nerve. Among 40 patients undergoing microvascular decompression, 75% rated the relief as excellent and 15% as good about 11 years later.[160]

Pro: After an unsuccessful trial with medication, glycerol rhizolysis may offer the patient relief. Success relies on appropriate diagnosis of neuropathic pain.

Con: Side effects may develop. Posterior fossa exploration with microvascular decompression is the recommended procedure if rhizolysis fails.

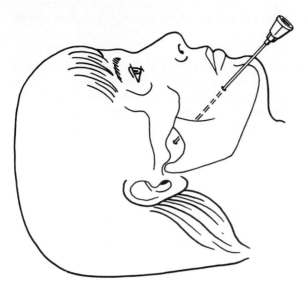

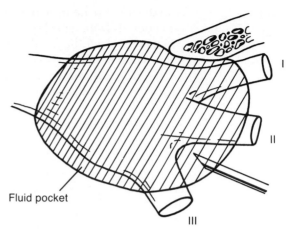

Fluid pocket

Figure 9-16.
Placement of the needle for injection of glycerol around the trigeminal nerve. (Courtesy of K. S. Sahni, Richmond, VA.)

Figure 9-17.
Tip of the needle is placed into the fluid pocket surrounding the trigeminal nerve. (Courtesy of K. S. Sahni, Richmond, VA.)

Occlusal Rehabilitation

There is widespread use of occlusal adjustment in the treatment of TMD. Adjustment is listed as the second most common form of treatment (30%) for MPD in a survey of 2143 general practitioners belonging to the American Dental Association.[161] Traditional practitioners argue that adjustment reduces or ultimately eliminates symptoms of TMD. Unfortunately, clinical judgments made without appropriate controls are often misleading. Even worse is the neglect of reading the literature on the part of some practitioners.

Results with adjustment procedures fail to validate the need for reduction of prematurities to relieve pain.[162] There is a strong placebo response. Mock adjustment completed on 25 MPD patients showed that 16 reported almost total relief of symptoms.[163] Thirteen patients remained free of symptoms for 29 months.

Recently, a double-blind study of 51 patients treated by adjustment of mediotrusive interferences and significant slides between retruded contact position and intercuspal position failed to confirm that this procedure differed from the placebo effect obtained by mock adjustment.[164]

Although there is no reason to adjust teeth for relief of tenderness in the masticatory muscles of patients with TMD, this procedure has been done with that purpose in mind.[165] The removal of prematurities during a period of variable muscular activity is questionable.

Pro: The primary reason for adjustment is to prevent, reduce, or eliminate lateral stresses on teeth. Improvements can be made in directing occlusal loading along the long axis of teeth. If one joint degenerates so severely that no occlusal contact occurs on the contralateral side, adjustment may stablize the occlusion on the affected side. Restoration of teeth on the contralateral side is an alternative. If unilateral surgery is required, adjustment may be needed on the affected side to improve the final occlusal contacting relation.

Con: Adjustment should not be made with an anticipation of pain relief.

PROTOCOLS OF SIMULATED PATIENTS

A few examples are described so that the practitioner may gain experience in the clinical management of selected cases of head and neck complaints. The treatment sequences begin with patients suffering from a primary complaint and build to management of patients having multiple complaints. No modality should be considered definitive.

Muscular Symptoms of the Jaw

Patient: #1
Chief complaint: Preauricular pain radiating along the left mandible
Past history: Fatigue and soreness in the jaw over the past 2 weeks
Examination: Localized tenderness of the masseter muscle with pain on palpation, absence of joint tenderness and sounds, voluntary opening and lateral mandibular motions within normal limits, TMJ radiograph within normal limits
Diagnosis: Localized myalgia
Treatment: Home care program as described above
Follow-up: Office visit after 1 week, interview and palpation of the area for tenderness, continued home care therapy for at least 1 week as required
Patient: #2
Chief complaint: Generalized bilateral orofacial pain, occasional neck pain
Past history: Periodic soreness and stiffness widely scattered over the face, neck, and shoulders for the past 5 years. Pain diffuse and aching in character, no history of joint sounds
Examination: Palpable tenderness of masticatory, neck, and shoulder muscles, voluntary opening >30 mm, lateral jaw movements >7 mm, TMJ radiograph within normal limits
Diagnosis: Generalized myofascial pain
Treatment: Home care program as described above
Follow-up: Office visit after 1 week, interview, palpation for tenderness; if no improvement, intraoral appliance, medication (antidepressant or diazepam), physical therapy

TM Joint Symptoms

Patient: #1
Chief complaint: Annoying clicking in the joints
Past history: Bilateral joint sounds for more than 2 years, which are bothersome during eating, no history of pain

Examination: Voluntary opening of 48 mm, lateral mandibular movements exceed 7 mm, minor tenderness on palpation of the temporalis tendons, bilateral reciprocal clicking, TMJ radiograph within normal limits

Diagnosis: Bilateral disk disorder with reduction

Treatment: Restriction of mandible on opening, yawning, and eating; chew small food portions bilaterally

Follow-up: If the patient is severely impaired, consider diagnostic arthroscopy including lavaging of the TMJ with irrigation solutions

Patient: #2

Chief complaint: Inability to open the mouth wide

Past history: Noise in the right joint for the past 6 weeks which disappeared suddenly during yawning; sharp pain on locking as voluntary opening decreased; present pain dull, aching

Examination: Restricted opening <30 mm, left lateral movement 4 mm, right lateral movement 8 mm, deviation of the mandible to the right on opening, localized tenderness on palpation of the right joint

Diagnosis: Right-side disk disorder without reduction

Treatment: Home care program with emphasis on stretching of the jaw

Follow-up: Office visit if no improvement within 1 week, measurements of voluntary opening and lateral motions, vapocoolant spray and manual manipulation of the mandible if opening <30 mm. Continuation of home care program with emphasis on stretching of the jaw. Stretching can be achieved with tongue depressors. Repeat office visit 1 week later using same treatment if minimal progress. Recommend physical therapy (moist heat, ultrasound, and manual manipulation), consider diagnostic arthroscopy with irrigation if condition become chronic

Patient: #3

Chief complaint: Limited voluntary opening, chronic pain in the left joint, recurrent headache

Past history: Grating sound in the left joint over the past year, mandible tends to hang during opening, recurrent dull pain that wakes the patient at night

Examination: Palpable tenderness in the left shoulder, neck, and masticatory muscles with a rating of 2 or more on a scale of 0 to 3, left joint with crepitus on opening and lateral movements, jaw deviates to left on opening, TMJ radiograph positive for joint erosion

Diagnosis: Left TMJ arthritis with arthralgia, headache, myofascial pain

Treatment: Initiate home care program, medication (antidepressant, medication to induce sleep, or both), begin fabrication of intraoral appliance

Follow-up: Office examination after 1 week for palpable pain and tenderness. Delivery of intraoral appliance. Another follow-up in 1 to 2 weeks to check on health of patient and status of appliance.

Patient: #4

Chief complaint: Mouth locks open and jaw cannot close, sharp pain in left TMJ

Past history: Frequent subluxation over the past year occasionally requiring assistance to reduce opening, recurrent pain on locking

Examination: Maximum voluntary opening 60 mm, right lateral movement 17 mm, left lateral movement 8 mm, tenderness of left TMJ and temporalis tendon, TMJ radiograph with possible flattened eminence of the left TMJ

Diagnosis: Left TMJ hypermobility

Treatment: Referral to an oral surgeon for TMJ surgery, likely arthroscopic cauterization of the posterior attachment to restrict movement

TMJ Arthrotomy

Chief complaint: Recurrent pain and extreme restriction of mouth opening following surgery for ankylosed left condyle

Past history: Ankylosis developed after trauma to the mandible resulting from a motor vehicular accident, loss of voluntary opening to 15 mm, left lateral mandibular movement 6 mm, right lateral movement 1 mm, no prior history of pain or limitation of mandibular movement

Examination: Mouth opening immediately after surgery 34 mm, left lateral movement 7 mm, right lateral movement 5 mm

Diagnosis: Bony ankylosis of left condyle

Treatment: Analgesics, diet instructions for soft or semisolid foods, program of physical therapy to maintain or improve voluntary opening and mandibular movement produced by surgery. Daily program of moist heat and ultrasound followed by active and passive exercises to facilitate protrusive, lateral and full opening activities. Home exercises with emphasis on compliance to reinforce instructions from physical therapist

Follow-up: Assessment of condition, restoration of joint and occlusal therapy as needed

Dentofacial Deformity and TMD Symptoms

Chief complaint: Upper jaw too large and lower jaw too small, pain around the right ear, and sounds in the right jaw joint

Past history: Congenital growth problems of face, preauricular pain radiating to the neck, joint sounds present for 5 years, no history of trauma

Examination: Voluntary opening of 44 mm, right and left lateral mandibular motions of 8 mm, generalized, muscular tenderness on palpation in neck and jaw bilateral in nature, unilateral popping in the right TMJ on opening but no functional pain, occlusion class II, TMJ radiograph within normal limit

Diagnosis: Myofascial pain, disk disorder with reduction, and class II skeletal and dental malocclusion

Treatment: Program of home care

Referral: Oral surgeon, orthodontist, and counseling for pain and esthetic changes in profile

Follow-up: Office visit following interviews by referral clinicians, continued treatment of pain by intraoral appliance and medication as needed

Confusing Symptoms

Patient: #1

Chief complaint: Limited voluntary opening, feeling of swelling and slight numbness in the right mandible

Past history: Opening and lateral jaw motions had decreased slowly within the past 2 months, perception of swelling along the angle of the mandible appeared with loss of opening, diffuse pain localized within the area of the lower second molar

Examination: Voluntary opening of 22 mm, left lateral movement 3 mm, right lateral movement 10 mm, tenderness on palpation along the ramus and angle of the mandible, absence of tenderness in masticatory muscles, gingiva surrounding the second molar healthy, tooth slightly tender to percussion, but no decay or restorations present determined clinically and radiologically, pulp test within normal limits, tooth not sensitive to ice or heat, TMJ radiograph with questionable radiolucency present near angle of of the right mandible

Diagnosis: Because history reveals no record of recent fracture, recommend bone scan of the mandible to rule out possible tumor; if positive bone scan, plain film of the mandible and bone biopsy

Treatment: If tumor confirmed, localized radiation or surgical excision

Follow-up: Program of physical therapy program to improve mouth opening and lateral jaw functions, monitoring of oral hygiene

Patient: #2

Chief complaint: Inability to open wide, persistent pain of the left mandible

Past history: Visited dentist 1 week ago for toothache, report of three shots in the lower left jaw, some numbness lasting over 2 hours, sharp pain present once anesthesia disappeared, no history of joint sounds

Examination: Maximum voluntary opening of 15 mm, left lateral movement 6 mm, right lateral movement 2 mm, well-defined tenderness on palpation along the angle of the left mandible and in the anterior fibers of the temporalis, no joint sounds, radiographs within normal limits

Diagnosis: Postinjection trismus

Treatment: Vapocoolant spray to left TMJ and masticatory muscles followed by manual manipulation of the mandible, analgesics

Follow-up: Office visit after 1 week; if no improvement repeat spray and manipulation, program of physical therapy to improve opening and lateral jaw motions

Patient: #3

Chief complaint: Generalized head and neck pain

Past history: Series of 12 root canals on upper and lower teeth with residual tooth pain inconsistent with pattern of decay and periodontal status; brain scans and magnetic resonance imaging of head and neck within normal limits; overconcern with minor aches; family problems

Examination: Absence of joint sounds and tenderness of TMJs, masticatory, neck, and shoulder muscles on palpation; treated teeth slightly sensitive to percussion; voluntary opening and mandibular movements within normal limits; radiographs and bone scan within normal limits

Diagnosis: Possible somatoform pain disorder

Treatment: Referral to psychologist or psychiatrist for evaluation and behavioral management

Follow-up: Office visit to reevaluate patient outcome once diagnosis is confirmed by psychological testing

Patient: #4

Chief complaint: Localized continuous pain in the region of lower second molar

Past history: Pain present for longer than 4 months, associated hyperesthesia localized to site of pain, unsuccessful root canal therapy including apicoectomy followed by extraction

Examination: Gingiva within normal limits, hyperesthesia at extraction site evoked by palpation, anesthesia block equivocal, radiographs within normal limits

Diagnosis: Atypical odontalgia

Treatment: Medication (antidepressant)

Follow-up: Interview for compliance with medication

Neuropathic Symptoms

Chief complaint: Short bursts of pain, unilateral in mandible
Past history: Health history unremarkable until 60 years of age, then pain localized to the molar area of the right mandible lasting for 10 seconds; rubbing the lower lip evokes pain
Examination: Absence of tenderness on palpation of TMJ, masticatory, and neck muscles, teeth with minor fillings and negative to testing, gingiva healthy, radiographs within normal limits, pressure on trigger points of lip causes repeated painful episodes, diagnostic anesthesia confirms referral of trigeminal pain
Diagnosis: Trigeminal neuralgia
Treatment: Baclofen or carbamazepine; if no relief, glycerol neurolysis or microvascular decompression

Headache

Chief complaint: Severe unilateral orbital or temporal pain or both lasting 15 to 180 minutes if untreated
Past history: Headache with pulsating quality, pain moderate to severe intensity, frequency from 1 every other day to 8 each day, aggravated by routine physical activity; nausea or vomiting, accompanied by lacrimation, nasal congestion, forehead and facial sweating, ptosis
Examination: Brain scan and physical symptoms within normal limits, no obvious pathology, oxygen inhalation aborts pain
Diagnosis: Cluster headache
Treatment: Oxygen inhalation, prophylactic regimen of sumatriptan or subcutaneous injection in emergencies

References

1. Glass EG, McGlynn FD, Glaros AG. A survey of treatments for myofascial pain dysfunction. J Craniomandib Pract 1991;9:165.
2. Le Resche L, Truelove EL, Dworkin SF. Temporomandibular disorders: a survey of dentists' knowledge and beliefs. J Am Dent Assoc 1993;124:90.
3. Greene CS. Managing TMD patients: initial therapy is the key. J Am Dent Assoc 1992;123:43.
4. Core Curriculum For Professional Education. In Fields HL et al (eds). Pain. International Association for the Study of Pain, Task Force on Professional Education. Seattle: IASP Publications, 1991.
5. Management of acute pain: a practical guide. International Association for the Study of Pain, Task Force on Acute Pain. Seattle: IASP Publications, 1992.
6. Toller P. Temporomandibular joint injection with cortisone. Br Dent J 1973;134:223.
7. Fricton JR, Schiffman EL, Haley DP. Natural progression of masticatory myofascial pain. Seventh World Congress on Pain, International Association for the Study of Pain. Seattle: IASP Publications, 1993:52. Abstract 142.
8. Magni G, Marchetti M, Moreschi C, Merskey H, Luchini SR. Chronic musculoskeletal pain and depressive symptoms in the National Health and Nutrition Examination: epidemiologic follow-up study. Pain 1993;53(pt 1):163.

9. Wright WJ. Temporomandibular disorders: occurrence of specific diagnoses and response to conservative management. J Craniomandib Pract 1986;4:149.

10. Keith D. Orofacial pain. In Warfield CA (ed). Principles and practice of pain management. New York: McGraw-Hill, 1993:99.

11. Gangarosa LP, Mahan PE. Pharmacologic management of TMJ-MPDS. Ear Nose Throat J 1982;61:670.

12. Ridder T. Orofacial physiotherapy after radiotherapy in the head and neck region. J Craniomandib Pract 1993;11:242.

13. Nelson SJ, Ash MM Jr. An evaluation of a moist heating pad for the treatment of TMJ/muscle pain dysfunction. J Craniomandib Pract 1988;6:355.

14. Nelson SJ, dos Santos J Jr, Barghi N. Using moist heat to treat acute temporomandibular muscle pain and dysfunction. Compend Contin Educ Dent 1991;12:808.

15. Belitsky RB, Odam SJ, Hubley-Kozey C. Evaluation of the effectiveness of wet ice, dry ice and cryogen packs in reducing skin temperature. Phys Ther 1987;67:1080.

16. Uriell P, Bertolucci L, Swaffer C. Physical therapy in the postoperative management of temporomandibular joint arthroscopic surgery. J Craniomandib Pract 1989;7:27.

17. Burgess JA, Sommers EE, Truelove EL, Dworkin SF. Short-term effect of two therapeutic methods on myofascial pain and dysfunction of the masticatory system. J Prosthet Dent 1988;60:606.

18. Gregg JM. Pharmacological management of myofascial pain dysfunction. In Laskin DM et al (eds). The President's Conference on the Examination, Diagnosis and Management of Temporomandibular Disorders. Chicago: American Dental Association, 1983:167.

19. Fricton JR. Recent advances in temporomandibular disorders and orofacial pain. J Am Dent Assoc 1991;122:25.

20. Berndt C, Maier C, Schutz H-W. Polymedication and medication compliances in patients with non-malignant pain. Pain 1993;52:331.

21. Stanko JR. A review of oral skeletal muscle relaxants for the craniomandibular disorder (CMD) practitioner. J Craniomandib Pract 1990;8:234.

22. Jaeschke R, Adachi J, Guyatt G, Keller J, Wong B. Clinical usefulness of amitriptyline in fibromyalgia. J Rheumatol 1991;18:447.

23. Gessel AH. Electromyographic biofeedback and tricyclic antidepressants in myofascial pain-dysfunction syndrome: psychological predictors of outcome. J Am Dent Assoc 1975;91:1048.

24. Pilowsky I, Barrow CG. A controlled study of psychotherapy and amitriptyline used individually and in combination in the treatment of chronic intractable, 'psychogenic' pain. Pain 1990;40:3.

25. Schnitzer TJ. Osteoarthritis treatment update: minimizing pain while limiting patient risk. Postgrad Med 1993;93:89.

26. Block SL, Laskin DM. The effectiveness of ibuprofen in treatment of temporomandibular joint pain. J Dent Res 1980;59(special issue):305. Abstract 152.

27. Cady RK, Wendt JK, Kirchner JR, Sargent JD, Rothrock JF, Skaggs H Jr. Treatment of acute migraine with subcutaneous Sumatriptan. JAMA 1991; 265:2831.

28. The Oral Sumatriptan Dose-Defining Study Group. Sumatriptan: an oral dose-defining study. Eur Neurol 1991;31:300.

29. Ekbom K, Waldenlind E, Cole J, Pilgram A, Kirkham A. Sumatriptan in chronic cluster headache: results of continuous treatment for eleven months. Cephalalgia 1992;12:254.

30. Mongini F, Bona G, Garnero M, Gioria A. Efficacy of meclofenamate sodium versus placebo in headache and craniofacial pain. Headache 1993;33:22.

31. Schokker RP, Hansson TL, Ansink BJ. The result of treatment of the masticatory system of chronic headache patients. J Craniomandib Disord Fac Oral Pain 1990;4:126.

32. Dionne RA. New approaches to preventing and treating postoperative pain. J Am Dent Assoc 1992;123:27.

33. Oleson J (ed). Headache Classification Committee of the International Headache Society: classification and diagnostic criteria for headache disorders, cranial neuralgias and facial pain. Cephalalgia 1988;8(suppl 7):1.

34. Merrill RL, Graff-Radford SB. Trigeminal neuralgia: how to rule out the wrong treatment. J Am Dent Assoc 1992;123:63.

35. Gibbs CH, Mahan PE, Mauderli A, Lundeen HC, Walsh EK. Limits of human bite strength. J Prosthet Dent 1986;56:226.

36. Robson FC. Practical management of internal derangements of the temporomandibular joint in partially and completely edentulous patients. J Prosthet Dent 1991;65:828.

37. Abbott DA, Bush FM, Butler JH. Occlusal appliances. In Clark JW (ed). Clinical dentistry. Vol 2. Philadelphia: Harper & Row, 1987.

38. Greene CS, Laskin DM. Splint therapy for myofascial pain dysfunction (MPD) syndrome: a comparative study. J Am Dent Assoc 1972;84:624.

39. Feine JS, Lavigne G, Lund JP, Dao TTT, Charbonneau A. An assessment of patient reports of relief from chronic orofacial pain. Seattle, WA: International Association for the Study of Pain. 1993:586. Abstract 1571.

40. Boero RP. The physiology of splint therapy: a literature review. Angle Orthod 1989;59:165.

41. Lund TW, Cohen JI. Trismus appliances and indications for their use. Quintessence International 1993;24:275.

42. Bush FM. Occlusal etiology of myofascial pain dysfunction syndrome. In Laskin D, Greenfield W, Gale E et al (eds). The President's Conference On The Examination, Diagnosis And Management Of Temporomandibular Disorders. Chicago: American Dental Association, 1983:95.

43. Tsuga K, Akagawa Y, Sakaguchi R, Tsuru H. A short-term evaluation of the effectiveness of stabilization-type occlusal splint therapy for specific symptoms of temporomandibular joint dysfunction syndrome. J Prosthet Dent 1989; 61:610.

44. Carlson N, Moline D, Huber L, Jacobson J. Comparison of muscle activity between conventional and neuromuscular splints. J Prosthet Dent 1993; 70:39.

45. Levitt SR, Mckinney MW, Willis WA. Measuring the impact of a dental practice on TMD disorder symptoms. J Craniomandib Pract 1993;11:211.

46. Naeije M. Short-term effect of the stabilization appliance on masticatory muscle activity in myogenous craniomandibular disorder patients. J Craniomandib Disord Fac Oral Pain 1991;5:245.

47. Humsi ANK, Naeije M, Hippe JA, Hansson TL. The immediate effects of a stabilization splint on muscular symmetry in the masseter and anterior tem-

poral muscles of patients with a craniomandibular disorder. J Prosthet Dent 1989;62:339.

48. Turk DC, Zaki HS, Rudy TE. Effects of intraoral appliance and biofeedback/ stress management alone and in combination in treating pain and depression in patients with temporomandibular disorders. J Prosthet Dent 1993;70:158.

49. Anderson GC, Schulte JK, Goodkind RJ. Comparative study of two treatment methods for internal derangement of the temporomandibular joint. J Prosthet Dent 1985;53:392.

50. Lundh H, Westesson PL, Eriksson I, Brooks SL. Temporomandibular joint disk displacement without reduction. Oral Surg Oral Med Oral Pathol 1992;73:655.

51. Okeson JP. Nonsurgical management of disc-interference disorders. Dent Clin North Am 1991;35:29.

52. Lobbezoo D, van der Glas HW, van Kampen FMC, Bosman F. The effect of an occlusal stabilization splint and the mode of visual feedback on the activity balance between jaw-elevator muscles during isometric contraction. J Dent Res 1993;72:876.

53. Wilkinson T, Hansson TL, McNeill C, Marcel T. A comparison of success of 24-hour occlusal splint therapy versus nocturnal occlusal splint therapy in reducing craniomandibular disorders. J Craniomandib Disord Fac Oral Pain 1992;6:64.

54. Roberts CA, Tallents RH, Katzberg RW, Sanchez-Woodworth RE, Mazionnne JV, Espeland MA, Handelman SL. Clinical and arthrographic evaluation of temporomandibular joint sounds. Oral Surg Oral Med Oral Pathol 1986;62: 373.

55. Manco LG, Messing SG. Splint therapy evaluation with direct sagittal computed tomography. J Oral Surg 1986;61:5.

56. Okeson J. Long-term treatment of disk-interference disorders of the temporomandibular joint with anterior repositioning occlusal splints. J Prosthet Dent 1988;60:611.

57. Tallents RH, Katzberg RW, Macher DJ, Roberts CA. Use of protrusive splint therapy in anterior disk displacement of the temporomandibular joint: a 1- to 3-year follow-up. J Prosthet Dent 1990;63:336.

58. Orenstein ES. Anterior repositioning appliances when used for anterior disk displacement with reduction: a critical review. J Craniomandib Pract 1993; 11:141.

59. Roberts CA, Tallents RH, Katzberg RW, Sanchez-Woodworth RE, Espeland MA, Handelman SL. Clinical and arthrographic evaluation of the location of temporomandibular joint pain. Oral Surg Oral Med Oral Pathol 1987;64:6.

60. Abbott DM, Bush FM. Occlusions altered by removable appliances. J Am Dent Assoc 1991;122:79.

61. Winkelstern SS. Three cases of iatrogenic intrusion of the posterior teeth during mandibular repositioning therapy. J Craniomandib Pract 1988;6:77.

62. Lerman MD. The hydrostatic appliance: a new approach to treatment of the TMJ pain dysfunction syndrome. J Am Dent Assoc 1974;89:1343.

63. Block SL, Apfel M, Laskin DM. The use of a resilient latex rubber bite appliance in the treatment of MPD syndrome. J Dent Res 1978;57(special issue):69. Abstract 71.

64. Harkins S, Marteney JL, Cueva O, Cueva L. Application of soft occlusal splints in patients suffering from clicking temporomandibular joints. J Craniomandib Pract 1988;6:71.

65. Singh BP, Berry DC. Occlusal changes following use of soft occlusal splints. J Prosthet Dent 1985;54:711.

66. Kraus H. Muscle spasm. In Kraus H (ed). Diagnosis and treatment of muscle pain. Chicago: Quintessence, 1988:11.

67. Haley D, Schiffman E, Baker C, Belgrade M. The comparison of patients suffering from temporomandibular disorders and general headache population. Headache 1993;33:210.

68. Barnes JF. Myofascial release emphasized. Craniocomments. J Craniomandib Pract 1987;5:311.

69. Prudden B. Myotherapy: complete guide to pain-free living. New York: Ballantine, 1984.

70. Eisen AG, Kaufman A, Greene CS. Evaluation of physical therapy for MPD syndrome. J Dent Res 1984;63(special issue):344. Abstract 1561.

71. Makofsky HW, August BF, Ellis JJ. A multidisciplinary approach to the evaluation and treatment of temporomandibular joint and cervical spine dysfunction. J Craniomandib Pract 1989;7:205.

72. Tegelberg A, Kopp S. Short-term effect of physical training on temporomandibular joint disorder in individuals with rheumatoid arthritis and ankylosing spondylitis. Acta Odontol Scand 1988;46:49.

73. Ayer WA, Levin MP. Theoretical basis and application of massed practice therapy exercises for elimination of tooth grinding habits. J Periodontol 1975;46:306.

74. Waide FL, Bade DM, Lovasko J, Montana J. Clinical management of a patient following temporomandibular joint arthroscopy. Phys Ther 1992;72:355.

75. Rocabado M. Arthrokinematics of the temporomandibular joint. Dent Clin North Am 1983;27:573.

76. Kraus SS. Cervical spine influences on the craniomandibular region. In Kraus SL (ed). TMJ disorders: management of the craniomandibular complex. New York: Churchill-Livingstone, 1988.

77. Osborne JJ. A physical therapy protocol for orthognathic surgery. J Craniomandib Pract 1989;7:132.

78. Morrone L, Makofsky H. TMJ home exercise program. Clinical Management 1991;11:20.

79. Jette DV, Falkel JE, Brombly C. Effect of intermittent supine cervical traction on the myoelectric activity of the upper trapezius muscle in subjects with neck pain. Phys Ther 1985;65:1173.

80. Pennie BW, Agambar LJ. Whiplash injuries: a trial of early management. J Bone Joint Surg (Br) 1990;72:277.

81. Beckerman H, Bouter LM, van der Heijden GJ, de Bie RA, Koes BW. Efficacy of physiotherapy for musculoskeletal disorders: what can we learn from research? Br J Gen Pract 1993;43:73.

82. Danzig WN, Van Dyke AR. Physical therapy as an adjunct to temporomandibular joint therapy. J Prosthet Dent 1983;49:96.

83. Clark GT, Adachi NY, Dornan MR. Physical medicine procedures affect temporomandibular disorders: a review. J Am Dent Assoc 1990;121:151.

84. Mohl ND, Ohrbach RK, Crow HC, Gross AJ. Devices for the diagnosis and treatment of temporomandibular disorders: thermography, ultrasound, electrical stimulation, and electromyographic biofeedback. J Prosthet Dent 1990;63(pt 3):472.

85. Erickson RI. Ultrasound: a useful adjunct in temporomandibular joint therapy. Oral Surg Oral Med Oral Pathol 1964;18:176.

86. Murphy GJ. Electrical physical therapy in treating TMJ patients. J Craniomandib Pract 1983;1:67.

87. Jospe M. The placebo effect in healing. Lexington, MA: Lexington Books, 1978.

88. Thorsteinsson G, Stonnington HH, Stillwell GK, et al. The placebo effect of transcutaneous electrical stimulation. Pain 1978;5:31.

89. Grieder A, Vinton DN, Cinotti WR, Kangur TT. An evaluation of ultrasonic therapy for temporomandibular joint dysfunction. Oral Surg 1971;31:25.

90. Esposito CJ, Veal SJ, Farman AG. Alleviation of myofascial pain with ultrasonic therapy. J Prosthet Dent 1984;51:106.

91. Talaat AM, El-Dibany MM, El-Garf A. Physical therapy in the management of myofascial pain dysfunction syndrome. Ann Otol Rhinol Laryngol 1986;95:225.

92. Braun BL. The effect of physical therapy intervention on incisal opening after temporomandibular joint surgery. Oral Surg Oral Med Oral Pathol 1987; 64:544.

93. Brooke RI. Secondary osteoarthrosis (osteoarthritis) of the temporomandibular joint. J Can Dent Assoc 1977;43:323.

94. Marchand S, Charest J, Li J, Chenard J-R, Lavignolle B, Laurencelle L. Is TENS purely a placebo effect? a controlled study of chronic low back pain. Pain 1993;54:99.

95. Chee EK, Walton W. Treatment of triggerpoints with microamperage transcutaneous electrical nerve stimulation (TENS). J Manipulative Physiol Ther 1986;9:131.

96. Shambaugh P. Treatment of trigger points with microamperage transutaneous electrical nerve stimulation (TENS: the Electro-Acuscope 80). J Manipulative Physiol Ther 1987;10:31.

97. Shealy CN. Transcutaneous nerve stimulation to control pain. Pain 1975;2:1.

98. Wessberg GA, Carroll WL, Dinham R, Wolford LM. Transcutaneous electrical stimulation as an adjunct in the management of myofascial pain-dysfunction syndrome. J Prosthet Dent 1981;45:307.

99. Terezhalmy GT, Ross GR, Holmes-Johnson E. Transcutaneous electrical nerve stimulation treatment of TMJ-MPDS patients. Ear Nose Throat J 1982;61:22.

100. Block SL, Laskin DM. The effectiveness of transcutaneous nerve stimulation (TENS) in the treatment of unilateral MPD syndrome. J Dent Res 1980; 59(special issue):519. Abstract 999.

101. Gold N, Greene CS, Laskin DM. TENS therapy for treatment of MPD syndrome. J Dent Res 1983;62(special issue):244. Abstract 676.

102. Clarke MS, Silverstone LM, Lindenmuyth J, Hicks MJ, Averbach RD, Kleier DJ, Stoller NH. An evaluation of the clinical analgesia/anesthesia efficacy on acute pain using the high frequency neural modulator in various dental settings. Oral Surg Oral Med Oral Pathol 1987;63:501.

103. Niv D, Ben-Ari S, Rapport A, Goldofski S, et al. Postherpetic neuralgia: clinical experience with a conservative treatment. Clin J Pain 1989;5:295.

104. Graff-Radford SB, Reeves JL, Baker RL, Chiu D. Effects of transcutaneous electrical stimulation on myofascial pain and trigger point sensitivity. Pain 1989;37:1.

105. Hansson P, Ekblom A. Transcutaneous electrical nerve stimulation (TENS) as compared to placebo (TENS) for the relief of acute oro-facial pain. Pain 1983;15:157.

106. Møystad A, Krogstad BS, Larheim TA. Transcutaneous nerve stimulation in a group of patients with rheumatic disease involving the temporomandibular joint. J Prosthet Dent 1990;64:596.

107. Lander J, Fowler-Kerry S. TENS for children's procedural pain. Pain 1993;52:209.

108. Taylor K, Newton RA, Personius WJ, Bush FM. Effect of interferential current stimulation for treatment of subjects with recurrent jaw pain. Phys Ther 1987;67:346.

109. Beckerman H, de Bie RA, Bouter LM, De Cuyper HJ, Oostendorp RA. The efficacy of laser therapy for musculoskeletal and skin disorders: a criteria-based meta analysis of randomized clinical trials. Phys Ther 1992;72:483.

110. Waylonis GW, Wilke S, O'Toole D, Waylonis DA, Waylonis DB. Chronic myofascial pain: management by low-output helium-neon laser therapy. Arch Phys Med Rehabil 1988;69:1017.

111. Thorsen H, Gam AN, Svensson BH, Jess M, Jenssen MK, Piculelli I, Schack LK, Skjott K. Low level laser therapy for myofascial pain in the neck and shoulder girdle: a double-blind, cross over study. Scand J Rheumatol 1992; 21:139.

112. Olavi P, Pekka R, Pertti K, Pekka P. Effects of the infrared laser therapy at treated and non-treated trigger points. Acupunct Electrother Res 1989;14:9.

113. Lark MR, Gangarosa LP, Sr. Iontophoresis: an effective modality for the treatment of inflammatory disorders of the temporomandibular joint and myofascial pain. J Craniomandib Pract 1990;8:108.

114. Schiffman EL, Braun BL. Effect of iontophoretic medication delivery on TMD signs and symptoms. J Dent Res 1993;72(special issue):337. Abstract 1869.

115. Grzesiak RC. Psychological consideration in temporomandibular dysfunction: a biopsychosocial view of symptom formation. Dent Clin North Am 1991; 35:209.

116. DePalma A-MC. The TMJ network: a support system for TMD patients. J Craniomandib Pract 1993;11:159.

117. Gatchel RJ. Managing anxiety and pain during dental treatment. J Am Dent Assoc 1992;123:37.

118. McGuigan FJ. Coping with stress through progressive relaxation. Basal Facts 1985;7:151.

119. Appleton SS, Sommers EE, Truelove EL, Le Resche L. Treating myofascial pain with occlusal splints and specific relaxation therapy. J Dent Res 1985;64(special issue):232. Abstract 514.

120. Holmes-Johnson E. Behavioral treatment of TMJ-MPDS patients. Ear Nose Throat J 1982;61:655.

121. Majewski RF, Gale EN. The effectiveness of relaxation training for TMJ/MPD patients. J Dent Res 1983;62(special issue). Abstract 150.

122. Gelb ML, Gale EN. Effects of home practice on biofeedback treatment of TMJ/MPD pain. J Dent Res 1983;62(special issue):186. Abstract 152.

123. Sorbi M, Tellegen BN, Du Long A. Long-term effects of training in relxation and stress coping in patients with migraine: a 3-year follow-up. Headache 1989;29:111.

124. Melis PML, Rooimans W, Spierings ELH, Hoogduin CAL. Treatment of chronic tension-type headache with hypnotherapy: a single-blind time controlled study. Headache 1991;31:686.

125. Cohen ES, Hillis RE. The use of hypnosis in treating the temporomandibular joint pain dysfunction syndrome. Oral Surg 1979;48:193.

126. Waese S. TMJ dysfunction: behaviour modification. Oral Health 1986;76:47.

127. Stam HJ, McGrath PA, Brooke RI, Cosier F. Hypnotizability and the treatment of chronic facial pain. Int J Clin Exp Hypn 1986;34:182.

128. Golan HP. Temporomandibular joint disease treated with hypnosis. Am J Clin Hypn 1989;31:269.

129. Dublin LL. The use of hypnosis for temporomandibular joint (TMJ). Psychiatr Med 1992;10:99.

130. Carlsson SG, Gale EN, Ohman A. Treatment of temporomandibular joint syndrome with biofeedback training. J Am Dent Assoc 1975;91:602.

131. Flor H, Turk DC. Psychophysiology of chronic pain: do chronic pain patients exhibit symptom-specific psychophysiological responses? Psychol Bull 1989; 105:215.

132. Dohrmann RJ, Laskin DM. An evaluation of electromyographic biofeedback in the treatment of myofascial pain-dysfunction syndrome. J Am Dent Assoc 1978;96:656.

133. Erlandson PM, Jr, Poppen R. Electromyographic biofeedback and rest position training of masticatory muscles in myofascial pain-dysfunction patients. J Prosthet Dent 1989;62:335.

134. Flor H, Birbaumer N. Efficacy of EMG-biofeedback, cognitive-behavior therapy, and medical treatment for chronic musculoskeletal pain. Biofeedback Self Regul 1991;16. Abstract 278.

135. Asfour SS, Khalil TM, Waly SM, Goldberg ML, Rosomoff RS, Rosomoff HL. Biofeedback in back muscle strengthening. Spine 1990;15:510.

136. Cott A, Parkinson W, Fabich M, Bedard M, Marlin R. Long-term efficacy of combined relaxation: biofeedback treatments for chronic headache. Pain 1992;51:49.

137. Arena JG, Hannah SL, Bruno GM, Meador KJ. Electromyographic biofeedback training for tension headache in the elderly: a prospective study. Biofeedback Self Regul 1991;16:379.

138. Middaugh SJ, Woods SE, Kee WG, Harden RN, Peters JR. Biofeedback-assisted relaxation training for the aging chronic pain patient. Biofeedback Self Regul 1991;16:361.

139. Raustia AM, Pohjola RT, Virtanen KK. Acupuncture compared with stomatognathic treatment for TMJ dysfunction: a randomized study. J Prosthet Dent 1985;54(pt 1):581.

140. List T. Acupuncture in the treatment of patients with craniomandibular disorders: comparative, longitudinal and methodological studies. Swed Dent J 1992;87(suppl):1.

141. Lapeer GL. Postsurgical myofascial pain resolved with dry-needling: treatment protocol and case report. J Craniomandib Pract 1989;7:243.

142. Melzack R, Katz J. Auriculotherapy fails to relieve chronic pain. J Am Med Assoc 1984;251:1041.

143. Johnson MI, Hajela VK, Ashton CH, Thompson JW. The effects of auricular transcutaneous electrical nerve stmulation (TENS) on experimental pain threshold and autonomic function in health subjects. Pain 1991;46:3737.

144. Fricton JR. Clinical care for myofascial pain. Dent Clin North Am 1991;35:1.

145. Graff-Radford SB. Headache problems that can present as toothache. Dent Clin North Am 1991;35:155.

146. Dieppe PA, Sathapat B, Jones HE, Bacon PA, Ring ETJ. Intra-articular steroids in osteoarthritis. J Rheumatol Rehabil 1980;19:19:212.

147. Shupak R, Tietel J, Garvey MB, Freedman J. Intraarticular methylpredniso-lone therapy in hemophilic arthropathy. Am J Hematol 1988;27:26.

148. Panavene DP. Bandzhivlene SIU, Iokimaitus KG, Dadoneme IG. The effect of intra-articular treatment with corticosteroids, polyvinyl pyrrolidone and di-methyl sulfoxide on the composition of the synovial fluid in patients with rheu-matoid arthritis. Ter Arkh 1989;61:116.

149. Fauno P, Andersen HJ, Simonsen O. A long-term follow-up of the effect of repeated corticosteroid injections for stenosing tenovaginitis. J Hand Surg (Br) 1989;14:242.

150. Kopp S, Wenneberg B. Effects of occlusal treatment and intraarticular injec-tions on temporomandibular joint pain and dysfunction. Acta Odontol Scand 1981;39:87.

151. Lynch MC, Taylor JF. Facet joint injection for low back pain: a clinical study. J Bone Joint Surg (Br) 1986;68:138.

152. Balogh K. The histological appearance of corticosteroid injection sites. Arch Pathol Lab Med 1986;110:1168.

153. Kopp W, Wenneberg B, Haraldson T, Carlsson GE. The short-term effect of intra-articular injections of sodium hyaluronate and corticosteroid on tempo-romandibular joint pain and dysfunction. J Oral Maxillofac Surg 1985; 43:429.

154. Kopp S, Carlsson GE, Haraldson T, Wenneberg G. Long-term effect of intra-articular injections of sodium hyaluronate and corticosteroid on temporoman dibular joint arthritis. J Oral Maxillofac Surg 1987;45:929.

155. Fader KW, Grummons DC, Maijer R, Christensen LV. Pressurized infusion of sodium hyaluronate for closed lock of the temporomandibular joint: a case study. J Craniomandib Pract 1993;11(pt 1):68.

156. Bertolami CN, Gay T, Clark GT, Rendell J, Shetty V, Liuv C, Schwann DA. Use of sodium hyaluronate in treating temporomandibular joint disorders: a randomized double-blind, placebo-controlled clinical trial. J Oral Maxillofac Surg 1993;51:232.

157. Mejersjö C, Kopp S. Effect of corticosteroid and sodium hyaluronate on in-duced joint lesions in guinea-pig knee. Int J Oral Maxillofac Surg 1987;16:194.

158. Burchiel KJ. Surgical treatment of trigeminal neuralgia: minor and major op-erative procedures. In Fromm GH (ed). The medical and surgical management of trigeminal neuralgia. New York: Futura, 1987:71, 101.

159. Sahni KS. Trigeminal glycerol rhizolysis: a book for patients. Available from author, 1469 Johnston Willis Drive, Richmond, VA 23235.

160. Tronnier VM, Wirtz CR, Steiner HH, Kunze ST. Long-term efficacy of micro-vascular decompression in trigeminal neuralgia. Seattle, WA: International As-sociation for the Study of Pain. 1993:53. Abstract 145.

161. Glass EG, Glaros AG, McGlynn FD. Myofascial pain dysfunction: treatments used by ADA members. J Craniomandib Pract 1993;11:25.

162. Bush FM. Occlusal therapy in the management of chronic orofacial pain. An-esthesia Progress 1984;31:10.

163. Goodman P, Greene CS, Laskin DM. Response of patients with myofascial pain dysfunction syndrome to mock equilibration. J Am Dent Assoc 1976;92:755.

164. Tsolka P, Morris RW, Preiskel HW. Occlusal adjustment therapy for craniomandibular disorders: a clinical assessment by a double-blind method. J Prosthet Dent 1992;68:957.

165. Long JH, Jr. Occlusal adjustment as treatment for tenderness in the muscles of mastication in category 1 patients. J Prosthet Dent 1992;676:519.

The Temporomandibular Joint and Related Orofacial Disorders,
by Francis M. Bush and M. Franklin Dolwick.
J.B. Lippincott Company, Philadelphia, © 1995.

10

Surgery of the Temporomandibular Joint

Surgery of the TMJ plays a small but significant role in the management of TMD. The most undisputed application of surgery is found in management of the least common TMJ disorders, such as ankylosis, growth disorders, recurrent dislocation, and neoplasia. Indications are less clear for more common disorders, such as internal derangements. Experience suggests that about 5% of all patients undergoing treatment for TMD require some surgical intervention.

A wide spectrum of surgical procedures is used for treatment of TMJ disorders. The procedures range from simple irrigation of the joint to complex open joint procedures. Surgical success depends on the appropriate selection of cases.

This chapter presents the indications, outcomes, and complications associated with some common surgical procedures. Extensive detail is beyond the scope of this chapter. Some procedures are briefly described to improve the reader's comprehension of problems faced by patients and by the practitioners who treat them.

Indications for Surgery

Individuals with genuine TMJ disorders suffer various afflictions. Surgery may be necessary if the symptoms are resistant to conservative, nonsurgical treatment. Most surgeries are performed for the following reasons:

Internal derangement
Osteoarthrosis (osteoarthritis)
Ankylosis (fibrous and bony)

357

Hypermobility, dislocation
Growth disorders (hyperplastic versus hypoplastic)
Condylar trauma
Infections
Neoplasia

Terminology of Surgical Techniques

Arthrotomy involves open surgery to expose and dissect structures of the joint.

Debridement concerns the removal of devitalized tissue by mechanical means.

Perforations imply holes in the disk or junction of the disk with the posterior attachment.

Disk repair involves procedures used to repair perforations or tears in the disk.

Disk repositioning is a procedure to move a displaced disk into a normal anatomic relation with respect to the condyle and fossa.

Diskectomy (sometimes inappropriately termed meniscectomy) refers to surgical removal of the disk.

Eminectomy involves removal of the eminence; *eminoplasty*, recontouring of the eminence (Fig. 10-1A).

Condylectomy involves total removal of the condyle (Fig. 10-1B).

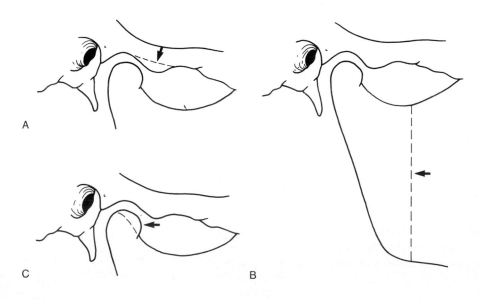

Figure 10-1.
Arrows show regions of bone dissection for different procedures. (A) Eminectomy. (B) Modified condylotomy. (C) High condylectomy.

Modified condylotomy is a variation of the vertical ramus osteotomy, whereby the condylar process is detached from the mandibular ramus. It is used in the treatment of internal derangement.

High condylectomy refers to limited bony recontouring of the head of the condyle (Fig. 10-1C). This procedure is sometimes called a "condylar shave." It is used to remove the diseased articular surface of the condylar head.

Arthroscopic surgery refers to operative procedures performed with fine instruments during telescopic penetration of a joint cavity for diagnostic and therapeutic reasons. The surgery is performed using a rigid endoscope (arthroscope). Arthroscopic surgery is less invasive than arthrotomy.

The scopes have an average external diameter of 2.5 mm and a lens diameter of about 2.0 mm (Fig. 10-2). The image is magnified from 1 to 15 times. The joint anatomy can be visualized, surgically altered if needed, and the procedure recorded by an attached cinecamera or videorecorder.

Anatomic details seen after insertion of the arthroscope into the healthy joint are the position of the disk, the articular surfaces, and the synovial membrane of the upper joint space.[1] Arthroscopy permits a viewing of pathologic changes in the joint, including degree of inflammation (eg, hyperemia, edema, synovitis), adhesion, fibrillation, fibrosis, disk displacement and rupture, and perforations. Bony irregularities may be visible.

Arthrocentesis refers to needle puncture of the joint space (Fig. 10-3). Usually, this procedure is combined with lavage. *Lavage* involves irrigation of the joint. After lavage, the mandible is gently manipulated to evaluate motion.

Lysis refers to mechanical or hydraulic techniques designed to loosen adhesions.

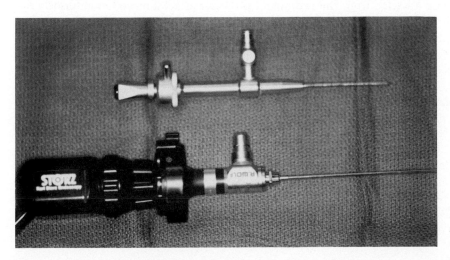

Figure 10-2.
Arthroscope used to view internal anatomy of the joint.

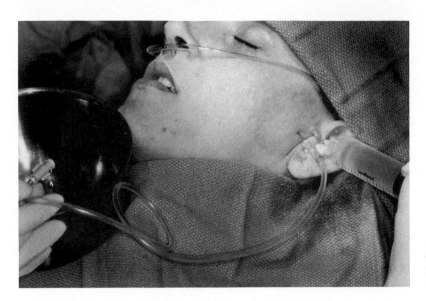

Figure 10-3.
Arthrocentesis followed by lavage is used for treatment of a patient with diskal displacement without reduction.

Anterior release (anterior band release) is a procedure used for freeing up fibrous tissue anterior to the disk. It helps to increase the mobility of the disk and may be accomplished with arthroscopic scissors or by electrocautery.

Posterior cauterization refers to electrocautery of the posterior attachment. The procedure is used primarily for symptomatic hypermobility with chronic condylar dislocation and hypertrophied synovial tissue. Proof is lacking for its value in retaining the posterior positioning of a disk freed by anterior release. *Synovial cauterization* is used if control of oozing and hemorrhage is required. Some surgeons use sutures to reposition the disk.

Plication involves folding or taking a tuck to reduce the size of the disk. It consists of removing a wedge from the redundant posterior attachment of an anteriorly displaced disk. The segments are sutured together (Fig. 10-4). *Partial-thickness plication* involves repositioning the disk without violating the lower joint space. *Full-thickness plication* means repositioning the disk by surgically exposing the lower joint space.

Arthroplasty generally involves recontouring the articular surface of the mandibular condyle or articular eminence. Another material may be inserted after surgical excision to replace some part of the joint.

This replacement may be made with either with an *autogenous* or *homogenous* tissue or with an *alloplastic* material. Autogenous tissue is obtained from the same individual and may include dermis, temporal fascia, or cartilage of the ear. Homogenous tissue is derived from another animal, such as collagen or lyophilized cartilage. An alloplast is a prosthesis made from a nonbiologic substance.

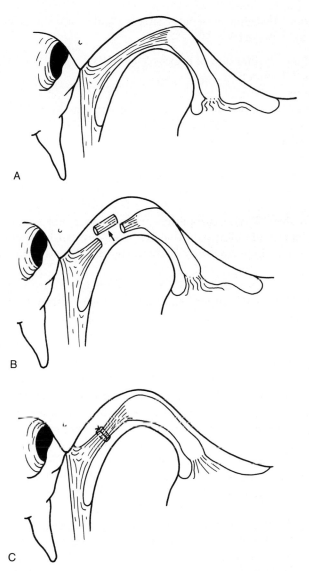

Figure 10-4.
Plication procedure used to reposition an anteriorly displaced disk. (A) Disk is anteriorly displaced. (B) A wedge is removed from the posterior attachment. (C) The disk is retracted posteriorly, and the ends are sutured.

Complications that may arise after surgery and require management mostly fall into the following categories:

- Neurologic dysfunction of nerves V and VII
- Auditory dysfunction
- Infections
- Limited mandibular movement from scarring and fibrosis
- Pain
- Hemorrhage

Rationale for Surgery

The patient with TMJ arthropathy may present to the surgeon with a generalized complaint of chronic joint pain that has been present for 6 months or longer. There may be hypo- or hypermobility of the mandible. No other jaw pathology is evident.

Experience has shown that most TMD patients benefit from appropriate nonsurgical treatment. Thus, TMJ surgery should rarely be performed before nonsurgical treatment has been attempted and found to be ineffective.[2–7]

Criteria for Successful Outcome

The patient considering TMJ surgery should understand that the surgery is an optional treatment. Details of each procedure should be thoroughly discussed between the surgeon and the patient and an agreement reached on what is interpreted as a "successful outcome." The patient or surgeon may interpret either improved motion or loss of pain as successful. There remains the possibility that the surgery may make the patient worse. Thus, specific treatment goals must be well defined and accepted by both parties before surgery.

Most surgical outcomes have been judged by their short-term results. Little information exists about long-term outcome for specific procedures. Most findings been have based on testimonials, either from patients' written reports or from verbal patient judgments interpreted by surgeons. Few surgical criteria have been identified that would serve as a "gold standard" for success or failure of treatment. Recent attempts have been made to establish some measure of assessment. These criteria can be summarized as follows:

1. Patient's sense of improvement
   a. Improvement in chewing and talking
   b. Reduction in pain
   c. Reduction in joint sounds
2. Surgeon's sense of improvement
   a. Improved range of motion, greater than 35 mm vertical opening and 5 mm protrusively and laterally
   b. Avoidance of postoperative complications
   c. Imaging or radiographic appearance of TMJs within normal limits

Patient's Interpretation of Pain

A Committee on TMJ Arthoscopy formed by the American Association of Oral and Maxillofacial Surgeons in 1988 has published the surgical findings from 12 multicenters across the United States.[8] Among the findings were degree of success or failure and outcome with different procedures employed.

Summary of patients' interpretations showed that 91% rated **pain response on palpation** as excellent to good (Table 10-1). An excellent response was rated as minimal to no pain, good as minimal pain, and poor as significant pain. An excellent to good **sense of improvement** was found in 90% of patients. An excellent rating meant a significant sense of improvement; good, a moderate improvement; and poor, a persistent disability. Similar findings were found for eating and dietary habits.

These data compare favorably with findings from another study of TMD patients treated with arthroscopic surgery who were followed for up to 3 years.[9] Procedures included lysis, lavage, debridement of the superior joint space, and mobilization of the joint. Treatment of the 109 TMD patients (150 arthroscopies) showed that three fourths rated the level of pain at 2 postoperatively, compared with 7 to 10 preoperatively. Ninety-three percent of the patients with pain managed it easily. Headache decreased from 83% preoperatively to 40% postoperatively. Chewing was significantly improved, and 90% reported that they could eat a regular diet after the surgery.

In studies concerned with arthrotomy, 80% of 83 patients considered the status of their TMJ as better.[10] About 70% reported being free of pain. Comparable success of 84% was claimed for 27 open surgical cases.[11] Ten percent of patients reported no relief of pain, and 6% described it as worse. Among 14 patients treated arthroscopi-

Table 10-1

Summary of Interpretations of Patients and Surgeons on Success of Surgery

Parameter	No. of Joints (j) or Patients (p)	Rating		
		Excellent	*Good*	*Poor*
Patient				
Palpable pain	4,736 j	71	20	9
Improvement	1,411 p	58	34	8
Eating/diet	2,978 p	51	40	9
Surgeon				
Range of motion	3,031 p	56	36	8

Modified from McCain JP, Sanders B, Koslin MG, Quinn JD, Peters PB, Indresano AT. Temporomandibular joint arthroscopy: a 6-year multicenter retrospective study of 4,831 joints. J Oral Maxillofac Surg 1992;50:926.

cally, one half reported less frequent and reduced pain intensity and one half had little to no change.

Questionnaires returned from 150 of 237 patients treated by different surgical procedures revealed that 146 had improved significantly (Table 10-2). The failure rate was highest in the few patients treated by diskectomy.[12] Overall, most stated that they would have the surgery again if needed.

Computation of results from another study of 77 patients (152 joints) treated arthroscopically found that 71% achieved excellent to very good results.[13] These patients had no pain and followed a diet without restrictions. Twenty-four percent were judged as good to fair because of occasional to slight discomfort. The treatment was considered to have failed in the remaining 5% of patients with unrelenting pain. The patients were followed for 2 to 31 months.

Significance: Collectively, the studies support the view that surgery is a meaningful option for management of patient's pain or dysfunction.

Table 10-2

Summary of Findings for Specific Treatments of 237 Patients Subjected to TMJ Surgery

Treatment	No. of Patients	Failure Rate	Success Rate
High condylectomy	38	16	84
Condylotomy	8		100
Eminectomy	6	33	67
Disk Repair			
Diskoplasty	23	9	91
Diskoplasty with condylar reduction	37	24	76
Diskoplasty with eminence reduction	12		100
Diskoplasty with condylar and eminence reduction	24	29	71
Diskectomy			
No implant	3	33	66
With Silastic fossa implant	69	9	91
With Silastic for 3–6 months	8	25	75
With Proplast-Teflon implant	4		100
With dermal graft	5	20	80

Modified from Merrill RG. Historical perspectives and comparisons of TMJ surgery for internal disk derangements and arthropathy. J Craniomandib Pract 1986;4:74.

Surgeon's Interpretation of Range of Motion and Tenderness

The findings obtained from the multicenter study revealed that a high percentage of surgeons were satisfied with the surgical outcome (see Table 10-1). A summary of the surgeons' interpretations showed that 92% rated patients' range of motion as excellent or good. This decision was based on an excellent rating of maximal vertical opening as 40 mm or more, good as 30 to 40 mm, and poor as less than 30 mm.

These data compare favorably with findings from another study of patients treated with arthroscopic surgery.[9] Seventy-five percent of of 109 patients had a maximal voluntary opening of 40 mm or more and similar improvement in lateral motions after surgery, where 47% had opening less than 35 mm prior to treatment. Additionally, muscular tenderness on palpation dropped from about 50% preoperatively to 29% postoperatively, and the discomfort was described as less severe.

Another study of 237 patients treated with different surgical procedures produced 83% success.[12] The author assessed the success from clinical and radiologic findings. The level of pain was determined by patient response to treatment. Absence of major complication was considered a surgical criterion. Success was judged by the specific procedure performed: bone reduction, 85%; disk repositioning and repair, 81%; and diskectomy, 89%. Length of follow-up was not stated.

Based on studies of 77 patients treated arthroscopically, another surgeon judged excellent to very good results as an interincisal opening of 35 mm or more and good mandibular function as an absence of joint noises.[13] Good to fair success was judged as minimal joint sounds, interincisal opening of 35 mm or more, and good mandibular function. Such patients had close follow-up, stress management, or physical therapy. Outcomes were judged as failures in patients who required further surgery because of pain or dysfunction.

Significance: Collectively, these studies support the view that surgeons interpret surgeries as worthwhile options for patients with chronic TMJ pain or dysfunction resistant to conservative therapy.

Diagnosis

Successful TMJ surgery depends on an accurate diagnosis. The diagnosis is derived after evaluation of the patient's chief complaint, history of the complaint, and the clinical findings.

The chief complaint must be severe or bothersome enough to constantly interfere with activities of daily living. The history should include some prior conservative therapies resulting in unfavorable outcomes.

Clinical examination relies on finding pain localized to the TMJ that is tender to palpation and painful when the joint is loaded. Mechanical interference of mandibular movement (locking, clicking, or popping) may be present.

Osseous changes may be visible by radiographic analysis. TMJ arthrographic or magnetic resonance imaging (MRI) evaluations of soft tissues help identify some deranged structures, but these evaluations should not be considered definitive diagnostically.

Surgical Dilemmas: Selected Opinions About TMJ Surgery

The surgeon should select operative procedures with the greatest potential for success and lowest possibility of complication. However, there is controversy within the profession about definitions of and need for TMJ surgery.[14] Sampling by postal questionnaire of 100 international "experts on temporomandibular joint surgery" revealed some degree of consensus for certain questions but disagreement for others (Table 10-3).

Length of Conservative Therapy

Opinions differed on the minimal time conservative therapy should be judged ineffective before surgery is attempted. Fifty-one percent of the surgeons designated as "experts" agreed on 6 months, and 34% agreed on 2 months.

Table 10-3
Summary of Opinions of 100 Experts on TMJ Surgery

Opinion	Definition	Agree/Disagree (%)
Internal derangement	Localized mechanical fault of joint that interferes with its smooth action	73/27
Osteoarthrosis	Noninflammatory disorder of a movable joint with deterioration and abrasion of the articular connective tissue and formation of new bone at the articular surfaces	80/20
Internal derangement leads to arthrosis		61/39
Stages of internal derangement (overall)		87/13
Early	Painless, early reciprocal clicking, no inflammation, disk slightly forward	30/70
Early-intermediate	Loud clicking, locking, mild inflammation, early deformed disk slightly forward	95/5
Intermediate	Major inflammation, marked disk deformity partially or completely forward	96/4
Intermediate-late	Clinical chronicity, disk completely forward, bony degeneration, remodeling	97/3
Late	Clinical chronicity, disk completely forward, perforated at posterior attachment, deformity of bony and soft tissues	100/0

Modified from Goss AN. The opinions of 100 international experts on temporomandibular joint surgery: a postal questionnaire. Int J Oral Maxillofac Surg 1993;22:66.

Definitions

Support among the "experts" was lowest for the statement that internal derangement led to arthrosis. Thirty-nine percent disagreed with this statement. The statement with the next to lowest support was the definition of internal derangement as a localized mechanical fault.

Surgery and Stage of Derangement

Five stages of progressively worsening internal derangement were defined, and 87% of the surgeons accepted them. Just 30% agreed that surgery should be performed in the earliest stage. Nearly complete agreement was found for performing surgery on patients in the early-intermediate to intermediate-late stages, and complete agreement for the latest stage. The preference for specific treatments at each of the five stages is outlined below:

Early: none

Early-intermediate: lysis and lavage with arthroscopy or disk repositioning with arthrotomy

Intermediate: disk repositioning or diskectomy with arthrotomy or lysis and lavage with arthroscopy

Late-intermediate: disk repositioning, diskectomy, or condylar shave with arthrotomy or lysis and lavage with arthroscopy (Few surgeons recommended lysis and lavage, but if arthroscopy was performed, some bony recontouring and repair were recommended.)

Late: diskectomy primarily with or without replacement during arthrotomy.

Relief of Pain

Eighty surgeons estimated surgical success for relief of pain at 70%. Other successes included relief from locking (60%), clicking (63%), and limitation of opening (77%).

But when the experts were questioned about failures, the ratings did not match the reciprocal percentages. Ratings for failures were estimated as continued pain (14%), locking (35%), clicking (10%), and limitation of opening (16%).

Postoperative Complications

Little difference was found in postoperative complications for surgery performed by arthroscopy or by arthrotomy. For as many as 10% of patients presenting with complications, surgical estimates for complications with arthroscopy were 65% for persistent pain and 82% for temporary facial weakness. For arthrotomy, the estimate was 61% for each, respectively.

Significance: A major criticism of the survey is that few oral surgeons were sampled from North America. The response rate was highest for surgeons from Asia, with 87% responding.

The relation of pain to stages of diskal disorder, particularly in light of the absence of neural tissue within the disk, is unclear.

For internal derangements, arthroscopic surgery was preferred by experts for its diagnostic and therapeutic values. Clinicians interested in arthroscopic surgery may review the excellent photographs of intra-articular morphology in *Diagnostic Arthroscopy of the TMJ* by Murakami and colleagues.[1]

History of TMJ Surgery and Related Procedures

Internal Derangement and Treatment

Since the introduction of surgery for disk repositioning,[15] surgical treatment of internal derangement has undergone major changes. Until the middle of the 1980s, most TMJ pain and dysfunction was attributed to diskal displacement and deformity.[16–22] Displaced, deformed disks were reshaped and repositioned after arthrotomy. Diskectomy and condylotomy were alternative procedures used then and later.[23–25]

Because open joint procedures failed to achieve expected results, surgeons sought alternative procedures. The surgical management of internal derangement was revolutionized by the introduction of TMJ arthroscopy.[26–30] The observation that lavage and lysis of adhesions done only within the upper joint compartment resulted in less pain and improved function raised important questions about the need to reposition the disk.[31] Recent observations after arthrocentesis with lavage makes the significance of diskal displacement as a cause of TMJ pain and dysfunction even more doubtful.

Most internal derangements in North America are managed arthroscopically. Others require arthrotomy, and still others may be performed with either procedure (Table 10-4). In most cases of arthrotomy, this decision is not made until the condition of

Table 10-4
Recommended Procedures for Specific Stages of Internal Derangement

Stage of Condition	Procedure
Disk Displacement With Reduction	
Mechanical interference	Arthrotomy
Smooth movement	Arthrotomy or modified condylotomy
Disk Displacement Without Reduction	
Acute	Arthrocentesis, lavage, and manipulation or arthroscopy with lavage, lysis
Chronic	Arthrotomy or arthroscopy with lavage, lysis
Disk Displacement With Performation	
	Arthrotomy

After Dolwick MF, Dimitroulis G. Is there a role for temporomandibular joint surgery? Br J Oral Maxillofac Surg 1994;32:1.

Table 10-5

Recommended Treatment of Diskal Disorders Based on Inspection at the Time of Operation

Disk Condition	Criteria	Procedure
Distinct zones, morphology smooth	Little change in shape, no adhesions	Repositioning or possible disk/articular surface recontouring
Morphology grossly deformed	Shortened anterioposteriorly, loss of resiliency, surface rough, color abnormal	Diskectomy, high condylectomy, with or without an implant in the inferior compartment
Degenerated with arthrosis	Perforations, adhesions, significant degeneration of articular surfaces	Diskectomy, with articular surface recontouring, high condylectomy with or without an implant in the inferior compartment

Modified from the 1984 Committee on TMJ Surgery, American Association of Oral and Maxillofacial Surgeons. See Merrill RG. Historical perspective and comparisons of TMJ surgery for internal disk derangements and arthropathy. J Craniomandib Pract 1986;4:74.

the disk is inspected at the time of the operation (Table 10-5). This difference in management is demonstrated by a review of the findings from patients treated at 12 multicenters across the United States (Table 10-6).

Differences between the diagnosis and severity of the disorders explain the variation in the procedures elected (see Table 10-6). Lysis and lavage have been the preferred treatment for patients suffering from arthralgia and disk disorder without reduction. Nearly three fourths of the surgeons applied this modality if pain was present, or if there was disk disorder without reduction. The next most often selected modality was anterior release, posterior cauterization without sutures for disk disorder without

Table 10-6

Summary of the Average Treatment of Patients With Specific Joint Disorders

Disorder	No. of Patients	Lysis/Lavage	Procedure (%) Anterior Release, Posterior Cautery		Debridement With Hand or Motors (d)/Synovial Cautery (s)
			Suture	No Suture	
Disk disorder without reduction	114	73	2	25	
Disk disorder with painful click	71	51	3	46	
Arthralgia	13	77			23s
Osteoarthritis	46	44			56d
Fibrous ankylosis	11	6			94d

Modified from McCain JP, Sanders B, Koslin MG, Quinn JD, Peters PB, Indresano AT. Temporomandibular joint arthroscopy: a 6-year multicenter retrospective study of 4,831 joints. J Oral Maxillofac Surg 1992;50:926.

reduction and for painful clicking. Synovial cauterization was preferred for arthralgia. Debridement was chosen for the treatment of fibrous ankylosis. Debridement and then lysis and lavage were applied for osteoarthritis.

About 6.1% (194/3146) of the patients developed complications. A temporary fifth nerve deficit accounted for 3.6% of the problems, followed by temporary seventh nerve paresis, and then partial hearing loss, respectively.

The frequencies of the follow-ups conducted were as follows: 6 months, 18%; 6 to 12 months, 18%; 12 to 18 months, 16%; 18 to 24 months, 19%; and more than 24 months, 29%.

Rationale for Treatment

There are several options for surgery of internal derangements. Because randomized prospective studies have not been conducted, a procedure should be selected based on available clinical data and the surgeon's experience. The prudent surgeon selects the procedure with the highest probability for success and the lowest probability of morbidity for each patient.

Surgeons should inform patients that although the derangement may progress anatomically, pain and dysfunction frequently diminish in the absence of treatment.[2,32,33]

The decision to perform surgery should be predicated on severity of the patient's symptoms, not on the degree of anatomic derangement. Because little is known about whether surgery is better than the natural course of the disorder, it should not be performed for preventive reasons.

Indication

Surgical treatment is indicated for the patient who presents with severe TMJ pain and dysfunction that has proved refractory to nonsurgical management.

Diagnostic Criteria

The best surgical candidate localizes the pain and dysfunction specifically in the TMJ, has a TMJ tender to palpation, and experiences increased TMJ pain when the joint is loaded. Mechanical interference such as locking or clicking may be demonstrable.

TMJ arthrography or magnetic resonance imaging may prove helpful in identifying certain deranged structures, but the lack of correlation between imaging findings and pain lessens their usefulness.[34–39] Although arthrography and imaging provide accurate images of the anatomy, they have proved disappointing for differentiating patients with TMJ pain from non-TMJ individuals.[40–42]

Further evidence confirms that MRI findings would be an inaccurate "gold standard" for predicting the presence of internal derangements.[43] Comparison of MRI findings with symptoms observed for right-side and left-side joints showed that the sensitivity was 68% and specificity was 82% for right-side joints. For left-side joints, these symptoms were 47% and 64%, respectively. Thus, over-reliance on the diagnostic value of imaging may lead to overdiagnosis and overtreatment.

Risks

Physical risks accompany surgery for internal derangements. It is not known whether the progression of anatomic derangement is altered by surgery.

Procedures

ARTHROSCOPY. TMJ arthroscopy was popularized in the late 1980s. It allowed observation of internal anatomy of the joint, led to improvement in diagnosis, and reduced the maneuvers required to perform surgery of the joint, particularly internal derangements. Clinical experience with arthroscopy raised serious questions as to whether it was necessary to reposition the disk to resolve pain and treat dysfunction.[46,47]

TMJ arthroscopy usually is performed with the patient under general anesthesia. The cannula attached to the rigid arthroscope is inserted into the upper joint compartment, and the arthroscope is connected to a television camera equipped with a video monitor. The upper joint compartment is thoroughly examined either directly through the ocular or indirectly from the monitor.

The most common procedures performed by arthroscopy are lavage and lysis of adhesions. Lavage of the compartment makes exploration easier and more effective. Probing at this time permits determination of tissue characteristics. Adhesions are lysed with instruments manipulated through a second cannula inserted in the compartment. Biopsy forceps or motorized devices fitted with different blades may be used to resect excess tissue.

Results with arthroscopy have been good. Improvement in range of mandibular motion and decreased pain have been judged successful in 79% to 93% of cases.[27,30,46,49–51] Retrospective studies confirmed that lavage and lysis of adhesions performed during arthroscopy are as effective as arthrotomy for treatment of chronic painful limited hypomobility.[46,52]

Some complications may develop during and after arthroscopy. Breaking of instruments within the compartment is a complication unique to arthroscopy. Mobility of the joint may be reduced after arthroscopy, which often requires an aggressive regimen of physical therapy.

Significance: Arthroscopy has both diagnostic and therapeutic value.[30,48–51] Surgery can be performed for all stages of internal derangement and has proved most effective in treating painful diskal disorders without reduction. Presumably, the disk adheres to the fossa, eminence, or both and fails to reduce. The immobility of the disk apparently results from changes in the synovial fluid or articular connective tissues, or is caused by a vacuum effect that develops between the disk and fossa.

ARTHROCENTESIS. Arthrocentesis coupled with lavage and manipulation has become the procedure of choice for many surgeons. Once the joint is anesthetized by local anesthesia, and the patient is under conscious sedation, a 20-gauge needle is placed in the upper joint compartment about 1 cm in front of the ear (see Fig. 10-

3). Hydraulic pressure is created by injecting about 2 mL of lactated Ringer's solution into the upper compartment.[44] A second 20-gauge needle is placed about 1 cm anterior to the first needle, and the joint is irrigated with 50 to 100 mL of the Ringer's solution.

The outflow needle is intermittently occluded to create hydraulic pressure within the compartment.[45] The mandible is gently manipulated to evaluate motion.

Arthrocentesis with irrigation has been used successfully without the need to reposition the disk. These steps proved effective in "unlocking" eight patients with diskal displacement without reduction.[46]

The mean interincisal opening was 22 mm preoperatively and 38 mm postoperatively. Furthermore, the procedure improved the range of mandibular motion and reduced pain in 17 patients with severely limited mouth opening.[47] Comparison of preoperative and postoperative measures showed that pain as measured by the visual analogue scale decreased from 9 to 2, and the frequency of clicking decreased from 12 to 4 patients. Mean voluntary opening increased from 24 to 43 mm and mean lateral motions from 4 to 11 mm. Overall success was 91% in patients followed for 4 to 14 months.

Significance: Surgeons can treat sudden, severely limited opening with arthrocentesis and lavage in patients with diskal displacement without reduction. Patients can expect low morbidity and few complications. Postoperative therapy requires repetitive opening and excursive exercises to main and improve function.

ARTHROTOMY. Arthrotomy may be indicated for all stages of internal derangement. Disk repositioning and diskectomy have been the most frequent procedures managed by open joint surgery.

The skin incision requires a preauricular, endaural, or postauricular approach. The decision of where to locate the incision is based on the surgeon's experience. Once the incision is made, the underlying soft tissue is dissected with care to avoid cutting the facial nerve. Internal components of the joint are evaluated after reflection of the capsule. Either disk repositioning or diskectomy is performed depending on clinical presentation of the joint.

Disk Repositioning. The healthy disk is free of tension and can be repositioned to a normal anatomic relation with the condyle and the fossa. During surgical exposure, the healthy disk is white and glistens. It is firm when manipulated.

Surgical management may entail a partial-thickness plication procedure (see Fig. 10-4), which does not require entrance into the lower synovial compartment.[53] A full-thickness plication is needed if entry is required to the lower compartment.[54]

Osseous recontouring of the condyle, achieved by high condylectomy, may be done to remove any bony irregularity or impingement. Usually this surgery is performed in the lateral third of the joint. Another option is eminoplasty to remove additional mechanical interference.

Surgery to reposition the disk was first used in 1979.[15] Studies concerned with success of disk repositioning have been mixed. Of 152 patients treated between 1980 and 1988, excellent results were reported by 52% and good results by 28%.[55] Nonetheless, about 5% to 10% of the patients reported no improvement or described their dysfunction as worse after the procedure. These findings confirmed the results of other studies.[15,53,56-58]

A serious complication after repair has been the formation of fibrous adhesions between the disks and regions of osseous reduction, particularly the condyle.[59] Relief of pain may occur. Some complaints, including joint sounds or reduced jaw motion, may remain. Temporary weakness of the facial nerve occurs in less than 5% of patients and is usually limited to temporal branches. Many patients experience occlusal changes. Infection develops in less than 1% of cases.

Significance: Disk repositioning is a conservative joint surgery because joint structures are preserved. This procedure is the most technically precise and requires careful postoperative management, especially attention to the occlusion. Long-term prognosis is considered excellent because joint structures are maintained.

Diskectomy. The decision to remove the disk is made in situations in which the disk is so deranged that few options exist. Instability of the disk because of perforation, fragmentation, loss of elasticity, or persistent pain after disk repositioning may require diskectomy.

Once the joint is exposed, the disk is excised, leaving as much synovium as possible. The articular surfaces are then recontoured conservatively if irregularities exist.

Diskectomy is an old procedure.[60] Many surgeons have been reluctant to perform diskectomy and the procedure remains controversial.[61,62] In a review of historical perspectives, excision without replacement was common between 1900 to 1960.[12] The trend in North America then shifted to replacement with an interpositional implant, although presently most surgeons do not use implants.

Outcomes with diskectomy have been equivocal. A comprehensive review described successful relief of pain in some cases, but long-term osseous changes and significant loss of motion were sequelae.[4] Histopathologic changes have been found after experimental diskectomy was performed in the joints of rabbits and baboons.[12]

Favorable results have been reported. No replacement proved effective in the hands of one orthopedic surgeon.[61] A total of 212 diskectomies performed without replacement and conducted over 32 years showed only 4% of the patients developed significant arthropathy. Evaluation of another 15 patients treated by diskectomy between 1947 and 1960 revealed all were pain free and just 1 opened less than 39 mm. Radiographic changes have been observed, primarily in the condyle.[62a] They tend to stabilize after 18 months. Presumably, these changes represent adaptation between the condyle and fossa.

Significant risks exist with diskectomy. Paresis of the facial nerve may occur in up to 5% of cases after diskectomy.[59] Heterotopic bone formation may cause ankylosis, which tends to follow extensive osseous recontouring. Condylar resorption may occur if multiple operations have been done. Significant malocclusion may develop and can be managed by occlusal adjustment.

Significance: Diskectomy is a valid surgical option. Nonetheless, surgeons have been reluctant to accept it because of perceived complications.

Modified Condylotomy. Condylotomy originated in 1957 as a procedure for treatment of painful TMJ.[63] A closed subcondylar incision was made through the neck of the condyle. Because of potential for hemorrhage and injury of the facial nerve, the original procedure was modified.[64] A current indication is for treatment of chronic refractory TMJ pain associated with a reducing disk.[65]

The procedure is performed under general anesthesia on an outpatient basis. The lateral aspect of the mandibular ramus is exposed through a transoral incision. A vertical cut extending from the sigmoid notch to the angle is made parallel to the posterior border of the mandible (Fig. 10-5). The osteotomized border of the proximal segment is smoothed and then is placed next to the distal segment. The incision is closed once the teeth are placed in maxillomandibular fixation. The mandible is

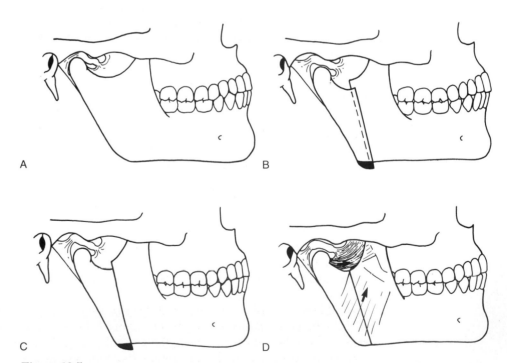

Figure 10-5.
Modified condylotomy used for treating a painful joint with reduction. (A) Disk anteriorly positioned that reduces. (B) Dissected proximal segment overlaps laterally as it moves inferiorly and anteriorly. (C) Union of proximal and distal segments. (D) Arrows show direction of pull produced by the lateral and medial pterygoid muscles. (Hall HD, Nickerson JW, McKenna SJ. Modified condylotomy for treatment of the painful temporomandibular joint with a reducing disc. J Oral Maxillofac Surg 1993;51:133.)

immobilized for 2 to 6 weeks. Training elastics are used to avoid significant malocclusion.

Surgical results have been reported as excellent.[64,66,67] About 92% of 207 patients (251 joints) treated in this manner have been considered successful.[33] These patients had little or no pain and an improved range of motion. A retrospective study of 400 patients followed over 9 years showed that 90% received pain relief from this procedure.[65] The authors claimed that clicking and locking were mostly eliminated.

Significance: Apparently, favorable outcome results because the condyle sags after surgery. This sag increases the space between the condyle, disk, and fossa. An unfavorable malocclusion may follow if the sag is excessive. Minor occlusal changes have been observed in 1% to 2% of patients. There is some possibility of injury to the inferior alveolar nerve during the surgery.[64]

Interpositional Implants. After diskectomy, many kinds of interpositional implants have been inserted to improve joint function. Implants used since 1960 include polycaps for the condyle, dermal or ear cartilage grafts, silicone (Silastic), polytef (Teflon), and Proplast implants, and chrome-cobalt (Vitallium) eminence prostheses.[12]

Replacement by alloplastic materials has been uniformly bad,[68–71] although some studies reported short-term success. Improvement has been reported by patients treated with Vitallium and Vitallium-and-Silastic implants;[72] a success rate of 85% was claimed in eliminating or significantly improving symptoms.

Some alloplasts have produced severe consequences. Foreign body reaction and synovitis were observed initially after Silastic implantation.[7] Other significant changes have included increased pain, bony resorption, and malocclusion. Clinical and radiographic studies were conducted on 43 patients who had diskectomies for chronic pain.[23] Twenty-two received a silicone implant, and 21 received no implant. Condylar erosion was found in 8 patients with implants. The outcome was judged poor in 5 patients; all had implants. Condylar erosion was found in 8 patients with implants. Recent evidence supports the negative long-term effects of these implants. Postinsertional symptoms developed about 4 years after surgery in 12 of 15 patients who received 23 implants.[73]

Proplast-Teflon implants were introduced as interpositional materials in 1976. Short-term results demonstrated favorable outcomes in about 90% of cases, and thousands of patients subsequently received these implants. However, deleterious side effects arguing against their use continued to emerge. Severe condylar and fossa degeneration developed in 90% of cases.[68,71,74] The implants have been unable to withstand functional loading and gradually disintegrated. A foreign body giant cell reaction with subsequent bony erosion and lymphadenopathy appeared within a few years.[75–77] Anterior open bite developed in some cases.[72]

Some measure of success has been accomplished with dermal grafts[78] and grafts consisting of cartilage procured from the ear.[79,80] Twenty patients (26 joints) with irreparable disks unsuitable for posterior plication were treated by diskectomy.[80] These disks were replaced with a $2 \times 2 \times 3$ cm piece of autogenous auricular cartilage sutured against the fossa. Seventeen patients had significant or total resolution of pain. Based on a scale of 0 to 3 (no pain to severe pain), the preoperative level of pain dropped from 2.8 to 0.4 postoperatively. An 85% success rate was claimed for increased range of motion. Maximum voluntary opening averaged 31 mm preoperatively and was 39 mm postoperatively with a follow-up of about 2 years.

Studies involving disk replacement with temporalis muscle pericranial flaps have been limited. The average preoperative opening increased from about 21 mm to 35 mm in 13 patients treated in this manner and followed for 15 months.[81]

Significance: Diskectomy without replacement is recommended over diskectomy with replacement. Long-term studies have not been evaluated in the small number of patients treated with dermal grafts, auricular cartilage grafts, and muscle flaps.

An implant alert concerning Proplast was issued by the Federal Drug Administration (FDA) in 1991. Since then, production for this purpose has ceased. Patients or clinicians concerned about individuals with Silastic or Teflon implants should consult an oral surgeon to see if the removal of implants is necessary. The consensus for symptomatic patients with Proplast-Teflon implants still in situ is for immediate removal. Radiographic follow-up is recommended every 6 months for asymptomatic patients. Information about alloplastic interpositional implants can be obtained from a special registry at the Medic Alert Foundation (800-344-3226). To report problems with these implants, notify the FDA (800-638-6725).

Hypermobility, Subluxation, and Dislocation

Hypermobility, dislocation, and subluxation represent a spectrum of disorders with various etiologies. Among TMD patients treated nonsurgically, 3% or less have a history of dislocation.[82]

The asymptomatic individual with a hypermobile mandible may lack the true pathology of the TMJ. Some hypermobile patients can smoothly translate the condyles horizontally and vertically beyond the peak of the eminence. Usually clicking, locking, and pain are absent as the condyles move to and from this extreme position.

Certain patients with hypermobility may not experience progressive osteoarthritis with advancing age. Thirteen subjects with bilateral hypermobility who were treated non-surgically were matched for gender and age against 13 patients who received routine dental care.[83] The hypermobile group was evaluated 30 years after treatment. Clinical and functional evaluation showed no significant difference between the two groups. Examination of transpharyngeal radiographs disclosed some sclerosis in the joints of the hypermobile patients, which was absent in the dental patients. The authors concluded that some hypermobile joints may degenerate and others may not.

Subluxation is an incomplete condylar translation and should be considered a pathologic condition. The condyle is briefly trapped in a forward position by diskal obstruction or an irregular articular surface. It may spontaneously return to the fossa or the patient may self-reduce the affected joint. Generally, subluxation and ultimate reduction are irregular motions, characterized by sudden popping and some intermittent pain.

Dislocation (luxation) results when contact is absent between normal articulating surfaces. The condyle is locked forward to the anterior slope of the eminence. The individual is unable to reduce the lock because the condylar displacement is too severe. Frequently, tension and pain develop within the lateral pterygoid muscle. The dislocated condyle is characterized by a depression anterior to the tragus. The point of the chin deviates toward the contralateral side on unilateral dislocation.

Radiographs should be obtained to rule out possible mandibular fracture before attempts are made to manipulate the dislocated mandible. Local anesthesia of the TMJ, auricular nerve, and lateral pterygoid muscle has proved helpful before manipulation.[84] Intravenous injection with diazepam (5 to 10 mg intravenously, adult dose given incrementally) may help after unsuccessful attempts. In patients with closed head injury and long-standing bilateral dislocation, arthrotomy may be required. Occasionally, patients may present with dislocation secondary to acute dystonic phenothiazine reaction. Injection with diphenhydramine (25 mg intravenously, adult dose) minimizes extrapyramidal effects and should be given before manual reduction is attempted.

Dislocations that become recurrent are a nuisance for the patient. Procedures for correction are designed to limit condylar translation, eliminate mechanical blocking, or both.[82]

Correction for recurrent dislocation may be accomplished by eminoplasty. A 1.5-cm preauricular incision allows exposure of the eminence. The tubercle and eminence are excised with an osteotome and mallet. The procedure may be done unilaterally or bilaterally.[85] A modified Myrhaug operation has proved successful.[86] Care is taken to avoid opening into the upper joint compartment. A horizontal groove made in the lateral part of the tubercle allows resection of the tubercle and eminence without damaging the articular cartilage.

Retrospective study of 11 patients treated for chronic dislocation and followed for up to 27 months found that all improved with or were satisfied by eminectomy.[85] Satisfactory results were obtained for another 16 patients (31 joints) treated with the modified Myrhaug operation.[86] Nine patients had no recurrence of dislocation, 5 showed improvement, and 1 required a second operation. Ten patients were 100% satisfied, 4 were 90% satisfied, 1 was 50% satisfied, and 1 was dissatisfied. The patients were followed for 8 months to just over 9 years.

Condylar translation can be limited by tightening the laxity associated with the capsule or posterior attachment, tethering the condyle to an adjacent structure, detaching the lateral pterygoid muscle, or forming an anterior block (supraeminence).

In patients with redundant posterior attachment, a partial- or full-thickness plication can be performed. Modest reduction in the height of the eminence improves the chance for success. Sclerosing agents can be injected into the prominent oblique protuberance found in the posteromedial recess of the superior joint compartment.

The patient's teeth should be placed in maxillomandibular fixation for 1 month to limit mandibular movement when these procedures are performed.

Chronic dislocation can be prevented by performing an osteotomy of the zygomatic arch. A slanted osteotomy is made in the posterior arch, and the anterior arch is distracted laterally and partially fractured into place below the intact posterior edge.[87] This surgery creates a large bony eminence.

Another procedure is insertion of a free autogenous bone graft or homologous graft to build up the eminence.[82] The technique has an important advantage because the graft is secured to the eminence with metal plates and screws. Thus, immediate postoperative forces are resisted. This fixation allows long-term healing of the graft to the eminence.

Significance: Eminoplasty appears to be a useful procedure for habitual dislocation. There is no interference with the articular or condylar surfaces or the capsule of the joint. The procedure most likely prevents dislocation because of fibrosis between the roughened surface of the eminence and the internal joint structures.[56] Other modalities, such as injection of sclerosing solution,[89] scarification of the temporalis tendon, or plication, require further study involving larger samples of patients to prove their long-term value.

Hypomobility Unrelated to Internal Derangement

Limited mandibular opening caused by ankylosis of the joint can be debilitating. Individuals experience problems with mastication, speech, and oral hygiene that make management difficult. Hypomobility arises from either extracapsular or intracapsular origins.[90]

Extracapsular Origin

Limited opening of extracapsular origin is termed *pseudoankylosis*. These patients often present with a history of soft tissue injury and scarring related to trauma. Some cases of hypomobility result from enlargement of the coronoid process. The patient typically presents with a gradual loss of opening with advancing age and has no history of trauma, orofacial pain, or TMJ disorder.

The treatment for extracapsular limited opening is generally scar release or coronoidectomy. Once the incision is made over the coronoid, part of the coronoid process is excised to prevent reattachment of the bony ends.[91]

Intracapsular Origin

Limited opening of intracapsular origin is termed *true ankylosis*. Some are bony, others are fibrous, and combinations of the two are termed *fibro-osseous ankylosis*. The primary cause of fibrous ankylosis is trauma. Less common causes are infection, neoplasia, and, rarely, growth disorders.

The procedure for correction of ankylosis is referred to as *gap arthroplasty*. An autogenous graft of temporal muscle or dermis may be positioned between the dissected surfaces to fill the gap.

Significance: Pain is rarely a feature of ankylosis, yet hypomobility may require extensive surgery. Frequent, aggressive physical therapy is required to restore and maintain the normal range of motion.

Skeletal and Dental Malocclusion

Severe cases of dental and skeletal malocclusion are correctable by means of orthognathic surgery. Beneficial effects include correction of the malocclusion, improvement in aesthetics, and reduction of the load on the TMJs. Few studies have assessed the effect of this surgery in TMD patients.

A retrospective study of 75 symptomatic and asymptomatic subjects who had undergone orthognathic surgery showed that 36 had preoperative TMD symptoms.[92] Among treated TMD patients, 89% improved, 8% developed more symptoms, and 3% remained unchanged. About 8% of patients who were asymptomatic before surgery developed some dysfunction postoperatively. The prevalence of dysfunction was greater in patients with class II than class III relations, but function improved in both groups after surgery.

Comparison of 53 retrognathic patients with class II, division I malocclusion treated by mandibular advancement showed that the surgery neither increased nor reduced the risk for TMD.[93] Findings obtained by means of a craniomandibular index confirmed that the signs and symptoms did not differ significantly between the preoperative condition and the condition 1 year after the surgery.

Significance: These limited outcome studies suggest that the surgery led to improvement in symptomatic individuals. Little to no short-term disability resulted.

References

1. Murakami K-I, Matsuki M, Iizuka T, Ono T. Diagnostic arthroscopy of the TMJ: differential diagnoses in patients with limited jaw opening. J Craniomandib Pract 1986;4:117.
2. Boering G. Temporomandibular joint arthrosis: an analysis of 400 cases. Leiden: Staflen, 1966.
3. Toller PA. Osteoarthrosis of the mandibular condyle. Br Dent J 1973;134:223.
4. Carlsson GE, Kopp S, Lindstrom J, Lindqvist S. Surgical treatment of temporomandibular disorders. Ear Nose Throat J 1982;61:679.
5. Greene CS, Laskin DM. Long term evaluation of treatment for myofascial pain-dysfunction syndrome. J Am Dent Assoc 1983;107:235.
6. Mejersjo C, Carlsson GE. Long term results of treatment for temporomandibular pain-dysfunction. J Prosthet Dent 1983;49:809.
7. Carlsson GE. Long term effects of treatment of craniomandibular disorders. J Craniomandib Pract 1985;3:337.
8. McCain JL, Sanders B, Koslin MG, Quinn JD, Peters PB, Indresano AT. Temporomandibular joint arthroscopy: a 6-year multicenter retrospective study of 4,831 joints. J Oral Maxillofac Surg 1992;50:926.
9. Mosby EL. Efficacy of temporomandibular joint arthroscopy: a retrospective study. J Oral Maxillofac Surg 1993;51:17.

10. Bronstein SL, Tomasetti BJ. Temporomandibular joint surgery: patient-based assessment and evaluation. J Am Dent Assoc 1985;110:485.

11. Hodges JH. Managing temporomandibular joint syndrome. Laryngoscope 1990;100:60.

12. Merrill RG. Historical perspectives and comparisons of TMJ surgery for internal disk derangements and arthropathy. J Craniomandib Pract 1986;4:74.

13. Tarro AW. TMJ arthroscopic diagnosis and surgery: clinical experience of 152 procedures over a 2-one-half year period. J Craniomandib Pract 1991;9:107.

14. Goss AN. The opinions of 100 international experts on temporomandibular joint surgery: a postal questionnaire. Int J Oral Maxillofac Surg 1993;22:66.

15. McCarty WL, Farrar WB. Surgery for internal derangements of the temporomandibular joint. J Prosthet Dent 1979;42:191.

16. Farrar WB. Diagnosis and treatment of anterior dislocation of the articular disc. N Y J Dent 1971;41:348.

17. Isberg AM, Westesson P-L. Movement of the disc and condyle in temporomandibular joints with clicking: an arthrographic and cineradiographic study of autopsy specimens. Acta Odontol Scand 1982;40:151.

18. Dolwick MF, Katzberg RW, Helms CA. Internal derangements of the temporomandibular joint: fact or fiction? J Prosthet Dent 1983;49:415.

19. Eriksson L, Westesson P-L. Clinical and radiological study of patients with anterior disc displacement of the temporomandibular joint. Swed Dent J 1983;7:55.

20. Scapino RP. Histopathology associated with malposition of the human temporomandibular joint disc. Oral Surg Oral Med Oral Pathol 1983;55:382.

21. Westesson P-L, Rohlin M. Internal derangement related to osteoarthrosis in temporomandibular joint autopsy specimens. Oral Surg Oral Med Oral Pathol 1984;57:17.

22. Hall MB, Brown RW, Baughman RA. Histologic appearance of the bilaminar zone in internal derangement of the temporomandibular joint. Oral Surg Oral Med Oral Pathol 1984;58:375.

23. Eriksson L, Westesson P-L. Temporomandibular joint diskectomy. No positive effect of temporary silicone implant in a 5-year follow-up. Oral Surg Oral Med Oral Pathol 1992;74:259.

24. Hall HD, Link J. Diskectomy alone and with ear cartilage in joint reconstruction. Oral Maxillofac Surg Clin North Am 1989;1:329.

25. Nickerson JW, Veaco NS. Condylotomy in surgery of the temporomandibular joint. Oral Maxillofac Surg Clin North Am 1989;1:303.

26. Ohnishi M. Arthroscopy of the temporomandibular joint. Journal of the Japanese Stomatological Society 1975;42:207.

27. Sanders B. Arthroscopic surgery of the temporomandibular joint: treatment of internal derangement with persistent closed lock. Oral Surg Oral Med Oral Pathol 1986;62:361.

28. Holmlund A, Hellsing G, Wredmark T. Arthroscopy of the temporomandibular joint: a clinical study. Oral Surg Oral Med Oral Pathol 1986;15:715.

29. McCain JP. Arthroscopy of the human temporomandibular joint. J Oral Maxillofac Surg 1988;46:648.

30. Sanders B, Buoncristiani RD. A 5-year experience with arthroscopic lysis and lavage for the treatment of painful temporomandibular hypomobility. In Clark GT, Sanders B, Bertomali CN (eds). Advances in diagnostic and surgical ar-

throscopy of the temporomandibular joint. Philadelphia: WB Saunders, 1993:31.

31. Nitzan DW, Dolwick MF, Heft MW. Arthroscopic lavage and lysis of the temporomandibular joint: a change in perspective. J Oral Maxillofac Surg 1990; 48:798.

32. Rasmussen DC. Description of population and progress of symptoms in a longitudinal study of temporomandibular arthropathy. Scand J Dent Res 1981; 89:196.

33. Nickerson JW, Boering G. Natural course of osteoarthrosis as it relates to internal derangement of the temporomandibular joint. Oral Maxillofac Surg Clin North Am 1989;1:27.

34. Wilkes CH. Arthrography of the temporomandibular joint in patients with TMJ pain dysfunction syndrome. Minn Med 1978;61:645.

35. Wilkes CH. Structure and function alterations of the temporomandibular joint. Northwest Dent 1978;57:287.

36. Dolwick MF, Katzberg RW, Helm CA, Bales CA. Arthrotomographic evaluation of the temporomandibular joint. J Oral Surg 1979;34:793.

37. Farrar WB, McCarty WL Jr. Inferior joint space arthrography and characteristics of condylar paths in internal derangements of the TMJ. J Prosthet Dent 1979;41:458.

38. Katzberg RW, Dolwick MF, Bales DJ, Helms CA. Arthrotomography of the temporomandibular jont: new technique and preliminary observations. AJR Am J Roentgenol 1979;132:949.

39. Blaschke D, Solberg W, Sanders B. Arthrography of the temporomandibular joint: review of current status. J Am Dent Assoc 1980;100:388.

40. Westesson P-L, Ericksson L, Kuista K. Reliability of a negative clinical temporomandibular joint examination: prevalence of disk displacements in asymptomatic temporomandibular joints. Oral Surg Oral Med Oral Pathol 1989;68:551.

41. Hatala MP, Westesson P-L, Tallents RH, Katzberg RW. TMJ disc displacement in asymptomatic volunteers detected by MR imaging. J Dent Res 1991;79(special issue):278. Abstract 100.

42. Tasaki MM, Westesson P-L. Temporomandibular joint: diagnostic accuracy with sagittal and coronal MR imaging. Head Neck Radiol 1993;186:723.

43. Schiffman E, Haley D. Sensitivity and specificity of diagnostic criteria for temporomandibular internal derangements. J Dent Res 1994;73(special issue):440. Abstract 2701.

44. Dolwick MF, Dimitroulis G. Is there a role for temporomandibular joint surgery? Oral Maxillofac Surg 1994;32:1.

45. Murakami K-I, Matsuki M, Iizuka T, Ono T. Recapturing the persistent anteriorly displaced disk by mandibular manipulation after pumping and hydraulic pressure to the upper joint cavity of the temporomandibular joint. J Craniomandib Pract 1987;5:17.

46. Nitzan DW, Dolwick MF, Heft MW. Arthroscopic lavage and lysis of the temporomandibular joint: a change in perspective. J Oral Maxillofac Surg 1990; 48:798.

47. Nitzan DW, Dolwick MF, Martinez GA. Temporomandibular joint arthrocentesis: a simplified treatment for severe, limited mouth opening. J Oral Maxillofac Surg 1991;49:1163.

48. Moses JJ, Poker I. TMJ arthroscopic surgery: an analysis of 237 patients. J Oral Maxillofac Surg 1989;47:790.

49. Clark GT, Moody DG, Sanders B. Arthroscopic treatment of temporomandibular joint locking resulting from disc derangement: two-year results. J Oral Maxillofac Surg 1991;49:157.

50. Davis CL, Kaminishi RM, Marshall MW. Arthroscopic surgery for treatment of closed lock. J Oral Maxillofac Surg 1991;49:704.

51. Montgomery MT, Van Sickles JE, Harms S. Success of temporomandibular joint arthroscopy in disk displacement with and without reduction. Oral Surg Oral Med Oral Pathol 1991;71:651.

52. Zeitler DS, Porter BT. A retrospective study comparing arthroscopic surgery with arthrotomy and disk repositioning. In Clark GT, Sanders B, Bertomali CN (eds). Advances in diagnostic and surgical arthroscopy of the temporomandibular joint. Philadelphia: WB Saunders, 1993:47.

53. Hall MB. Meniscoplasty of the displaced temporomandibular meniscus without violating the inferior joint space. J Oral Maxillofac Surg 1984;42:788.

54. Dolwick MF, Sanders B. TMJ internal derangement and arthrosis: surgical atlas. St Louis: CV Mosby, 1985.

55. Dolwick MF, Nitzan DW. TMJ disk surgery: 9 year followup evaluation. Fortschritt der Kiefer- und Gesicht-Chirurgie 1991;35:162.

56. Mercuri LG, Campbell RL, Shamaskin RG. Inter-articular meniscus dysfunction surgery: a preliminary report. Oral Surg Oral Med Oral Pathol 1982;54:613.

57. Marciani RD, Seigler RC. Temporomandibular joint surgery: a review of 51 operations. Oral Surg Oral Med Oral Pathol 1983;56:472.

58. Kerstens JCJ, Tuinzing DB, Van der Kwast WAM. Eminectomy and discoplasty for correction of the displaced temporomandibular joint disc. J Oral Maxillofac Surg 1989;47:150.

59. Vallerand WP, Dolwick MF. Complications of temporomandibular joint surgery. Oral Maxillofac Clin North Am 1990;2:481.

60. Lanz AB. Dictis mandibularis. Zentrabl Chir 1909;36:289.

61. Silver CM. Long-term results of meniscectomy of the temporomandibular joint. J Craniomandib Pract 1984;3:46.

62. Buckley MJ, Merrill RG, Braun TW. Surgical management of internal derangement of the temporomandibular joint. J Oral Maxillofac Surg 1993;51(suppl 1):20.

62a. Eriksson L, Westesson P–L. Long–term evaluation of diskectomy of the temporomandibular joint: a follow–up study. J Oral Maxillofac Surg 1985;43: 263.

63. Ward TG, Smith DG, Sommar M. Condylotomy for mandibular joints. Br Dent J 1957;103:147.

64. Nickerson JW, Veaco NS. Condylotomy in surgery of the temporomandibular joint. Oral Maxillofac Surg Clin North Am 1989;1:303.

65. Hall HD, Nickerson JW, Jr, McKenna SJ. Modified condylotomy for the treatment of the painful temporomandibular joint with a reducing disk. J Oral Maxillofac Surg 1993;51:133.

66. Tasanen A, von Konow L. Closed condylotomy in the treatment of idiopathic and traumatic pain-dysfunction syndrome of the temporomandibular joint. Int J Oral Maxillofac Surg 1973;2:102.

67. Upton LG, Sullivan SM. The treatment of temporomandibular joint internal

derangements using the modified open condylotomy: a preliminary report. J Oral Maxillofac Surg 1991;49:578.

68. Timmis DP, Aragon SB, Van Sickels JE, Aufdemorte TB. Compressive study of alloplastic materials for temporomandibular joint replacement in rabbits. J Oral Maxillofac Surg 1986;44:541.

69. Westesson P-L, Ericksson L, Lindstrom C. Destructive lesions of the mandibular condyle following discectomy with temporary silastic implants. Oral Surg Oral Med Oral Pathol 1987;63:143.

70. Kaplan PA, Tu HK, Williams SM. Erosive arthritis of the temporomandibular joint caused by Teflon-Proplast implants: plain film features. AJR Am J Roentgenol 1988;151:337.

71. Ryan DE. Alloplastic implants in the temporomandibular joint. Oral Maxillofac Surg Clin North Am 1989;1:427.

72. Morgan DH. Evaluation of alloplastic TMJ implants. J Craniomandib Pract 1988;6:224.

73. Feinerman DM, Piecuch JF. Long-term retrospective analysis of twenty-three Proplast-Teflon temporomandibular joint interpositional implants. Int J Oral Maxillofac Surg 1993;22:16.

74. Schellhas KP, Wilkes CH, El Beeb M. Permanent Proplast temporomandibular joint implants: MR imaging of destructive complications. AJR Am J Roentgenol 1988;151:731.

75. Dolwick MF, Aufdemorte TB. Silicone-induced foreign body reaction and lymphadenopathy after temporomandibular joint arthroplasty. Oral Surg Oral Med Oral Pathol 1985;59:449.

76. Lagrotteria L, Scapino R, Granston AS, Felgenhauer D. Patient with lymphadenopathy following temporomandibular joint arthroplasty with Proplast. J Craniomandib Pract 4:172.

77. Wagner JD, Mosby EL. Assessment of Proplast-Teflon disk replacements. J Oral Maxillofac Surg 1990;48:1140.

78. Gerogiade N. The surgical correction of temporomandibular joint dysfunction by means of autogenous dermal grafts. Plast Reconstr Surg 1962;30:68.

79. Witsenberg B, Freihofer HPM. Replacement of pathological temporomandibular articular disc using autogenous cartilage of the ear. Int J Oral Surg 1984;13:401.

80. Pincock JL, Dann JJ. Auricular cartilage grafting after disectomy of the temporomandibular joint. J Oral Maxillofac Surg 1993;51:256.

81. Feinberg SE, Larsen PE. The use of a pedicled temporalis muscle-pericranial flap for replacement of the TMJ disc. J Oral Maxillofac Surg 1989;47:142.

82. Merrill RG. Mandibular dislocation and hypermobility. In Merrill RG (ed). Disorders of the TMJ: arthrotomy. Oral Maxillofac Surg Clin North Am 1989;1(pt 2):399.

83. Dijkstra PU, de Bont LGM, de Leeuw R, Stegenga B, Boering G. Temporomandibular joint osteoarthrosis and temporomandibular joint hypermobility. J Craniomandib Pract 1993;11:268.

84. Littler BO. The role of local anaesthetic in the reduction of long-standing dislocation of the temporomandibular joint. Br J Oral Surg 1980;18:81.

85. Lovely FW. Surgery for recurrent TMJ dislocation. Ear Nose Throat J 1982;61:694.

86. Blankestign J, Boering G. Myrhaug's operation for treating recurrent dislocation of the temporomandibular joint. J Craniomandib Pract 1985;3:245.

87. LeClerc G, Girarde G. Un nouveau procede de butee dans le traitement chirurgical de la luxation recidivante de la machoire inferior. Mem Acad Chir 1943;69:451.

88. Mercuri LG. Eminectomy and discoplasty for correction of the displaced mandibular joint disc. J Oral Maxillofac Surg 1989;47:153.

89. Kopp S, Wenneberg B, Haraldson T, Carlsson GE. The short-term effect of intra-articular injections of sodium hyaluronate and corticosteroid on temporomandibular joint pain and dysfunction. J Oral Maxillofac Surg 1985;43:429.

90. Henny FA. The temporomandibular joint. In Kruger GO (ed). Textbook of oral surgery. St Louis: CV Mosby, 1984:436.

91. Bronstein SL, Osborne JJ. Mandibular limitation due to bilateral coronoid enlargement: management by surgery and physical therapy. J Craniomandib Pract 1985;3:58.

92. White CS, Dolwick MF. Prevalence and variance of temporomandibular dysfunction in orthognathic surgery patients. Int J Adult Orthod Orthognath Surg 1992;7:7.

93. De Boever A, Bays R, Keeling SD, Tiner BD, Flaharty CD, Clark GM, Rugh JD. Influence of mandibular advancement surgery on TM signs and symptoms. J Dent Res 1994;73(special issue):439. Abstract 2699.

The Temporomandibular Joint and Related Orofacial Disorders,
by Francis M. Bush and M. Franklin Dolwick.
J.B. Lippincott Company, Philadelphia, © 1995.

11

Record Keeping, Litigation, and Insurance

Nature of the TMD Complaint

The TMD complaint may mimic symptoms common to medical or dental disorders. This unique feature complicates matters for the patient, the practitioner, the health care insurer, and the attorney who is confronted with establishing or negating "probable cause" between the complaint and an injury. The patient may visit a physician who identifies some of the musculoskeletal symptoms and diagnoses the disorder as "TMJ." To confirm the diagnosis, the physician may refer the patient for dental consultation. After initial consultation, the dentist may recognize need for further diagnosis and treatment. Although patients usually have medical insurance, insurers may be reluctant to reimburse them for services rendered by a dentist. Physical therapists have similar problems. Often, the plaintiff's attorney who seeks judgment for a client has difficulty in arranging payment by the insurer for treatment of the client. Conflicts develop from lack of comprehension on the part of all parties concerned.

Impairment and Disability

TMD patients suffer varying degrees of impairment associated with their disorders. *Impairment* is reflected in symptom presentation and overt illness behavior exhibited by the patient. The impairment may lead to disability. *Disability* concerns the inability to engage in gainful (daily living) activities because of the impairment.[1]

Proof of impairment is confirmed by the findings of many epidemiologic studies around the world. Less is known about what degree disability results from impairment. Attempts have been made to determine the extent of this problem.

385

Disability produced by TMD has been estimated to range from 65% to 80%.[2] This conclusion was based on studies using an index that measured symptom intensity and frequency and the level of functional impairment. Comparable studies conducted on nonpatients showed a range of values from 5% to 10% with the same index. The assumption, then, is that 55% to 70% of the patients suffered some disability.

Other evidence confirms that TMD patients suffer significant disability. Judged from an index concerned with activities of daily living, the level of disability produced by TMD pain alone was estimated to be less by a factor of two when compared with levels described for some other musculoskeletal pain disorders.[3] Other impairments, such as joint noise and limited opening, were not measured, although they contribute significantly to disability.

The compensation system available to TMD patients can promote psychological stress and alter their impairments. Among low back pain patients, compensated recipients receiving regular payments showed more signs of emotional distress, had greater difficulty coping with pain, and reported more disruption in life events than subjects who had settled their claims.[4] Nonetheless, some patients who had settled claims continued to have severe pain. The authors recommended that the compensation system promote patient employment as soon as possible after injury.

Quality Assurance

The chief problem in quality assurance is protection of the patient from misdiagnosis and mistreatment. In many medical specialties, diagnostic tests have proved reliable, and treatment protocols have become standardized. In contrast, few well-defined, valid protocols exist for assessment and management of TMD patients. Thus, the quality of health care received by patients varies greatly. Because there is no speciality in "TMJ," clinicians' opinions differ depending on geographic location and the kind of training acquired at their respective schools. Analysis of the consensus among practitioners about diagnosis and methods of treatment reflects such differences.

No independent agency is empowered to monitor credentials or practices of the various clinicians who manage TMD patients. Instead, practitioners are governed by the same standards of care provided by other practitioners within the same community. A. V. Pearson, attorney, described the standards of care test in a speech before the Loyola University of Chicago Law School: "Practitioners should possess minimum common skills possessed by the vast majority of dentists, use these skills with care and reasonable diligence and apply good judgement."[5,6] American courts consider statements of this kind as the basis for the *professional standards test*.[7,8]

Equally important is the need to notify patients of the considerations involved in (1) diagnosis, (2) reasons for treatment, (3) nature of care and treatment, (4) prognosis, (5) risks, (6) alternatives, and (7) likely outcome for nontreatment.[8] Such information embraces the *prudent patient risk test*. The standard is based on the information needed by a prudent patient to decide whether to undergo a proposed treatment.[7]

Attempts have been made to improve standards of care for TMD patients. In 1982, the American Dental Association (ADA) endorsed some limited guidelines in the *Report of the President's Conference on the Examination, Diagnosis and Management of Temporomandibular Disorders*.[9] The ADA missed a major opportunity to update these guidelines at another conference held in 1988. The meeting between a panel of "TMD experts" selected by the ADA and certain community practitioners around the United States led to so much discord little of importance resulted."[10]

After this conference, members of the American Academy of Craniomandibular Disorders sought the aid of other reputable TMD practitioners to evaluate present guidelines.[11] Important changes were made. Most noteworthy was the formulation of a system of diagnostic classification. The main subjects addressed were diagnosis and treatment.[12] Health care use, impairment and disability, and the possibility of TMD developing secondarily from injury were briefly discussed. These modified guidelines have not been endorsed by ADA members or non-ADA practitioners.

Thus, patients are protected by professional standard and prudent patient risk tests. The duty of practitioners is to enforce these standards until more definitive guidelines are accepted by the profession.

Litigation

Clinicians have become subject to lawsuits because of the greater public awareness about TM disorders. Unwarranted legal action has been brought against clinicians by patients. The patients assume negligence (malpractice) and seek legal redress.

Cases have evolved from negligence alleged by plantiffs concerning unsatisfactory diagnosis and treatment for TMD,[7] as well as for periodontal disease and for root resorption attributed to orthodontic therapy.[13]

Two medicolegal presentations have been found by a study of 731 facial pain cases at London's Eastman Dental Hospital. These concerned the failure to diagnose or treat the patient's facial pain appropriately.[14] Pain developed spontaneously in some patients and became unremitting after unsuccessful treatment with traditional dental procedures. The patients claimed that the dental treatment caused the pain. Clinicians failed to recognize the presence of psychiatric illness in the second presentation. The authors concluded that all patients should have been treated initially with appropriate medication.

Other litigation has focused on the possibility of TMD developing secondarily following whiplash or overt trauma within the TMJ region. Drawing conclusions about this potential etiology and recovery of the patient during active litigation has proved perplexing.

Consider some current opinions of dentists about this dilemma. A survey led to the conclusion that if TMD symptoms appeared within 2 months of the injury, there was probably a relation.[15] If the duration was longer, then the probable cause lessens.

The authors discussed these findings as a basis for compensation by the insurance industry and by worker's compensation.

During active litigation, there is the presumption that injured patients would be less likely to report relief of symptoms and have poorer treatment outcome. Studies conducted on 53 TMD patients with ongoing litigation for overt trauma or whiplash and 43 other nonlitigating TMD patients produced mixed findings (Tables 11-1 and 11-2). Certain parameters were significantly higher in litigating patients than in nonlitigating patients.[16] More litigating patients reported facial and neck pain and endorsed more pain sites than nonlitigating patients. Other findings were less impressive. The level of pain determined by visual analogue scale (VAS), the duration of pain, and the affective pain dimension as assessed by the McGill Pain Questionnaire did not differ significantly between groups. The pressure pain threshold for the left masseter and frontal muscles was significantly higher in nonlitigating patients than in litigating patients, but no significant differences existed between groups for

---

Table 11-1

Statistically Significant Differences Between Litigating and Nonlitigating TMD Patients

Parameter	Litigating	Nonlitigating	Probability (*P* value <)
Pain			
No. total sites*	5.6	3.9	0.01
Facial pain (%)	92	31	0.04
Neck pain (%)	55	26	0.01
Pressure Pain Threshold			
Frontal*	2.3	2.6	0.01
Left masseter*	1.4	1.8	0.006
Endorsement (%)			
Overt trauma (%)	12	52	0.0001
Whiplash (%)	88	49	0.0001
Sleep problem (%)	67	40	0.03
Symptom Checklist 90 Scores			
Somatization	1.08	0.76	0.008
Treatment Outcome			
Duration (weeks)*	18.4	12.7	0.05
Clinical sessions*	7.5	4.6	0.002
Post VAS (%)	24.9	15.3	0.001
Change VAS (%)	43.9	10.7	0.001
Improvement (%)	67.0	87.8	0.001

Modified from Burgess JA, Dworkin SF. Litigation and post-traumatic TMD: how patients report treatment outcome. J Am Dent Assoc 1993;124:105.

*Mean.
VAS, visual analogue scale.

the pressure pain threshold of the right masseter, passive range of motion, and joint clicking.

Although the somatization score was higher in litigating than nonlitigating patients, the depression and anxiety scores were not. Significant improvement was observed in VAS pain, range of motion, and pressure pain thresholds for masseter muscle after treatment of both groups. Litigating patients reported less overall improvement. The authors concluded that the interaction between litigation and TMD symptoms remains unclear.

These conclusions support the findings of another study regarding TMD and trauma.[17] Based on analysis of 230 patients diagnosed into six TMD subgroups, the authors concluded that specific trauma may not initiate TMD symptoms but may have an important cumulative effect.

Table 11-2
Nonstatistical Differences Between Litigating and Nonlitigating TMD Patients

Parameter	Litigating	Nonlitigating
Pain		
VAS	57.7*	45.9
MPQ affective	4.8*	3.6
Pain duration	13.4*	15.9
Pressure Pain Threshold		
Right masseter	1.5*	1.7
Other Clinical Indices		
Passive ROM	37.3*	38.7
Clicking (%)	22	14
Symptom Checklist 90 Score		
Depression	0.86	0.67
Anxiety	0.66	0.54
Treatment Outcome		
ROM*	44.6	44.9
Change ROM (%)	−33.2	−28.1
Frontalis (%)	−9.7	−1.6
Left masseter (%)	−46.0	−29.8
Right masseter (%)	−57.3	−46.3

Modified from Burgess JA, Dworkin SF. Litigation and posttraumatic TMD: how patients report treatment outcome. J Am Dent Assoc 1993;124:105.

*Mean.
VAS, visual analogue scale; MPQ, McGill Pain Questionnaire; ROM, range of motion.

Prevention of Litigation

Effective communication helps clinicians avoid litigation. Legal action may result from poor interpersonal relationships between clinicians and patients. Many lawyers practicing professional negligence law agree that keeping good rapport with patients reduces the chance of lawsuits.[18] Most dissatisfaction concerns inadequate financial agreement, appointment failures, broken appliances, and faulty restorative or prosthetic treatment.

Several practical suggestions have been made by E. J. Zinman, dentist-attorney, to improve rapport.[19] He recommended that clinicians be honest and fair, listen to the patient, be prompt, and explain thoroughly.

Myths

Many questions asked by the TMD patient are the same ones asked by attorneys and the patient's insurer. Practitioners can help dispel some of the myths and fears associated with "TMJ." Some of the fallacies that require clarification follow.

- **Fallacy:** *Can a diagnosis be trusted if many clinical findings have proved negative?* Patients expect quick diagnosis and aggressive treatment of their complaints. The fact is that even with accurate diagnosis, existing treatment may fail. Accurate diagnosis does not always lead to a rational choice of therapies. Some diagnoses cannot be treated successfully.
- **Fallacy:** *Early TMD progresses to a worse condition.* Even within TMD clinical populations in which patients share common diagnoses, the timing and stage of the disorder makes prediction of progression difficult. Consider the findings of 262 TMD patients followed independently for either pain or clicking. Just 61% eventually had some limitation of mandibular motion.[20]

  Some patients have several symptoms simultaneously. Also, they may erroneously relate the appearance of new symptoms with preexisting symptoms. Consider the long-standing belief, promulgated in Costen's trilogy of TMJ, that jaw pain coincides with nonpainful symptoms of tinnitus and dizziness. Clinicians have perpetuated such myths because they have had limited information. Statistical analysis showed no significant relation among these three symptoms.[21,22]
- **Fallacy:** *An injured TM joint causes pain in the neck, shoulder, and back.* Some patients tell clinicians that pain within the TM joint radiates down into the shoulder or back. The fact is that if there is a connection, it is in the other direction. Pain originating from the back, the shoulders, and the neck is likely to have a common origin within muscles. Pain may radiate from the neck to the head or face. Muscular pain in the jaw represents part of the overall muscular dysfunction.
- **Fallacy:** *TMD and headache are caused by hormonal changes.* This notion has been exaggerated. Well-meaning clinicians have told patients about these potential relations. Insurers and patients have spent fortunes trying to associate symptoms with hormonal changes. Proof is lacking of a direct link even between headache and menstrual changes in hormone levels. Future monies should be appropriated for well-designed research protocols designed to study chemical triggers or potential psychological factors that may contribute to these conditions.

- **Fallacy:** *A diagnosis of "TMJ" means that there is a psychological problem.* In reality, clinicians have not been able to establish a clear connection between psychological factors and pain of more debilitating musculoskeletal disorders, such as "bad back." Studies conducted on 75 adult patients admitted to a TMD clinic showed that 31% suffered from depression.[23] The depression was positively and significantly related to limitations in activities in daily living as a result of pain or neuroticism. But even if these patients required psychological therapy, 69% would not.

  Patients benefit from psychological counseling when interpersonal or family problems are causing stress and might worsen their condition. Careful screening improves the chance of locating these problems.

- **Fallacy:** *Women are more prone to TMD than men; they suffer more intense and more frequent pain than men.* No one has established why women register more health complaints than men. TMD is no exception. Analysis of patients visiting TMD clinics across the world shows that the ratio of women to men is about 4 to 1.[24] The disparity is not related to the degree of pain suffered. Women are probably more aware of their bodies than are men, whereas men may be more likely than women to disregard symptoms.

- **Fallacy:** *TMD can be inherited.* Some patients with TM joint sounds or jaw pain report to practitioners that a close relative has similar joint noise or pain. In truth, definitive answers are lacking about familial relations for many musculoskeletal syndromes.

  One suspects that the inheritance pattern of TMD patients with myofascial pain is similar to the inheritance pattern of patients with primary fibromyalgia. Both share clinical manifestations of pain and muscular tenderness. Primary fibromyalgia seems to be an autosomal dominantly inherited condition with a variable latent period before clinical expression of the disorder.[25]

- **Fallacy:** *Clinicians can cure TMD.* Wrong. Most recoveries occur naturally. The vast majority of musculoskeletal disorders resolve with little or no care. Most recalcitrant cases can be managed with home care, medication, and dental or physical therapy. Few require surgical treatment.

- **Fallacy:** *Certain dental treatments cause TMD.* Evidence of deleterious effects is lacking even in cases of orthodontic therapy that has continued for several years. Most litigation cases of patients blaming dentists for causing TMD have been related to complaints involving occlusal adjustment or faulty bridgework.[7]

  Careful screening and examination of patients saves practitioners needless grief. Many patients have TMD signs and symptoms before treatment is initiated. The dental records should detail their occurrence. Patients should be warned of their existence.

- **Fallacy:** *Adjustment of the occlusion solves most TMD complaints.* If the teeth are suspected as triggering complaints, the patient should be fitted with an intraoral appliance before more extensive treatment is begun. Many patients have been overtreated by adjusting their teeth. Most jaw pain originates from tender muscles that limit normal mandibular motion. The patient reports this displacement. Overzealous grinding at the peak of the complaint makes no sense. Home care, medication, and an intraoral appliance ease most problems.

- **Fallacy:** *Most TMD patients seek or abuse narcotic medications.* The reality is that most TMD patients refuse even less potent medications. Many patients can obtain significant relief by following a regimen of appropriate medication.

Some patients would benefit by taking medication more powerful than nonsteroids to reduce the pain. Some practitioners have been slow to recognize this opportunity. If substance abuse is suspected, practitioners should communicate with pharmacists in the area where the patient lives. They are more than willing to disclose potential abuse.

- **Fallacy:** *Disk disorders diagnosed by magnetic resonance imaging means TMJ surgery will be successful.* Being tested generally is not helpful. Surgery is performed on the TM joints because some patients demand further treatment once they discover minor problems early in the course of the disorder. Early diagnosis extends the time the patient is aware of the problem. This awareness may produce excessive worry and aggravate the condition.

- **Fallacy:** *Wearing an anterior repositioning appliance eliminates joint sounds.* Certain patients may show improvement in joint sounds by wearing this appliance. There is high probability of altering the patient's occlusion unless the appliance is designed and fitted appropriately and adjusted regularly. Relief of pain may result, but often the patient becomes "appliance dependent." Other useful protocols are available with less destructive potential.

Threat of Litigation

According to Dr. D. A. Hatfield, dentist-attorney, practitioners should conduct a self-assessment regarding TMD.[26] Practitioners may be asked to:

1. Demonstrate competence or experience to diagnose and treat TMD.
2. Provide documentation of the patient's informed consent.
3. Describe the diagnostic records.
4. Provide the basis for treatment and for the kind of treatment rendered.

Some of these concerns have been described elsewhere.[14] Practitioners also may be asked to describe the reason for treating rather than referring the patient. Strategies for coping with litigation have been suggested for the clinician who is sued.[27] Recommended strategies include the following: don't take the case personally, get a good attorney, and learn about the legal process. Additionally, some litigation may lead to initiation of an investigation by the State Dental Board within the clinician's geographic region.[28] This action delays the chance of settlement for the practitioner's negligence insurance carrier. The clinician pays for his or her legal fees caused by action of State Boards.

Records

Clinicians may avoid legal actions by keeping complete, high-quality records of the patient's health. Primary among these records should be a document of *patient consent*. There are two forms of consent: *plain* and *informed*.[7] Plain consent concerns valid exemption from liability for battery. Informed consent concerns apprisal of the nature and risks of a medical procedure.

The document of *informed consent*, to be agreed upon verbally and signed by the patient, should advise the patient that current TMD signs and symptoms may remain after treatment. Although improvement may be expected after treatment, the patient

Informed Consent Treatment Report
PART I
Information
"The purpose of this report is to inform you _____. Once you fully understand
  your TMD situation, you will be asked to provide the appropriate signatures on the endorse-
  ment pages."
Specific sections
Patient complaint: "You first presented on _____ stating _____."
Medical history: Only that which pertains to this treatment
Dental history: Only that which pertains to this treatment
Synopsis: Helpful if the informed consent is long or complex
Examination: "Clinical and radiograph findings revealed _____."
Consultation: Requires findings from referrals
Recommended treatment: Benefits, risks
Treatment alternatives: Options, possible effect of nontreatment
General sections
Office Policy: Policy regarding appointments, photographs, video
Medication: Only that which pertains to treatment, including known side effects that need to be
  revealed
Psychological assessment: Analysis of interpersonal relationships and social history that per-
  tains to treatment
Physical therapy: General description of modality, benefits, risks
Dental therapy: General description of type, benefits, risks
Warranty: Describe adjustment periods and warranty policy, if any
Behavioral therapy: General description of kind, benefits, risks
Surgical procedure: General description of type, benefits, risks
Patient acceptance
"I understand the recommendations detailed in my chart and reviewed in this report _____
_____."
Endorsement
"Your endorsement of this report, Part I, indicates _____. These stipulations are
requested of all prospective patients so that at least one other opinion from an "interested"
party will be sought by you and that procedures will not be entered into without thorough delib-
eration on your part. If you have any questions concerning the recommended treatment, alternatives, benefits, procedures, limitations, possible complications, or any other information relative to your proposed treatment, please ask."

_____   _____
Patient signature   Date

_____   _____
Parent or legal guardian (if less than 18)   Date

_____   _____
Spouse or interested cosigner (optional)   Date

_____   _____
Witness (professional staff member)   Date

Figure 11-1.
*Sample of informed consent report. (Modified from Murrell GA, Sheppard GA. The
informed consent treatment report. J Prosthet Dent 1992;68:970.)*

(continued)

PART II

Financial

   "Fees in this office are based on the nature and complexity of the procedure. Once the schedule of treatment is _____."

Treatment sequence and cost estimate

1. Finalize diagnosis, consultations, review patient information, consent, appointments, coordinating speciality referrals, and financial arrangements. Dr._____; Fee $ _____.

2. Radiographs, CT scans, magnetic resonance imaging, conferences between Dr. _____ to finalize other therapy options and patient approval. Dr. _____; Fee: Separate

3. Psychological assessment and testing. Dr. _____; Fee: Separate

4. Dental therapy, including making impressions, preparation, and mounting of patient casts on an articulator. Dr. _____; Fee $ _____.

5. Fabrication of an intraoral appliance to fit the patient's teeth. Delivery of appliance to patient. Dr. _____; Fee $ _____.

6. Physical therapy as needed. Outpatient Physical Therapy Service _____ Fee $ _____; Separate

7. Behaviorial therapy management as needed. Dr. _____; Fee $ _____; Separate

8. Surgical evaluation and procedure as needed. Dr. _____; Fee $ _____; Separate

9. Conduct final review conferences with the patient to confirm the appropriate time for wearing appliance. Dr. _____; Fee $ _____.

   The total estimated fee for the recommended service described in this report is $ _____. This applies to services rendered in this office only and does not reflect any alternative treatment suggestions or any other referred services. The estimated treatment time is 6 months depending on the duration of other types of services (eg, dental therapies) being rendered. Except for major treatment changes or additional time or procedure requirements described earlier in this report, these fees will remain in effect if the treatment commences by _____, and is completed by_____.

_____
Patient signature   Date

_____
Witness   Date

Figure 11-1. (*Continued*)

should be notified that new discomfort may arise during and after treatment.[5,6] Informed consent may be recorded by video, as suggested by Dr. E. J. Zinman, a dentist-attorney who specializes in dental jurisprudence.[29]

No standard form exists for obtaining informed consent from TMD patients. Few would be totally inclusive. The sample form presented in Figure 11-1 has been modified from a document used to obtain informed consent from prosthodontic patients.[8] This modified form embodies much of the same format and embraces many of the original descriptions of prosthodontics. Practitioners are encouraged to add or delete items from this modified document.

Complete records should include a description of the patient's chief complaint,[5] history of the complaint, questionnaires, examination forms, findings of special tests, and treatment protocols, including a list of procedures from the initiation of diagnosis through treatment. Copies of referral letters or referral forms should be retained. Two examples of referral letters are presented for the practitioner: one to verify the presence of TMD and the other for surgical evaluation (Figs. 11-2 and 11-3).

Details of the progress notes should be written in a legible manner. The notes should show dated follow-ups and progress reviews involving post-treatment conferences. Information regarding vital signs and medical care should be recorded after each appointment.[30]

A simplified form has been developed that allows clinicians an opportunity to record the progress of TMD patients.[31] At the initial and subsequent appointments, patients list their symptoms according to the degree of severity (Fig. 11-4). They use this adjunct to rank the frequency and intensity of their complaint numerically at each appointment. Patients sign and date the form after each treatment. This progress report allows comparison of the patient's status from one treatment session to another.

Records need updating periodically. Updates should be conducted at least yearly. New or forgotten information may necessitate more frequent changes in informed consent, kind of medication, postoperative instructions, or progress notes.

Re: Patient's name
      Chart #
Dear Dr _____:
   This 38-year-old white male presented with left side jaw pain on April 12, 1993. He ignored the initial symptoms that developed during the middle of March, 1993, because they were so minor. There has been a steady progression of pain since onset.
   His health history is unremarkable for headache and neckache. Recently, he had a physical examination, with vital signs and blood tests within normal limits. He has no family history that suggests problems of this kind.
   Clinical examination showed muscle tenderness in the left masseter, medial pterygoid, and anterior fibers of the temporalis. There is some soft clicking in the left temporomandibular joint but no tenderness on palpation.
   The jaw motions are 45mm maximal voluntary opening. Right and left lateral and protrusive movements are 9 mm each. There is no deviation on opening.
   The dentition is in excellent condition. He has no restorations and the periodontal health is within normal limits. A panoramic radiograph of the jaws is within normal limits. His occlusion is Class I bilaterally with no major slide between retruded contact position and intercuspal position. There is wear along the anterior teeth. The right maxillary canine and right mandibular canine are severely worn from bruxism.
   Diagnostic impression is consistent with myalgia of the left temporomandibular joint region. A secondary diagnosis is diskal disorder with reduction in the left temporomandibular joint.

                                        Sincerely,

                                        _____ DDS

Figure 11-2.
Sample referral letter to verify the presence of TMD.

Referral for Surgical Evaluation of the TMJ

Re: Patient's name
      Chart #

Dear Dr_____:

    This 21-year-old white female presented on June 14, 1993 with right side temporomandibular joint pain. She noticed some clicking in the joint approximately 6 months ago. There was little pain initially, but after three episodes of locking, the pain worsened. Routine home-care therapy and delivery of a intraoral appliance have aided with the dysfunction.

    On January 2, 1993, she attempted to eat a bagel and was unable to open her mouth fully. Sharp pain ensued, so she visited the office immediately. An examination showed point tenderness in the left temporomandibular joint with some minor tenderness in the left temporalis tendon and masseter regions. Maximum voluntary opening was 8 mm. Lateral jaw motions were 2 mm laterally. Repeated efforts to unlock the joint have been unsuccessful.

    Previously, her health was excellent. She had a tonsillectomy as a child and an allergy to penicillin. She has just had a physical examination without evidence of problems.

    Based on clinical findings, the diagnosis was diskal displacement without reduction. Please evaluate for possible arthroscopic surgery.

                    Sincerely,

                  _____DDS

Figure 11-3.
Sample referral letter for surgical evaluation of the TMJ.

TMD Progress Report

Name:_____Patient no: _____

Directions: Rank your four main symptoms in decending order, with number 1 as the most
      severe.

Rating: Circle the frequency and intensity of your symptoms.
        Frequency (1) seldom, (2) occasional, (3) frequent
        Intensity: 0 to 10 (0 = no pain and 10 = the most severe pain)

Symptoms: (1)_____   (2)_____   (3)_____   (4)_____
Date:_____
Frequency   123   123   123   123
Intensity   12345678910   12345678910   12345678910   12345678910

_____Treatment_____
Signed
Symptoms: (1)_____   (2)_____   (3)_____   (4)_____
Date:_____
Frequency   123   123   123   123
Intensity   12345678910   12345678910   12345678910   12345678910

_____Treatment_____
Signed

Figure 11-4.
Sample TMD progress report. (Modified from Owen AH. Record keeping adjuncts for TMD therapy. J Craniomandib Pract 1991;9:39.)

According to D. A. Hatfield, attorney-dentist, clinicians can initiate and maintain complete patient records by using the SOAP (subjective, objective, assessment, plan) format.[26] SOAP formats promote safe practices.

Reimbursement and Insurance Plans

Who Should Be Reimbursed?

If the patient has a comprehensive health care plan, TMD services should be covered in the same way as other musculoskeletal disorders. Patients should be reimbursed fairly by insurers for the cost of services. Practitioners deserve compensation for providing standards of care equal to those of comparable disorders.[32]

Third-party plans continue to have an increasing role in the delivery of TMD care. Numerous states, including Georgia, Kentucky, Maryland, Minnesota, Nevada, New Mexico, North Dakota, Tennessee, Texas, Washington, and West Virginia, have passed legislation or issued directives for inclusion of TMD treatment in health policies.[33] Most have followed the mandate of Minnesota, which enacted a law (62A.043 subd 3) in 1987 requiring medical coverage for TMD if the treatment is administered or prescribed by a physician or dentist.[34]

On the whole, TMD reimbursements have lagged well behind claims paid for comparable disorders. Among hospital dental practices covered by Medicare, just 14% of dentists reported reimbursement for TMD surgical treatment and 11% for TMD nonsurgical treatment.[35]

If insured TMD care is unavailable, patients and practitioners should negotiate with insurers or seek legislative action to ensure coverage, especially reimbursement for nonsurgical care. Since enactment of the Minnesota legislation, the overall cost for insurers of TMD care has been reduced by about 14% because simpler, less costly treatments (eg, home care) have been used.[36] Fewer surgeries and other complex treatments have been needed, which has reduced costs.

Codes and Claims

Insurance codes pertaining to diagnosis and treatment of TMD are available in versions of the Physician's Current Procedural Terminology (CPT-4),[37] the International Classification of Diseases, Adapted For Use in the United States (ICD-9),[38] and the Code on Dental Procedures, Current Dental Terminology (CDT-1).[39] In contrast to the CPT-4 and ICD-9 codes, the first number of each dental code in the CDT-1 begins with "0."[39] These codes are revised about every 5 years.

Claims for diagnosis or treatment of TMD for insured patients may be submitted on dental or medical forms and must comply with the administrative requirements of each plan. The key factor in securing reimbursement is identifying the appropriate codes used by the patient's insurer.

The terminology used to describe the same treatment differs slightly in some cases between CPT-4 and CDT-1 codes. Other treatments lack codes that overlap. Claims submitted against these codes must be filed separately on the correct form. A well-documented narrative report to be prepared by the practitioner may be requested by the insurer (Fig. 11-5). A listing of codes most frequently used is provided in Table 11-3. These codes have been borrowed from the CPT-4, CDT-1, and ICD-9 systems.

Explanation of Benefits

Much valuable information is available by reviewing the explanation of benefits (EOB) sent to the patient by the insurer. Most claims are rejected for:[40]

1. Incorrect patient name or number.
2. Improper diagnostic code.
3. Submitting an unspecific code without a written explanation.
4. Diagnostic code disagrees with expected treatment.

Questionable Reimbursement

Disputes concerning reimbursement for certain services arise between patients and their insurers. Some guidelines have been proposed for settling these disagreements.[41] Recommended for review on a case by case basis are these criteria:

1. An independent consultant who is uninformed about the party making the request should be selected.

(text continues on p. 402)

LETTER IN RESPONSE TO REQUEST FROM INSURANCE CARRIER

Re: Patient's Name
       Chart #

Dear_____:

   Your customer was seen in this office on January 4, 1993, for grinding of his teeth. He has experienced several broken teeth during the past 2 years. These fractures were unrelated to eating foods tough to chew.

   An examination of the dentition revealed that most of the anterior teeth were abraded into the dentin. Teeth #3/30 and #14/19 had wear facets. Number 19 was crowned last year because of a previous fracture.

   Further examination showed muscular tenderness along the ramus of the left mandible, masseter, and temporalis muscle. All jaw functions were within normal limits.

   The diagnoses are noctural bruxism and myalgia.

   The treatment recommended is delivery of a full arch intraoral appliance that will cover all of the maxillary teeth. Expected outcomes will be management of bruxism and relief of muscular discomfort.

   Although an intraoral appliance is not included in the patient's explanation of benefits, the appliance is cost effective. Your company will save money because fewer teeth will be broken.

                                        Sincerely,

                                        _____DDS

Figure 11-5.
Sample letter in response to request from insurance carrier.

Table 11-3
Diagnosis and Treatment Codes Used by Different Insurers

	CPT-4 Codes		CDT-1 Codes
History and Examination			
New patient	90620		00110

Consultations	New Patient	Established Patient	
Limited	90600	90641	
Intermediate	90605	90642	
Extensive	90610		
Comprehensive	90620		09310

Radiographs/Scans/Magnetic Imaging		
Panoramic	70355	00330
Coronal, L & R condyles	76100	00321
Transcranial	70330	00321
Frontal skull (AP/PA)	70140	00290
Frontal sinus	70210	00290
Maxillary sinus	70140	00290
Lateral skull	70350	00290
Submentovertex	76499	
TMJ Tomographic		00322
Lft joint closed	76100	
Lft joint extended	76100	
Rt joint closed	76100	
Rt joint extended	76100	
Computerized axial tomography (CAT) face	70486	
Cervical		
Neutral position	72040	
Flexion	72052	
Extension	72052	
Lft oblique	72052	
Rt oblique	72052	
Anteroposterior	72040	
Bone (nuclear, limited)	78300	
Magnetic resonance imaging (MRI)		
TMJ	70336	
Face/neck	70540	
Radiologic consultation (x-rays made elsewhere)	76140	
Duplication of x-rays	76499	

Special Diagnostic Procedures		
Diagnostic molds (casts)	95999	00470
Muscle testing	95833	00990
Nerve block injection	20605	09212
Trigger point injection	20550	09210
TMJ injection	20605	09210
Manipulation of TMJ	97260	07830
Pulp vitality test		00460
Vapocoolant spray	97000C	09210
Photographs	95999	00471
Thermography	76300	
Electromyography	95867	

(continued)

Table 11-3   *(Continued)*

	CPT-4 Codes	CDT-1 Codes
Diagnosis (ICD-9 Codes)		
Ankylosis	718.5	
Articular cartilage disorder	718.0	
Atypical facial pain	350.2	
Bell's palsy	351.0	
Bone spur	726.91	
Carotidnia	337.0	
Cephalgia	784.9	
Cervical dysfunction	739.1	
Cervical torticollis	723.5	
Cervicalgia	723.1	
Chondroma	213.0	
Crepitus	719.6	
Degenerative arthritis	715.9	
Dislocation of jaw—closed	830.0	
Dislocation of jaw—open	830.1	
Displacement of meniscus—recurrent	718.3	
Displacement of meniscus—nonrecurrent	718.2	
Eagle's syndrome	728.3	
Glossopharyngeal neuralgia	352.1	
Headache, facial pain	784.0	
Headache, tension	307.81	
Hypermobility	728.5	
Inflammatory osteomyelitis of jaw	526.4	
Joint stiffness	719.5	
Loose body in joint	718.1	
Malocclusion, unspecified	524.4	
Masseter parotid hypertrophy	785.6	
Migraine, classical	346.0	
Migraine, common	346.1	
Migraine, unspecified	346.9	
Muscle spasm	728.85	
Myalgia/myositis	729.1	
Myofascial pain dysfunction	306.0	
Neutral entrapment	355.9	
Orofacial dyskinesia	333.82	
Osteoarthrosis of jaw	715.8	
Pain in jaw	526.9	
Posterior capsulitis	719.0	
Psoriatic arthritis	696.0	
Rheumatoid arthritis	716.9	
Steroid necrosis	526.4	
Synovitis/tenosynovitis	727.0	
Temporal arteritis	446.5	
Temporomandibular joint disorder	524.6	
Tinnitus	388.3	
Trauma to TMJ	959.0	
Traumatic arthritis	714.0	
Traumatic arthropathy	716.18	
Trigeminal neuralgia	350.1	
Trismus	718.4	
Unilateral condylar hypo/hyperplasia	526.89	

(continued)

Table 11-3   *(Continued)*

	CPT-4 Codes	CDT-1 Codes
Unspecified arthropathy/ arthritis	716.9	
Unspecified neuralgia/ neuritis	729.2	

Treatments (CPT-4 Codes)

Visits	New Patient	Established Patient	
Minimal		90030	
Brief	90000	90040	
Limited	90010	90050	
Intermediate	90015	90060	
Extended	90017	90070	
Comprehensive	90020	90080	09420

Appliances

Oral orthopedic	21110	07880
Cranial/mandibular orthopedic	21499	09940
Mandibular/maxillary orthopedic repositioning	20999	09940

Physical Therapies

Hot/cold pack	97010	
Massage	97024	
Spray/stretch	97124	
Manipulation of dislocated joint		
Without anesthesia	21480	
With local anesthesia	21485	
Mechanical traction	97012	
Muscle therapy, manual	97112	
Cranial/cervical/spinal manipulation	22500	
Neuromuscular reeducation (MFT)	97112	
Ultrasound	97128	
Diathermy	97024	
Iontophoresis	97120	
Transcutaneous neural stimulation (TENS)	64550	
Biofeedback	95868	09920
Electrogalvanic stimulation (EGS/HV)	97118	

Injections

Trigger point	20550	09210
Nerve block	20605	09212
TMJ	20605	09210

Surgery

Removal—foreign body reaction		07540
Arthrotomy of TMJ	21010	07860
Condylectomy	21050	07840

(continued)

Table 11-3   *(Continued)*

	CPT-4 Codes	CDT-1 Codes
Disectomy (meniscectomy)	21060	07850
Disk repair		07852
Arthroplasty		07870
Synovectomy		07854
Arthroscopy		
Diagnostic		07872
Surgical		07873
Coronoidectomy	21070	07991
Arthrocentesis	20605	07870
Joint reconstruction		07858
Excision—cyst or tumor of mandible	21040	07430
Excision—bone abscess	21025	07550
Excision—salivary gland		07981
Biopsy—muscle	20200	07852
Other		
Emergency service, office	99058	07899
Medical testimony	99075	
Special report, medical status, insurance form	99080	
Occlusal analysis— mounted casts		09950
Occlusal adjustment		
Limited		09951
Complete		09420

2. Diagnosis and treatment should be supported by valid studies from reputable publications. The value of assessment and modality should be judged by qualified practitioners.
3. Impairment should be based on a rating system, such as (a) disk derangement, (b) range of motion, and (c) arthropathy.
4. Commitment by the insurer for phase I treatment makes the insurer responsible for phase II treatment.
5. Insurers should recognize that treatment may require more than 6 months to achieve successful outcome.
6. Fees should be reasonable for the geographic location and degree of difficulty.

Adherence to these or similar guidelines form equitable grounds for settling disputes.

References

1. Guides to the evaluation of permanent impairment, 2nd ed. Chicago: American Medical Association, 1984.
2. Pullinger AG, Monteiro AA. Functional impairment in TMJ patient and non-patient groups according to a disability index and symptom profile. J Craniomandib Pract 1988;6:156.

3. Bush FM, Harkins SW, Laskin DM. An index of pain impairment: psychometric properties in TMD patients. J Dent Res 1992;71(special issue):192. Abstract 692.

4. Guest GH, Drummond PD. Effect of compensation on emotional state and disability in chronic back pain. Pain 1992;48:125.

5. Pearson AV. TMJ and malpractice: defining the standard of care. Lecture at the Third Dentistry and Law Conference, University of Chicago. November 9, 1991.

6. Jacob JA. Dentists can prevent TMD suits. ADA News 1991;22:21.

7. Ebersold LA. Malpractice: risk management for dentists. Tulsa: Penn-Well Books, 1986.

8. Murrell GA, Sheppard GA. The informed consent treatment report. J Prosthet Dent 1992;68:970.

9. Griffith RH. Report of the President's Conference on the Examination, Diagnosis and Management of Temporomandibular Disorders. J Am Dent Assoc 1983;106:75.

10. Nasedkin JN. TMJ conference flops. J Craniomandib Pract 1989;7:87.

11. McNeill C. Craniomandibular disorders: guidelines for evaluation, diagnosis, and management. Chicago: Quintessence, 1990.

12. Independent Medical and Dental Consultants (IMDC). TMJ Bulletin No. 6. Marlton, NJ: IMDC, 1990.

13. Machen DE. Orthodontic/TMD litigation increases. TMD Diary 1992;4:7.

14. Harris M, Feinmann C, Wise M, Treasure F. Temporomandibular joint and orofacial pain: clinical and medicolegal management problems. Br Dent J 1993;174:129.

15. Doerrer A, Figart F. TMJ syndrome: is it compensable? Rehabil Nurs 1991;16:23.

16. Burgess JA, Dworkin SF. Litigation and post-traumatic TMD: how patients report treatment outcome. J Am Dent Assoc 1993;124:105.

17. Pullinger AG, Seligman DA. Trauma history in diagnostic groups of temporomandibular disorders. Oral Surg Oral Med Oral Pathol 1991;71:529.

18. Moyers RE. Quality assurance in orthodontics. Am J Orthod Dentofacial Orthop 1990;97:3.

19. Zinman EJ. Dentists and the law. Dental Management 1991;31:52.

20. Greene CS, Lerman MD, Sutcher HD, Laskin DM. The TMJ pain-dysfunction syndrome: heterogeneity of the patient population. J Am Dent Assoc 1969; 79:1168.

21. Bush FM. Tinnitus and otalgia in temporomandibular disorders. J Prosthet Dent 1988;58:495.

22. Bush FM, Harkins SW. Costen's syndrome revisited: common non-painful symptoms in temporomandibular disorders (TMD). Seattle, WA: International Association for the Study of Pain, 1993:51. Abstract 141.

23. Bush FM, Harkins SW, Welleford EA. Depression in orofacial pain: relation to activities of daily living (ADL) and neuroticism. 7th World Congress on Pain. Paris: 1993:51. Abstract 141.

24. Bush FM, Harkins SW, Harrington WG, Price DD. Analysis of gender effects on pain perception and symptom presentation in temporomandibular pain. Pain 1993;53:73.

25. Pellegrino MJ, Waylonis GW, Sommer A. Inheritance of primary fibromyalgia. First International Symposium on Myofascial Pain and Fibromyalgia. Minne-

apolis, Minnesota, University of Minnesota Continuing Education and Extension, 1989. Abstract 37, p. 76.

26. Gerber PC. TMJ malpractice: are you at risk? Dental Management 1991;31:16.

27. Gerber PC. Malpractice: making the best of a bad situation. Dental Management 1991;31:22.

28. Machen DE. Legal aspects of orthodontic practice: risk management concepts. Am J Orthod Dentofacial Orthop 1990;97:88.

29. Spaeth D. Informed consent goes video. ADA News 1991;22:22.

30. Minden JM, Fast TB. The patient's health history form: how healthy is it? J Am Dent Assoc 1993;124:100.

31. Owen AH. Record keeping adjuncts for TMD therapy. J Craniomandib Pract 1991;9:39.

32. Cooper BC. Insurance reimbursement for the treatment of craniomandibular disorders. J Craniomandib Pract 1988;6:197. Guest Editorial.

33. Nierman R. Guidelines for mandatory coverage. TMD Diary 1991;3:20.

34. Uppgaard RO. Medical coverage for TMJ patients in Minnesota: a breakthrough. Cranio Communications. J Craniomandib Pract 1987;5:312.

35. Reagan JG, Rutkauskas JS, Conklin CE. Medicare: trends in reimbursing hospital dental practices. J Am Dent Assoc 1993;124:89.

36. Fricton JR, Gibilisco J. The effects of an insurance coverage mandate and care parameters for TMD in Minnesota. J Craniomandib Disord Facial Oral Pain 1991;5:7.

37. Physician's current procedural terminology CPT. Chicago: American Medical Association, 1993.

38. Karaffa MC. Practice Management. In ICD-9-CM. International Classificaiton of Diseases, Clinical Modification. 3rd ed. Los Angeles: Information Corporation, 1993.

39. Code on dental procedures and nomenclature: report from the council on dental care programs. J Am Dent Assoc 1991;122:91.

40. Nierman R. Four major reasons claims not paid. TMD Diary 1993;5:35.

41. Nierman RN. Proposed criteria for independent peer reviewers. J Craniomandib Pract 1990;8:171.

Index

Page numbers followed by *f* indicate figures; page numbers followed by *t* indicate tables.

A

Abscesses, periodontal, toothache from, 65
Accessory lymph nodes, anatomy of, 33*f*
Acupressure, 324–325
Acupuncture, 338–339
Adhesions, lysis of, arthroscopy for, 371
Adults
    temporomandibular disorders in,
        epidemiologic studies of, 142, 143*t*,
        144–145
    young, temporomandibular disorders in,
        epidemiologic studies of, 145*t*, 145–
        146
Age, and temporomandibular disorders,
        epidemiologic studies of, 137*t*–141*t*.
        See also specific symptoms, e.g.,
        Headache
Amitriptyline, for treatment of muscular pain,
    313
Analgesic spraying, 255*f*–257*f*, 255–263, 257*t*
Anesthesia, local, for treatment of
        temporomandibular disorders, 339
Ankylosis
    fibro-osseous, 378
    fibrous, surgical treatment of, 369*t*
    true, 378
Anterior jig, for emergency treatment of
        temporomandibular disorders, 319
Anticonvulsants, for treatment of
        temporomandibular disorders, 312*t*
Antidepressants, for treatment of
        temporomandibular disorders, 312*t*
Antihistamines, for treatment of
        temporomandibular disorders, 312*t*
Anti–inflammatory agents, for treatment of
        temporomandibular disorders, 312*t*

Anxiety, in patient with temporomandibular
        disorder, 70–71
Anxiolytics, for treatment of
        temporomandibular disorders,
        312*t*
Arteries, supplying temporomandibular joint,
        21*f*, 21–22
Arthralgia
    pathophysiology of, 51
    surgical treatment of, 369, 369*t*
    treatment of, intraoral appliances for, 317
Arthritic pain, 52–55, 53*t*
Arthritis, rheumatoid
    condyle in, 278*f*
    and predisposition to temporomandibular
        disorders, 53*t*, 54–55
Arthrocentesis, 360*f*, 371–372
Arthrography, in patient examination, 282,
        282*f*–285*f*
Arthroscope, 359*f*
Arthroscopic surgery, 358, 359*f*
Arthroscopy, 370–371
Arthrotomy, 358, 372–376
Articular capsule, anatomy of, 5, 8*f*
Articular disk
    anatomy of, 8, 9*f*–10*f*
    bands of, anatomy of, 11*f*
    zones of, 8, 10, 11*f*
Assessment instruments, in screening for
        temporomandibular disorders, 224,
        225*f*–229*f*
Atypical odontalgia, 60–62, 61*t*
Auricular lymph nodes, anatomy of, 29, 30*f*
Auriculotemporal nerve blocks, for evaluation
        of temporomandibular disorders,
        259–260, 261*f*